YOGA IN PRACTICE

PRINCETON READINGS IN RELIGIONS

Donald S. Lopez, Jr., Editor

TITLES IN THE SERIES

Religions of India in Practice edited by Donald S. Lopez, Jr.

Buddhism in Practice edited by Donald S. Lopez, Jr.

Religions of China in Practice edited by Donald S. Lopez, Jr.

Religions of Tibet in Practice edited by Donald S. Lopez, Jr.

Religions of Japan in Practice edited by George J. Tanabe, Jr.

Religions of Asia in Practice: An Anthology edited by Donald S. Lopez, Jr.

Religions of Late Antiquity in Practice edited by Richard Valantasis

Tantra in Practice edited by David Gordon White

Judaism in Practice: From the Middle Ages through the Early Modern Period edited by Lawrence Fine

Religions of the United States in Practice, Volumes 1 and 2 edited by Colleen McDannell

Religions of Asia in Practice: An Anthology edited by Donald S. Lopez, Jr.

Religions of Korea in Practice edited by Robert E. Buswell, Jr.

The Historical Jesus in Context edited by Amy-Jill Levine, Dale C. Allison Jr., and John Dominic Crossan

Medieval Christianity in Practice edited by Miri Rubin

Islam in South Asia in Practice edited by Barbara D. Metcalf

Yoga in Practice edited by David Gordon White

YOGA

IN PRACTICE

Edited by
David Gordon White

PRINCETON READINGS IN RELIGIONS

PRINCETON UNIVERSITY PRESS

PRINCETON AND OXFORD

Published by Princeton University Press, 41 William Street, Princeton, New Jersey 08540
In the United Kingdom: Princeton University Press, 6 Oxford Street,
Woodstock, Oxfordshire OX20 1TW

ISBN: 978-0-691-14085-8

ISBN (pbk.): 978-0-691-14086-5

Library of Congress Control Number: 2011934245

British Library Cataloging-in-Publication Data is available

This book has been composed in Adobe Caslon Pro with Charlemagne Std Display

Printed on acid-free paper ∞

press.princeton.edu

Printed in the United States of America

3 5 7 9 10 8 6 4

CONTENTS

CONTENTS BY TRADITION

Buddhism

Hinduism

Islam

Jainism

CONTENTS BY COUNTRY

Nepal

Tibet

United States

CONTRIBUTORS

Jason Birch is reading for a Ph.D. in Oriental Studies at Oxford University. He also teaches Hatha Yoga in Singapore, Japan, and Australia.

Christopher Key Chapple is Doshi Professor of Indic and Comparative Theology at Loyola Marymount University, Los Angeles.

Jacob P. Dalton teaches Tibetan and Buddhist Studies at the University of California, Berkeley.

Paul Dundas is a Reader in Sanskrit in the Department of Asian Studies at the University of Edinburgh, United Kingdom.

Carl W. Ernst is William R. Kenan, Jr., Distinguished Professor of Religious Studies at the University of North Carolina at Chapel Hill.

James L. Fitzgerald is the Das Professor of Sanskrit in the Department of Classics at Brown University, Providence, Rhode Island.

Ann Grodzins Gold is a professor in the Departments of Religion and Anthropology at Syracuse University, New York.

Daniel Gold teaches in the Department of Asian Studies at Cornell University, Ithaca, New York.

Paul G. Hackett holds a research position in the Center for Buddhist Studies at Columbia University, New York.

Glen Alexander Hayes teaches in the Religion Program at Bloomfield College, Bloomfield, New Jersey.

Roger Jackson is John W. Nason Professor of Asian Studies and Religion at Carleton College, Northfield, Minnesota.

Knut A. Jacobsen is professor in Religious Studies at the University of Bergen, Norway.

M. A. Jayashree is a research scholar at the Anantha Research Foundation in Mysore, India.

Gerald James Larson is Tagore Professor Emeritus, Indiana University, Bloomington, and Professor Emeritus, Religious Studies, University of California, Santa Barbara.

Angelika Malinar is Professor of Indology at the University of Zürich.

James Mallinson is an independent scholar living in England.

M. Narasimhan is a research scholar at the Anantha Research Foundation in Mysore, India.

William R. Pinch teaches in the Department of History at Wesleyan University, Middletown, Connecticut.

Olle Qvarnström teaches in the Department of History of Religions at the University of Lund, Sweden.

Jeffrey Clark Ruff teaches in the Department of Religious Studies at Marshall University, West Virginia.

Mark Singleton teaches at St. John's College, Santa Fe, New Mexico.

Sthaneshwar Timalsina teaches in the Department of Religious Studies at San Diego State University.

Somadeva Vasudeva is Assistant Professor of Sanskrit at Columbia University, New York.

Vesna Wallace teaches in the Department of Religious Studies at the University of California, Santa Barbara.

David Gordon White is the J. F. Rowny Professor of Comparative Religions at the University of California, Santa Barbara.

Dominik Wujastyk is a Research Fellow at the Institute of South Asian, Tibetan, and Buddhist Studies at the University of Vienna, Austria.

YOGA IN PRACTICE

Yoga, Brief History of an Idea

David Gordon White

Over the past decades, yoga has become part of the *Zeitgeist* of affluent western societies, drawing housewives and hipsters, New Agers and the old-aged, and body culture and corporate culture into a multibillion-dollar synergy. Like every Indian cultural artifact that it has embraced, the West views Indian yoga as an ancient, unchanging tradition, based on revelations received by the Vedic sages who, seated in the lotus pose, were the Indian forerunners of the flat-tummied yoga babes who grace the covers of such glossy periodicals as the *Yoga Journal* and *Yoga International*.[1]

In the United States in particular, yoga has become a commodity. Statistics show that about 16 million Americans practice yoga every year. For most people, this means going to a yoga center with yoga mats, yoga clothes, and yoga accessories, and practicing in groups under the guidance of a yoga teacher or trainer. Here, yoga practice comprises a regimen of postures (*āsana*s)—sometimes held for long periods of time, sometimes executed in rapid sequence—often together with techniques of breath control (*prāṇāyāma*). Yoga entrepreneurs have branded their own styles of practice, from Bikram's superheated workout rooms to studios that have begun offering "doga," practicing yoga together with one's dog. They have opened franchises, invented logos, packaged their practice regimens under Sanskrit names, and marketed a lifestyle that fuses yoga with leisure travel, healing spas, and seminars on eastern spirituality. "Yoga celebrities" have become a part of our vocabulary, and with celebrity has come the usual entourage of publicists, business managers, and

[1] In this introduction, names in [square brackets] refer to contributions found in this volume, while references in (parentheses) refer to works found in Works Cited at the end of this chapter.

lawyers. Yoga is mainstream. Arguably India's greatest cultural export, yoga has morphed into a mass culture phenomenon.

Many yoga celebrities, as well as a strong percentage of less celebrated yoga teachers, combine their training with teachings on healing, spirituality, meditation, and India's ancient yoga traditions, the Sanskrit-language *Yoga Sūtra* (YS) in particular. Here, they are following the lead of the earliest yoga entrepreneurs, the Indian gurus who brought the gospel of yoga to western shores in the wake of Swami Vivekananda's storied successes of the late nineteenth and early twentieth centuries.

But what were India's ancient yoga traditions, and what relationship do they have to the modern postural yoga (Singleton 2010) that people are practicing across the world today? In fact, the yoga that is taught and practiced today has very little in common with the yoga of the YS and other ancient yoga treatises. Nearly all of our popular assumptions about yoga theory date from the past 150 years, and very few modern-day practices date from before the twelfth century. This is not the first time that people have "reinvented" yoga in their own image. As the contributions to this volume demonstrate, this is a process that has been ongoing for at least two thousand years. Every group in every age has created its own version and vision of yoga. One reason this has been possible is that its semantic field—the range of meanings of the term "yoga"—is so broad and the concept of yoga so malleable, that it has been possible to morph it into nearly any practice or process one chooses.

When seeking to define a tradition, it is useful to begin by defining one's terms. It is here that problems arise. "Yoga" has a wider range of meanings than nearly any other word in the entire Sanskrit lexicon. The act of yoking an animal, as well as the yoke itself, is called yoga. In astronomy, a conjunction of planets or stars, as well as a constellation, is called yoga. When one mixes together various substances, that, too, can be called yoga. The word yoga has also been employed to denote a device, a recipe, a method, a strategy, a charm, an incantation, fraud, a trick, an endeavor, a combination, union, an arrangement, zeal, care, diligence, industriousness, discipline, use, application, contact, a sum total, and the Work of alchemists. But this is by no means an exhaustive list.

So, for example, the ninth-century *Netra Tantra*, a Hindu scripture from Kashmir, describes what it calls subtle yoga and transcendent yoga. Subtle yoga is nothing more or less than a body of techniques for entering into and taking over other people's bodies. As for transcendental yoga, this is a process that involves superhuman female predators, called *yoginīs*, who eat people! By eating people, this text says, the *yoginīs* consume the sins of the body that would otherwise bind them to suffering rebirth, and so allow for the "union" (*yoga*) of their purified souls with the supreme god Śiva, a union that is tantamount to salvation (White 2009: 162–63). In this ninth-century source, there is no discussion whatsoever of postures or breath control, the prime markers of yoga as we know it today. More troubling still, the third- to fourth-century CE YS and *Bhagavad Gītā* (BhG), the two most widely cited textual sources for "classical yoga," virtually ignore postures and breath control, each devoting a total of fewer than ten verses to these practices. They are far more concerned with the issue of human salvation, realized through the theory and practice of meditation (*dhyāna*) in the YS [Larson] and through concentration on the god Kṛṣṇa in the BhG [Malinar].

Indian Foundations of Yoga Theory and Practice

Clearly something is missing here. There is a gap between the ancient, "classical" yoga tradition and yoga as we know it. In order to understand the disconnect between then and now, we would do well to go back to the earliest uses of the term yoga, which are found in texts far more ancient than the YS or BhG. Here I am referring to India's earliest scriptures, the Vedas. In the circa fifteenth-century BCE *Ṛg Veda*, yoga meant, before all else, the yoke one placed on a draft animal—a bullock or warhorse—to yoke it to a plow or chariot. The resemblance of these terms is not fortuitous: the Sanskrit "yoga" is a cognate of the English "yoke," because Sanskrit and English both belong to the Indo-European language family (which is why the Sanskrit *mātṛ* resembles the English "mother," *sveda* looks like "sweat," *udara*—"belly" in Sanskrit—looks like "udder," and so forth). In the same scripture, we see the term's meaning expanded through metonymy, with "yoga" being applied to the entire conveyance or "rig" of a war chariot: to the yoke itself, the team of horses or bullocks, and the chariot itself with its many straps and harnesses. And, because such chariots were only hitched up (*yukta*) in times of war, an important Vedic usage of the term yoga was "wartime," in contrast to *kṣema*, "peacetime."

The Vedic reading of yoga as one's war chariot or rig came to be incorporated into the warrior ideology of ancient India. In the *Mahābhārata*, India's 200 BCE–400 CE "national epic," we read the earliest narrative accounts of the battlefield apotheosis of heroic chariot warriors. This was, like the Greek *Iliad*, an epic of battle, and so it was appropriate that the glorification of a warrior who died fighting his enemies be showcased here. What is interesting, for the purposes of the history of the term yoga, is that in these narratives, the warrior who knew he was about to die was said to become *yoga-yukta*, literally "yoked to yoga," with "yoga" once again meaning a chariot. This time, however, it was not the warrior's own chariot that carried him up to the highest heaven, reserved for gods and heroes alone. Rather, it was a celestial "yoga," a divine chariot, that carried him upward in a burst of light to and through the sun, and on to the heaven of gods and heroes.

Warriors were not the sole individuals of the Vedic age to have chariots called "yogas." The gods, too, were said to shuttle across heaven, and between earth and heaven on yogas. Furthermore, the Vedic priests who sang the Vedic hymns related their practice to the yoga of the warrior aristocracy who were their patrons. In their hymns, they describe themselves as "yoking" their minds to poetic inspiration and so journeying—if only with their mind's eye or cognitive apparatus—across the metaphorical distance that separated the world of the gods from the words of their hymns. A striking image of their poetic journeys is found in a verse from a late Vedic hymn, in which the poet-priests describe themselves as "hitched up" (*yukta*) and standing on their chariot shafts as they sally forth on a vision quest across the universe.

The earliest extant systematic account of yoga and a bridge from the earlier Vedic uses of the term is found in the Hindu *Kaṭhaka Upaniṣad* (KU), a scripture dating from about the third century BCE. Here, the god of Death reveals what is termed the "entire yoga regimen" to a young ascetic named Naciketas. In the course of his teaching, Death compares the relationship between the self, body, intellect, and so forth to the relationship between a rider, his chariot, charioteer, etc. (KU 3.3–9), a comparison which approximates that made in Plato's *Phaedrus*. Three elements of this text set the agenda for much of what constitutes yoga in the centuries that follow. First, it introduces a sort of yogic physiology, calling the body a "fort with eleven gates" and evoking "a person the size of a thumb" who, dwelling within, is worshiped by all the gods (KU 4.12; 5.1, 3). Second, it identifies the individual person within with the universal Person (*puruṣa*) or absolute Being (*brahman*), asserting that this is what sustains life (KU 5.5, 8–10). Third, it describes the hierarchy of mind-body constituents—the senses, mind, intellect, etc.—that comprise the foundational categories of Sāṃkhya philosophy, whose metaphysical system grounds the yoga of the YS, BhG, and other texts and schools (KU 3.10–11; 6.7–8). Because these categories were hierarchically ordered, the realization of higher states of consciousness was, in this early context, tantamount to an ascension through levels of outer space, and so we also find in this and other early Upaniṣads the concept of yoga as a technique for "inner" and "outer" ascent. These same sources also introduce the use of acoustic spells or formulas (*mantras*), the most prominent among these being the syllable OṂ, the acoustic form of the supreme *brahman*. In the following centuries, mantras would become progressively incorporated into yogic theory and practice, in the medieval Hindu, Buddhist, and Jain Tantras, as well as the *Yoga Upaniṣads*.

Following this circa third-century BCE watershed, textual references to yoga multiply rapidly in Hindu, Jain, and Buddhist sources, reaching a critical mass some seven hundred to one thousand years later. It is during this initial burst that most of the perennial principles of yoga theory—as well as many elements of yoga practice—were originally formulated. Toward the latter end of this period, one sees the emergence of the earliest yoga *systems*, in the YS; the third- to fourth-century scriptures of the Buddhist Yogācāra school and fourth- to fifth-century *Visuddhimagga* of Buddhaghoṣa; and the *Yogadṛṣṭisamuccaya* of the eighth-century Jain author Haribhadra. Although the YS may be slightly later than the Yogācāra canon, this tightly ordered series of aphorisms is so remarkable and comprehensive for its time that it is often referred to as "classical yoga." It is also known as *pātañjala yoga* ("Patañjalian yoga"), in recognition of its putative compiler, Patañjali.

The Yogācāra ("Yoga Practice") school of Mahāyāna Buddhism was the earliest Buddhist tradition to employ the term yoga to denote its philosophical system. Also known as Vijñānavāda ("Doctrine of Consciousness"), Yogācāra offered a systematic analysis of perception and consciousness together with a set of meditative disciplines designed to eliminate the cognitive errors that prevented liberation from suffering existence. Yogācāra's eight-stage meditative practice itself was not termed yoga, however, but rather "calmness" (*śamatha*) or "insight" (*vipaśyanā*) meditation (Cleary 1995). The Yogācāra analysis of consciousness has many points in common with the more or less coeval YS, and there can be no doubt that cross-pollination occurred across religious boundaries in matters of yoga (La Vallée Poussin, 1936–1937). The *Yogavāsiṣṭha* ("Vasiṣṭha's Teachings on Yoga")—a circa tenth-century Hindu work from Kashmir that combined analytical and practical teachings on "yoga" with vivid mythological accounts illustrative of its analysis of consciousness [Chapple]—takes positions similar to those of Yogācāra concerning errors of perception and the human inability to distinguish between our interpretations of the world and the world itself.

The Jains were the last of the major Indian religious groups to employ the term yoga to imply anything remotely resembling "classical" formulations of yoga theory and practice. The earliest Jain uses of the term, found in Umāsvāti's fourth- to fifth-century *Tattvārthasūtra* (6.1–2), the earliest extant systematic work of Jain philosophy, defined yoga as "activity of the body, speech, and mind." As such, yoga was, in early Jain parlance, actually an impediment to liberation. Here, yoga could only be overcome through its opposite, *ayoga* ("non-yoga," inaction)—that is, through meditation (*jhāṇa*; *dhyāna*), asceticism, and other practices of purification that undo the effects of earlier activity. The earliest systematic Jain work on yoga, Haribhadra's circa 750 CE *Yoga-*

dṛṣṭisamuccaya, was strongly influenced by the YS, yet nonetheless retained much of Umāsvāti's terminology, even as it referred to observance of the path as *yogācāra* (Qvarnström 2003: 131–33).

This is not to say that between the fourth century BCE and the second to fourth century CE, neither the Buddhists nor the Jains were engaging in practices that we might today identify as yoga. To the contrary, early Buddhist sources like the *Majjhima Nikāya*—the "Middle-length Sayings" attributed to the Buddha himself—are replete with references to self-mortification and meditation as practiced by the Jains, which the Buddha condemned and contrasted to his own set of four meditations (Bronkhorst 1993: 1–5, 19–24). In the *Aṅguttara Nikāya* ("Gradual Sayings"), another set of teachings attributed to the Buddha, one finds descriptions of *jhāyin*s ("meditators," "experientialists") that closely resemble early Hindu descriptions of practitioners of yoga (Eliade 2009: 174–75). Their ascetic practices—never termed yoga in these early sources—were likely innovated within the various itinerant *śramaṇa* groups that circulated in the eastern Gangetic basin in the latter half of the first millennium BCE.

Even as the term yoga began to appear with increasing frequency between 300 BCE and 400 CE, its meaning was far from fixed. It is only in later centuries that a relatively systematic yoga nomenclature became established among Hindus, Buddhists, and Jains. By the beginning of the fifth century, however, the core principles of yoga were more or less in place, with most of what followed being variations on that original core. Here, we would do well to outline these principles, which have persisted through time and across traditions for some two thousand years. They may be summarized as follows:

1. *Yoga as an analysis of perception and cognition*. Yoga is an analysis of the dysfunctional nature of everyday perception and cognition, which lies at the root of suffering, the existential conundrum whose solution is the goal of Indian philosophy. Once one comprehends the cause(s) of the problem, one can solve it through philosophical analysis combined with meditative practice.

At bottom, India's many yoga traditions are *soteriologies*, doctrines of salvation, concerning the attainment of release from suffering existence and the cycle of rebirths (*saṃsāra*). The problem of suffering existence and the allied doctrine of cyclic rebirth emerges about five centuries before the beginning of the common era, in the early Upaniṣads as well as the original teachings of the Jain founder Mahāvīra and the Buddhist founder Gautama Buddha. The same teachings that posit the problem of suffering existence also offer a solution to the problem, which may be summarized by the word "gnosis" (*jñāna* or *prajñā* in Sanskrit; *paññā* in Pali). As such, these are also to be counted among the earliest Indian *epistemologies*, philosophical theories of what constitutes authentic knowledge. Gnosis—transcendent, immediate, non-conventional knowledge of ultimate reality, of the reality behind appearances—is the key to salvation in all of these early soteriologies, as well as in India's major philosophical schools, many of which developed in the centuries around the beginning of the Common Era. As such, these are *gnoseologies*, theories of salvation through knowledge, in which to know the truth (i.e., that in spite of appearances, one is, in fact, not trapped in suffering existence) is to realize it in fact. The classic example of such a transformation is that of the Buddha: by realizing the Four Noble Truths, he became the "Awakened" or "Enlightened" One (*Buddha*), and so was liberated from future rebirths, realizing the extinction of suffering (*nibbāna*; *nirvāṇa*) at the end of his life.

In all of these systems, the necessary condition for gnosis is the disengagement of one's cognitive apparatus from sense impressions and base matter (including the matter of the body). An important distinguishing characteristic of all Indian philosophical systems is the concept that the mind or mental capacity (*manas*, *citta*) is part of the body: it is the "sixth sense," which, located in the heart, is tethered to the senses of hearing, seeing, tasting, touching, and smelling, as well as their associated bodily organs. What this means is that Indian philosophy rejects the mind-body distinction. In doing so, however, it does embrace another distinction. This is the distinction between the mind-body complex on the one hand, and a higher cognitive apparatus—called *buddhi* ("intellect"), *antaḥkaraṇa*, *vijñāna* (both translatable as "consciousness"), etc.—on the other. In these early sources, the term yoga is often used to designate the theory and practice of disengaging the higher cognitive apparatus from the thrall of matter, the body, and the senses (including mind). Yoga is a regimen or discipline that trains the cognitive apparatus to perceive clearly, which leads to true cognition, which in turn leads to salvation, release from suffering existence. Yoga is not the sole term for this type of training, however. In early Buddhist and Jain scriptures as well as many early Hindu sources, the term *dhyāna* (*jhāna* in the Pali of early Buddhist teachings, *jhāṇa* in the Jain Ardhamagadhi vernacular), most commonly translated as "meditation," is far more frequently employed. So it is that Hindu sources like the BhG and YS, as well as a number of Buddhist Mahāyāna works, frequently use yoga, *dhyāna*, and *bhāvanā* ("cultivation," "contemplation") more or less synonymously, while early Jain and Buddhist texts employ the term *dhyāna* in its various spellings exclusively. Both the YS and the Noble Eightfold Path of Buddhism also employ the term *samādhi* ("concentration") for the culminating stage of meditation (Sarbacker 2005: 16–21). At this stage, all objects have been removed from consciousness, which thereafter continues to exist in isolation (*kaivalyam*), forever liberated from all entanglements. *Kaivalyam* is also employed in Jain soteriology for the final state of the fully purified liberated soul.

The BhG, the philosophical charter of "mainstream" Hindu theism, uses the term yoga in the broad sense of "discipline" or "path," and teaches that the paths of gnosis (*jñāna-yoga*) and action *(karma-yoga)* are inferior to the path of devotion (*bhakti-yoga*) to an all-powerful and benevolent supreme being. However, here as well, it is the constant training of the cognitive faculties—to meditatively concentrate on God in order to accurately perceive Him as the source of all being and knowledge—that brings about salvation. In this teaching, revealed by none other than the supreme being Kṛṣṇa himself, the devotee whose disciplined meditation is focused on God alone is often referred to as a yogin. The BhG is possibly the first but by no means the last teaching to use the term yoga preceded by an adjective or modifier (*karma-*, *jñāna-*, *bhakti-*), thereby acknowledging—but also creating—a variety of yogas.

2. *Yoga as the raising and expansion of consciousness.* Through analytical inquiry and meditative practice, the lower organs or apparatus of human cognition are suppressed, allowing for higher, less obstructed levels of perception and cognition to prevail. Here, consciousness-raising on a cognitive level is seen to be simultaneous with the "physical" rise of the consciousness or self through ever-higher levels or realms of cosmic space. Reaching the level of consciousness of a god, for example, is tantamount to rising to that deity's cosmological level, to the atmospheric or heavenly world it inhabits. This is a concept that likely flowed from the experience of the Vedic poets, who, by "yoking" their minds to poetic inspiration, were empowered to journey to the farthest reaches of the universe. The physical rise of the dying *yoga-yukta* chariot warrior to the highest cosmic plane may have also contributed to the formulation of this idea.

Another development of this concept is the notion that the expansion of consciousness is tantamount to the expansion of the self to the point that one's body or self becomes coextensive with the entire universe. The 289th chapter of the twelfth book of the *Mahābhārata* concludes with a description of just such an expansion of a yogi's self [Fitzgerald], and one finds a similar description in the Jain Umāsvāti's fourth- to fifth-century *Praśamaratiprakaraṇa*. Several Mahāyāna Buddhist sources contain accounts of enlightened beings whose "constructed bodies" (*nirmāṇakāya*) expand to fill the universe; and the BhG's description of the god Kṛṣṇa's universal body (*viśvarūpa*), through which he displays his "masterful yoga," is of the same order (White 2009: 167–97).

Also in this regard, it should be noted that attention to the breath is a feature of the theory and practice of meditation from the earliest times. Mindfulness of one's breathing is introduced in such early sources as the *Majjhima Nikāya* as a fundamental element of Theravāda Buddhist meditation. In early Hindu sources as well, controlling and stilling the breath is a prime technique for calming the mind and turning it inward, away from the distractions of sensory perception. *Ātman*, the term for the "self" or "soul" in the classical Upaniṣads and later works, is etymologically linked to the Sanskrit verb **an*, "breathe," and it is via breath channels leading up from the heart—channels that merge with the rays of the sun—that the self leaves the body at death to merge with the Absolute (*brahman*) at the summit of the universe. These descriptions of the breath channels also lie at the origin of yogic or "subtle" body physiology, which would become fleshed out in great detail in India's medieval Tantric scriptures. In these and later works, the breath-propelled self's rise through the levels of the universe would become completely internalized, with the spinal column doubling as the universal axis mundi and the practitioner's own cranial vault becoming the place of the *brahman* and locus of immortality.

3. *Yoga as a path to omniscience.* Once it was established that true perception or true cognition enables a self's enhanced or enlightened consciousness to rise or expand to reach and penetrate distant regions of space—to see and know things as they truly are beyond the illusory limitations imposed by a deluded mind and sense perceptions—there were no limits to the places to which consciousness could go. These "places" included past and future time, locations distant and hidden, and even places invisible to view. This insight became the foundation for theorizing the type of extrasensory perception known as yogi perception (*yogipratyakṣa*), which is in many Indian epistemological systems the highest of the "true cognitions" (*pramāṇa*s), in other words, the supreme and most irrefutable of all possible sources of knowledge. For the Nyāya-Vaiśeṣika school, the earliest Hindu philosophical school to fully analyze this basis for transcendent knowledge, yogi perception is what permitted the Vedic seers (*ṛṣi*s) to apprehend, in a single panoptical act of perception, the entirety of the Vedic revelation, which was tantamount to viewing the entire universe simultaneously, in all its parts. For the Buddhists, it was this that provided the Buddha and other enlightened beings with the "*buddha*-eye" or "divine eye," which permitted them to see the true nature of reality. For the early seventh-century Mādhyamaka philosopher Candrakīrti, yogi perception afforded direct and profound insight into his school's highest truth, that is, into the emptiness (*śūnyatā*) of things and concepts, as well as relationships between things and concepts (MacDonald 2009: 133–46). Yogi perception remained the subject of lively debate among Hindu and Buddhist philosophers well into the medieval period.

It was a widely held precept among ascetic traditions that extrasensory insight into the ultimate nature of reality, a sort of omniscience, could be attained through meditative practice. Here, there were two schools of thought concerning the attainment of such insight. The Jains and a number of Hindu and Buddhist schools asserted that the soul, self, or mind was luminous by nature and innately possessed of perfect perception and insight, and that the path to liberation simply comprised the realization of one's innate qualities and capacities. Others, including Theravāda and Sarvāstivāda Buddhists, maintained that the path of asceticism and the practice of meditation were necessary to purge cognition of its inborn defilements, and that only once this difficult work had been completed could yogi perception and omniscience arise (Franco 2009, 4–5). In the former case, meditation was the means to realizing the divine within, one's innate Buddha nature, to see the universe as Self, and so forth. In the latter, the resulting extrasensory insight allowed the ontologically imperfect practitioner to clearly see and truly know a god or Buddha that nonetheless remained Wholly Other. Through such knowledge one could, in the parlance of many of the dualist Hindu Tantric schools, "become a god in order to worship god"—but one could never become god, which is what the non-dualist schools maintained.

4. *Yoga as a technique for entering into other bodies, generating multiple bodies, and the attainment of other supernatural accomplishments.* The classical Indian understanding of everyday perception (*pratyakṣa*) was similar to that of the ancient Greeks. In both systems, the site at which visual perception occurs is not the surface of the retina or the junction of the optic nerve with the brain's visual nuclei, but rather the contours of the perceived object. This means, for example, that when I am viewing a tree, a ray of perception emitted from my eye "con-forms" to the surface of the tree. The ray brings the image of the tree back to my eye, which communicates it to my mind, which in turn communicates it to my inner self or consciousness. In the case of yogi perception, the practice of yoga enhances this process (in some cases, establishing an unmediated connection between consciousness and the perceived object), such that the viewer not only sees things as they truly are, but is also able to directly see *through* the surface of things into their innermost being. For non-Buddhists, this applies, most importantly, to the perception of one's own inner self as well as the selves or souls of others. From here, it is but a short step to conceiving of the viewer possessed of the power of yogi perception—texts often call him a yogi—as possessing the power to physically penetrate, with his enhanced cognitive apparatus, into other people's bodies (White 2009: 122–66). This is the theory underlying the Tantric practice of "subtle yoga" described at the beginning of this introduction. But in fact, the earliest references in all of Indian literature to individuals explicitly called yogis are *Mahābhārata* tales of Hindu and Buddhist hermits who take over other people's bodies in just this way; and it is noteworthy that when yogis enter into other people's bodies, they are said to do so through rays emanating from their eyes. The epic also asserts that a yogi so empowered can take over several thousand bodies simultaneously, and "walk the earth with all of them." Buddhist sources describe the same phenomenon with the important difference that the enlightened being creates multiple bodies rather than taking over those belonging to other creatures. This is a notion already elaborated in an early Buddhist work, the *Sāmaññaphalasutta*, a teaching contained in the *Dīgha Nikāya* (the "Longer Sayings" of the Buddha), according to which a monk who has completed the four Buddhist meditations gains, among other things, the power to self-multiply. Several of the key terms found in this text reappear, with specific reference to yoga and yogis, in the 100 BCE–200 CE Indian medical classic, the *Caraka Saṃhitā* [Wujastyk].

The ability to enter into and control the bodies of other creatures is but one of the supernatural powers (*iddhi*s in Pali; *siddhi*s or *vibhūti*s in Sanskrit) that arise from the power of extrasensory perception (*abhiññā* in Pali; *abhijñā* in Sanskrit). Others include the power of flight, clairaudience, telepathy, invisibility, and the recollection of past lives—precisely the sorts of powers that the yogis of Indian legend have been said to possess.

Here, it is helpful to introduce the difference between "yogi practice" and "yoga practice," which has been implicit to South Asian thought and practice since the beginning of the Common Era, the period in which the terms "yogi" and "yogi perception" first appeared in the Indian scriptural record. On the one hand, there is "yoga practice," which essentially denotes a program of mind-training and meditation issuing in the realization of enlightenment, liberation, or isolation from the world of suffering existence. Yoga practice is the practical application of the theoretical precepts of the various yogic soteriologies, epistemologies, and gnoseologies presented in *analytical* works like the YS and the teachings of the various Hindu, Buddhist, and Jain philosophical schools. Yogi practice, on the other hand, concerns the supernatural powers that empower yogis to take over other creatures' bodies and so forth. Nearly every one of the earliest *narrative* descriptions of yogis and their practices underscore the axiom that the penetration of other bodies is the *sine qua non* of yoga.

The cleavage between these two more or less incompatible bodies of theory and practice can be traced back to early Buddhist sources, which speak of a rivalry between meditating "experimentalists" (*jhāyins*) and "speculatives" (*dhammayogas*). In medieval Tantra, the same division obtained, this time between practitioners whose meditative practice led to gnosis and identity with the divine on the one hand, and on the other, practitioners—referred to as yogis or *sādhakas*—whose goal was this-worldly supernatural power in one's now invulnerable, ageless, and adamantine human body. The gulf between yoga practice and yogi practice never ceased to widen over the centuries, such that, by the time of the British Raj, India's hordes of yogis were considered by India's elites to be little more than common criminals, with their fraudulent practices—utterly at odds with the "true" science of yoga, which, taught in the YS, was practiced by none—save perhaps for a handful of isolated hermits living high in the Himalayas (Oman 1908: 3–30).

These four sets of concepts and practices form the core and foundational vocabulary of nearly every yoga tradition, school, or system, with all that follow the fourth- to seventh-century watershed—of the YS and various foundational Buddhist and Jain works on meditation and yogi perception—simply variations and expansions on this common core.

Medieval Developments

YOGA IN THE TANTRAS

The Tantras are pivotal works in the history of yoga, inasmuch as they carry forward both the yoga and yogi practices and the gnoseological theory of earlier traditions while introducing important innovations in theory and practice. On the theoretical side, these medieval scriptures and commentarial traditions promulgate a new variation on the preexisting yoga soteriology. No longer is the practitioner's ultimate goal liberation from suffering existence, but rather self-deification: one *becomes* the deity that has been one's object of meditation. In a universe that is nothing other than the flow of divine consciousness, raising one's consciousness to the level of god-consciousness—that is, attaining a god's-eye view that sees the universe as internal to one's own transcendent Self—is tantamount to becoming divine. A primary means to this end is the detailed visualization of the deity with which one will ultimately identify: his or her form, face(s), color, attributes, entourage, and so on. So, for example, in the yoga of the Hindu Pāñcarātra sect, a practitioner's meditation on successive emanations of the god Viṣṇu culminates in his realization of the state of "consisting in god" (Rastelli 2009: 299–317). The Tantric Buddhist cognate to this is "deity yoga" (*devayoga*), whereby the practitioner meditatively assumes the attributes and creates the environment (i.e., the Buddha world) of the Buddha-deity he or she is about to become.

In fact, the term yoga has a wide variety of connotations in the Tantras. It can simply mean "practice" or "discipline" in a very broad sense, covering all of the means at one's disposal to realize one's goals. It can also refer to the goal itself: "conjunction," "union," or identity with divine consciousness. Indeed, the *Mālinīvijayottara Tantra*, an important ninth-century Śākta-Śaiva Tantra, uses the term yoga to denote its entire soteriological system (Vasudeva 2004). In Buddhist Tantra—whose canonical teachings are divided into the exoteric Yoga Tantras and the increasingly esoteric Higher Yoga Tantras, Supreme Yoga Tantras, Unexcelled (or Unsurpassed) Yoga Tantras, and Yoginī Tantras—yoga has the dual sense of both the means and ends of practice. Yoga can also have the more particular, limited sense of a program of meditation or visualization, as opposed to ritual (*kriyā*) or gnostic (*jñāna*) practice. However, these categories of practice often bleed into one another. Finally, there are specific types of yogic discipline, such as the *Netra Tantra*'s transcendent and subtle yogas, already discussed.

Indo-Tibetan Buddhist Tantra—and with it, Buddhist Tantric Yoga—developed in lockstep with Hindu Tantra, with a hierarchy of revelations ranging from earlier, exoteric systems of practice to the sex- and death-laden imagery of later esoteric pantheons, in which horrific skull-wielding Buddhas were surrounded by the same *yoginī*s as their Hindu counterparts, the Bhairavas of the esoteric Hindu Tantras. In the Buddhist Unexcelled Yoga Tantras, "six-limbed yoga" comprised the visualization practices that facilitated the realization of one's innate identity with the deity [Wallace]. But rather than simply being a means to an end in these traditions, yoga was also primarily an end in itself: yoga was "union" or identity with the celestial Buddha named Vajrasattva—the "Diamond Essence (of Enlightenment)," that is, one's Buddha nature. However, the same Tantras of the Diamond Path (Vajrayāna) also implied that the innate nature of that union rendered the conventional practices undertaken for its realization ultimately irrelevant [Dalton].

Here, one can speak of two principal styles of Tantric Yoga, which coincide with their respective metaphysics. The former, which recurs in the earliest Tantric traditions, involves exoteric practices: visualization, generally pure ritual offerings, worship, and the use of mantras. The dualist metaphysics of these traditions maintains that there is an ontological difference between god and creature, which can gradually be overcome through concerted effort and practice. The latter, esoteric, traditions develop out of the former even as they reject much of exoteric theory and practice. In these systems, esoteric practice, involving the real or symbolic consumption of forbidden substances and sexual transactions with forbidden partners, is the fast track to self-deification. However, given the non-dualist metaphysics of esoteric Tantra, which maintains that all creatures are innately divine or enlightened, such practices are considered ultimately unnecessary. A number of Tantric scriptures and commentaries underscore the complementarity of the exoteric and esoteric approaches, urging that the yogi's central task is to balance the two: this is the position taken, for example, by the Buddhist Mahāsiddha Saraha in his analysis of the doctrines and practices of the Yoginī Tantras [Jackson].

In the exoteric Tantras, visualization, ritual offerings, worship, and the use of *mantra*s were the means to the gradual realization of one's identity with the absolute. In later, esoteric traditions, however, the expansion of consciousness to a divine level was instantaneously triggered through the consumption of forbidden substances: semen, menstrual blood, feces, urine, human flesh, and the like. Menstrual or uterine blood, which was considered to be the most powerful among these forbidden substances, could be accessed through sexual relations with female Tantric consorts. Variously called *yoginī*s, *ḍākinī*s, or *dūtī*s, these were ideally low-caste human women who were considered to be possessed by, or embodiments of, Tantric goddesses. In the case of the *yoginī*s, these were the same goddesses as those that ate their victims in the practice of "transcendent yoga." Whether by consuming the sexual emissions of these forbidden women or through the bliss of sexual orgasm with them, Tantric yogis could "blow their minds" and realize a breakthrough into transcendent levels of consciousness. Once again, yogic consciousness-raising doubled with the physical rise of the yogi's body through space, in this case in the embrace of the *yoginī* or *ḍākinī* who, as an embodied goddess, was possessed of the power of flight. It was for this reason that the medieval *yoginī* temples were roofless: they were the *yoginī*s' landing fields and launching pads (White 2003: 7–13, 204–18).

In many Tantras, such as the eighth-century CE *Mataṇgapārameśvarāgama* of the Hindu Śaivasiddhānta school, this visionary ascent became actualized in the practitioner's rise through the levels of the universe until, arriving at the highest void, the supreme deity Sadāśiva conferred his own divine rank upon him (Sanderson 2006: 205–6). It is in such a context—of a graded hierarchy of stages or states of consciousness, with corresponding deities, mantras, and cosmological levels—that the Tantras innovated the construct known as the "subtle body" or "yogic body." Here, the practitioner's body became identified with the entire universe, such that all of the processes and transformations occurring to his body in the world were now described as occurring to a world inside his body. While the breath channels (*nāḍī*s) of yogic practice had already been discussed in the classical Upaniṣads, it was not until such Tantric works as the eighth-century Buddhist *Hevajra Tantra* and *Caryāgīti* that a hierarchy of inner energy centers—variously called *cakra*s ("circles," "wheels"), *padma*s ("lotuses"), or *pīṭha*s ("mounds")—were introduced. These early Buddhist sources only mention four such centers aligned along the spinal column, but in the centuries that follow, Hindu Tantras such as the *Kubjikāmata* and *Kaulajñānanirṇaya* would expand that number to five, six, seven, eight, and more. The so-called classical hierarchy of seven *cakra*s—ranging from the *mūlādhāra* at the level of the anus to the *sahasrāra* in the cranial vault, replete with color coding, fixed numbers of petals linked to the names of *yoginī*s, the graphemes and phonemes of the Sanskrit alphabet—was a still later development. So too was the introduction of the *kuṇḍalinī*, the female Serpent Energy coiled at the base of the yogic body, whose awakening and rapid rise effects the practitioner's inner transformation (White 2003: 220–34).

Given the wide range of applications of the term yoga in the Tantras, the semantic field of the term "yogi" is relatively circumscribed. Yogis who forcefully take over the bodies of other creatures are the villains of countless medieval accounts, including the tenth- to eleventh-century Kashmirian *Kathāsaritsāgara* ("Ocean of Rivers of Story," which contains the famous *Vetālapañcaviṃśati*—the "Twenty-five Tales of the Zombie") and the *Yogavāsiṣṭha*. In the seventh-century farce entitled *Bhagavadajjukīya*, the "Tale of the Saint Courtesan," a yogi who briefly occupies the body of a dead prostitute is cast as a comic figure. Well into the twentieth century, the term yogi continued to be used nearly exclusively to refer to a Tantric practitioner who opted for this-worldly self-aggrandizement over disembodied liberation. Tantric yogis specialize in esoteric practices, often carried out in cremation grounds, practices that often verge on black magic and sorcery. Once again, this was, overwhelmingly, the primary sense of the term "yogi" in pre-modern Indic traditions: nowhere prior to the seventeenth century do we find it applied to persons seated in fixed postures, regulating their breath or entering into meditative states.

HAṬHA YOGA

A new regimen of yoga called the "yoga of forceful exertion" rapidly emerges as a comprehensive system in the tenth to eleventh century, as evidenced in works like the *Yogavāsiṣṭha* and the original *Gorakṣa Śataka* ("Hundred Verses of Gorakṣa") [Mallinson]. While the famous *cakra*s, *nāḍī*s, and *kuṇḍalinī* predate its advent, *haṭha yoga* is entirely innovative in its depiction of the yogic body as a pneumatic, but also a hydraulic and a thermodynamic system. The practice of breath control becomes particularly refined in the hathayogic texts, with elaborate instructions provided concerning the calibrated regulation of the breaths. In certain sources, the duration of time during which the breath is held is of primary importance, with lengthened periods of breath stoppage corresponding to expanded levels of supernatural power. This science of the breath had a number of offshoots, including a form of divination based on the movements of the breath within and outside of the body, an esoteric tradition that found its way into medieval Tibetan and Persian [Ernst] sources.

In a novel variation on the theme of consciousness-raising-as-internal-ascent, *haṭha yoga* also represents the yogic body as a sealed hydraulic system within which vital fluids may be channeled upward as they are refined into nectar through the heat of asceticism. Here, the semen of the practitioner, lying inert in the coiled body of the serpentine *kuṇḍalinī* in the lower abdomen, becomes heated through the bellows effect of *prāṇāyāma*, the repeated inflation and deflation of the peripheral breath channels. The awakened *kuṇḍalinī* suddenly straightens and enters into the *suṣumṇā*, the medial channel that runs the length of the spinal column up to the cranial vault. Propelled by the yogi's heated breaths, the hissing *kuṇḍalinī* serpent shoots upward, piercing each of the *cakra*s as she rises. With the penetration of each succeeding *cakra*, vast amounts of heat are released, such that the semen contained in the *kuṇḍalinī*'s body becomes gradually transmuted. This body of theory and practice was quickly adopted in both Jain and Buddhist Tantric works. In the Buddhist case, the cognate of the *kuṇḍalinī* was the fiery *avadhūtī* or *caṇḍālī* ("outcaste woman"), whose union with the male principle in the cranial vault caused the fluid "thought of enlightenment" (*bodhicitta*) to flood the practitioner's body.

The *cakra*s of the yogic body are identified in hathayogic sources not only as so many internalized cremation grounds—both the favorite haunts of the medieval Tantric yogis, and those sites on which a burning fire releases the self from the body before hurling it skyward—but also as "circles" of dancing, howling, high-flying *yoginī*s whose flight is fueled, precisely, by their ingestion of male semen. When the *kuṇḍalinī* reaches the end of her rise and bursts into the cranial vault, the semen that she has been carrying has been transformed into the nectar of immortality, which the yogi then drinks internally from the bowl of his own skull. With it, he becomes an immortal, invulnerable, being possessed of supernatural powers, a god on earth.

Without a doubt, *haṭha yoga* both synthesizes and internalizes many of the elements of earlier yoga systems: meditative ascent, upward mobility via the flight of the *yoginī* (now replaced by the *kuṇḍalinī*), and a number of esoteric Tantric practices. It is also probable that the thermodynamic transformations internal to Hindu alchemy, the essential texts of which predate the *haṭha yoga* canon by at least a century, also provided a set of theoretical models for the new system (White 1996).

With respect to modern-day postural yoga, *haṭha yoga*'s greatest legacy is to be found in the combination of fixed postures (*āsanas*), breath control techniques (*prāṇāyāma*), locks (*bandhas*), and seals (*mudrās*) that comprise its practical side. These are the practices that isolate the inner yogic body from the outside, such that it becomes a hermetically sealed system within which air and fluids can be drawn upward, against their normal downward flow. These techniques are described in increasing detail between the tenth and fifteenth centuries, the period of the flowering of the *haṭha yoga* corpus. In later centuries, a canonical number of eighty-four *āsanas* would be reached (Bühnemann 2007).

Often, the practice system of *haṭha yoga* is referred to as "six-limbed" yoga, as a means of distinguishing it from the "eight-limbed" practice of the YS. What the two systems generally share in common with one another—as well as with the yoga systems of the late classical Upaniṣads, the later *Yoga Upaniṣads*, and every Buddhist yoga system—are posture, breath control, and the three levels of meditative concentration leading to *samādhi*. In the YS, these six practices are preceded by behavioral restraints and purificatory ritual observances (*yama* and *niyama*). The Jain yoga systems of both the eighth-century Haribhadra and the tenth- to thirteenth-century Digambara Jain monk Rāmasena are also eight-limbed [Dundas]. By the time of the fifteenth-century CE *Haṭhayogapradīpikā* (also known as the *Haṭhapradīpikā*) of Svātmarāman, this distinction had become codified under a different set of terms: *haṭha yoga*, which comprised the practices leading to liberation in the body (*jīvanmukti*) was made to be the inferior stepsister of *rāja yoga*, the meditative techniques that culminate in the cessation of suffering through disembodied liberation (*videha mukti*). These categories could, however, be subverted, as a remarkable albeit idiosyncratic eighteenth-century Tantric document makes abundantly clear [Vasudeva].

Here, it should be noted that prior to the end of the first millennium CE, detailed descriptions of *āsanas* were nowhere to be found in the Indian textual record. In the light of this, any claim that sculpted images of cross-legged figures—including those represented on the famous clay seals from third millennium BCE Indus Valley archeological sites—represent yogic postures are speculative at best (White 2009: 48–59).

THE NĀTH YOGĪS

All of the earliest Sanskrit-language works on *haṭha yoga* are attributed to Gorakhnāth, the twelfth- to thirteenth-century founder of the religious order known as the Nāth Yogīs, Nāth Siddhas, or simply, the yogis. The Nāth Yogīs were and remain the sole South Asian order to self-identify as yogis, which makes perfect sense given their explicit agenda of bodily immortality, invulnerability, and the attainment of supernatural powers. While little is known of the life of this founder and innovator, Gorakhnāth's prestige was such that an important number of seminal *haṭha yoga* works, many of which postdated the historical Gorakhnāth by several centuries, named him as their author in order to lend them a cachet of authenticity. In addition to these Sanskrit-language guides to the practice of *haṭha yoga*, Gorakhnāth and several of his disciples were also the putative authors of a rich treasury of mystic poetry, written in the vernacular language of twelfth- to fourteenth-century northwest India. These poems contain particularly vivid descriptions of the yogic body, identifying its inner landscapes with the principal mountains, river systems, and other landforms of the Indian subcontinent as well as with the imagined worlds of medieval Indic cosmology. This legacy would be carried forward in the later Yoga Upaniṣads as well as in the mystic poetry of the late medieval Tantric revival of the eastern region of Bengal [Hayes]. It also survives in popular traditions of rural north India, where the esoteric teachings of yogi gurus of yore continue to be sung by modern-day yogi bards in all-night village gatherings [Gold and Gold].

Given their reputed supernatural powers, the Tantric yogis of medieval adventure and fantasy literature were often cast as rivals to princes and kings whose thrones and harems they tried to usurp. In the case of the Nāth Yogīs, these relationships were real and documented, with members of their order celebrated in a number of kingdoms across northern and western India for having brought down tyrants and raised untested princes to the throne. These feats are also chronicled in late medieval Nāth Yogī hagiographies and legend cycles, which feature princes who abandon the royal life to take initiation with illustrious gurus, and yogis who use their remarkable supernatural powers for the benefit (or to the detriment) of kings. All of the great Mughal emperors had interactions with the Nāth Yogīs, including Aurangzeb, who appealed to a yogi abbot for an alchemical aphrodisiac; Shāh Alam II, whose fall from power was foretold by a naked yogi; and the illustrious Akbar, whose fascination and political savvy brought him into contact with Nāth Yogīs on several occasions [Pinch].

While it is often difficult to separate fact from fiction in the case of the Nāth Yogīs, there can be no doubt but that they were powerful figures who provoked powerful reactions on the part of the humble and mighty alike. At the height of their power between the fourteenth and seventeenth centuries, they appeared frequently in the writings of north Indian poet-saints (*sant*s) like Kabīr and Guru Nānak, who generally castigated them for their arrogance and obsession with worldly power. The Nāth Yogīs were among the first religious orders to militarize into fighting units, a practice that became so commonplace that by the eighteenth century the north Indian military labor market was dominated by "yogi" warriors who numbered in the hundreds of thousands (Pinch 2006)! It was not until the late eighteenth century, when the British quashed the so-called Sannyasi and Fakir Rebellion in Bengal, that the widespread phenomenon of the yogi warrior began to disappear from the Indian subcontinent.

Like the Sufi *fakir*s with whom they were often associated, the yogis were widely considered by India's rural peasantry to be superhuman allies who could protect them from the supernatural entities responsible for disease, famine, misfortune, and death. Yet, the same yogis have long been dreaded and feared for the havoc they are capable of wreaking on persons weaker than themselves. Even to the present day in rural India and Nepal, parents will scold naughty children by threatening them that "the yogi will come and take them away." There may be a historical basis to this threat: well into the modern period, poverty-stricken villagers sold their children into the yogi orders as an acceptable alternative to death by starvation.

THE YOGA UPANIṢADS

The Yoga Upaniṣads [Ruff] are a collection of twenty-one medieval Indian reinterpretations of the so-called classical Upaniṣads, that is, works like the *Kaṭhaka Upaniṣad*, quoted earlier. Their content is devoted to metaphysical correspondences between the universal macrocosm and bodily microcosm, meditation, mantra, and techniques of yogic practice. While it is the case that their content is quite entirely derivative of Tantric and Nāth Yogī traditions, their originality lies in their Vedānta-style non-dualist metaphysics (Bouy 1994). The earliest works of this corpus, devoted to meditation upon *mantra*s—especially OṂ, the acoustic essence of the absolute *brahman*—were compiled in north India some time between the ninth and thirteenth centuries. Between the fifteenth and eighteenth centuries, south Indian brahmins greatly expanded these works—folding into them a wealth of data from the Hindu Tantras as well as the *haṭha yoga* traditions of the Nāth Yogīs, including the *kuṇḍalinī*, the yogic *āsana*s, and the internal geography of the yogic body. So it is that many of the Yoga Upaniṣads exist both in short "northern" and longer "southern" versions. Far to the north, in Nepal, one finds the same influences and philosophical orientations in the *Vairāgyāṃvara*, a work on yoga composed by the eighteenth-century founder of the Josmanī sect. In some respects, its author Śaśidhara's political and social activism anticipated the agendas of the nineteenth-century Indian founders of modern yoga [Timilsina].

Modern Yoga

In Calcutta, colonial India's most important center of intellectual life, the late nineteenth century saw the emergence of a new "holy man" style among leaders of the Indian reform and independence movement. A prime catalyst for this shift was the 1882 publication of Bankim Chandra Chatterji's powerful and controversial Bengali novel *Ānandamath* (Lipner 2005), which drew parallels between the Sannyasi and Fakir Rebellion and the cause of Indian independence. In the years and decades that followed, numerous (mainly Bengali) reformers shed their Western-style clothing to put on the saffron robes of Indian holy men. These included, most notably, Swami Vivekananda, the Indian founder of "modern yoga" (De Michelis 2004: 91–180); and Sri Aurobindo, who was jailed by the British for plotting a *sannyāsī* revolt against the Empire but who devoted the latter part of his life to yoga, founding his famous *āśram* in Pondicherry in 1926. While the other leading yoga gurus of the first half of the twentieth century had no reform or political agenda, they left their mark by carrying the gospel of modern yoga to the west. These include Paramahamsa Yogananda, the author of the perennial best-selling 1946 publication, *Autobiography of a Yogi*; Sivananda, who was for a short time the guru of the pioneering yoga scholar and historian of religions Mircea Eliade; Kuvalayananda, who focused on the modern scientific and medical benefits of yoga practice (Alter 2004: 73–108); Hariharananda Aranya, the founder of the Kapila Matha [Jacobsen]; and Krishnamacharya [Singleton, Narasimhan, and Jayashree], the guru of the three *haṭha yoga* masters most responsible for popularizing postural yoga throughout the world in the late twentieth century.

Vivekananda's rehabilitation of what he termed "rāja yoga" is exemplary, for its motives, its influences, and its content. A shrewd culture broker seeking a way to turn his countrymen away from practices he termed "kitchen religion," Vivekananda seized upon the symbolic power of yoga as a genuinely Indian, yet non-sectarian, type of applied philosophy that could be wielded as a "unifying sign of the Indian nation . . . not only for national consumption but for consumption by the entire world" (Van der Veer 2001: 73–74). For Vivekananda, *rāja yoga*, or "classical yoga," was the science of yoga taught in the *Yoga Sūtra*, a notion he took from none other than the Theosophist Madame Blavatsky, who had a strong Indian following in the late nineteenth century. Following his success in introducing *rāja yoga* to western audiences at the 1892 World Parliament of Religions at Chicago, Vivekananda remained in the United States for much of the next decade (he died in 1902), lecturing and writing on the YS. His quite idiosyncratic interpretations of this work were highly congenial to the religiosity of the period, which found expression in India mainly through the rationalist spirituality of Neo-Vedānta. So it was that Vivekananda defined *rāja yoga* as the supreme contemplative path to self-realization, in which the self so realized was the supreme self, the absolute *brahman* or god-self within.

While Vivekananda's influence on present-day understandings of yoga theory is incalculable, his disdain for the means and ends of *haṭha yoga* practice were such that that form of yoga—the principal traditional source of modern postural yoga—was slow to be embraced by the modern world. It should be noted here that within India, the tradition of *haṭha yoga* had been all but lost, and that it was not until the publication of a number of editions of late *haṭha yoga* texts, by the Theosophical Society and others, that interest in it was rekindled. Indeed, none other than the great Krishnamacharya himself went to Tibet in search of true practitioners of a tradition he considered lost in India (Kadetsky 2004: 76–79). One of the earliest American practitioners to study yoga under Indian teachers and later attempt to market the teachings of *haṭha yoga* in the west, Theos Bernard died in Tibet in the 1930s while searching there for the yogic "grail" [Hackett].

Whatever Krishnamacharya found in his journey to Tibet, the yoga that he taught in his role of "yoga master" of the Mysore Palace was an eclectic amalgam of *haṭha yoga* techniques, British military calisthenics, and the regional gymnastic and wrestling traditions of southwestern India (Sjoman 1996). Beginning in the 1950s, his three leading disciples—B. K. S. Iyengar, K. Pattabhi Jois, and T.K.V. Desikachar—would introduce their own variations on his techniques and so define the postural yoga that has swept Europe, the United States, and much of the rest of the world. The direct and indirect disciples of these three innovators form the vanguard of yoga teachers on the contemporary scene. The impact of these innovators of yoga, with their eclectic blend of training in postures with teachings from the YS, also had the secondary effect of catalyzing a reform within the Śvetāmbara Jain community, opening the door to the emergence of a universalistic and missionary yoga-based Jainism in the United Kingdom in particular [Qvarnström and Birch].

In the course of the past thirty years, yoga has been transformed more than at any time since the advent of *haṭha yoga* in the tenth to eleventh centuries (Syman 2010). The theoretical pairing of yoga with mind-expanding drugs, the practice of "cakra adjustment," the use of crystals: these are but a few of the entirely original improvisations on a four-thousand-year-old theme, which have been invented outside of India during the past decades. Aware of this appropriation of what it rightly considers to be its own cultural legacy, Indians have begun to take steps to safeguard their yoga traditions. In 2001, the Traditional Knowledge Digital Library (TKDL) was founded in India as a tool for preventing foreign entrepreneurs from appropriating and patenting Indian traditions as their own intellectual properties. Spurred by the 2004 granting of a U.S. patent on a sequence of twenty-six *āsana*s to the Indian-American yoga celebrity Bikram Chaudhury, the TKDL has turned its attention to yoga. In the light of the history outlined in this introduction, the TKDL has a vast range of theories and practices to protect.

Works Cited

Alter, Joseph S. (2004). *Yoga in Modern India: The Body between Science and Philosophy*. Princeton, NJ: Princeton University Press.

Bouy, Christian (1994). *Les Nātha-yogin et les Upaniṣads*. Paris: De Boccard.

Bronkhorst, Johannes (1993). *The Two Traditions of Meditation in Ancient India*. Delhi: Motilal Banarsidass.

Bühnemann, Gudrun (2007). *Eighty-four Āsanas in Yoga. A Survey of Traditions (with Illustrations)*. New Delhi: D. K. Printworld.

Cleary, Thomas, tr. (1995). *Buddhist Yoga, A Comprehensive Course*. Boston and London: Shambhala.

De Michelis, Elizabeth (2004). *A History of Modern Yoga. Patañjali and Western Esotericism*. New York and London: Continuum.

Eliade, Mircea (2009). *Yoga: Immortality and Freedom*, 2d ed. Princeton, NJ: Princeton University Press.

Franco, Eli (2009). "Introduction." In *Yogic Perception, Meditation and Altered States of Consciousness*, ed. Eli Franco and Dagmar Einar, pp. 1–51. Vienna: Österreichische Akademie der Wissenschaften.

Kadetsky, Elizabeth (2004). *First There Is a Mountain: A Yoga Romance*. Boston, New York, and London: Little, Brown.

La Vallée Poussin, Louis de (1936–1937). "Le Bouddhisme et le yoga de Patañjali." *Mélanges chinois et bouddhiques* 5: 223–42.

Lipner, Julius J., tr. (2005). *Anandamath, or The Sacred Brotherhood: Translated with a Critical Introduction*. New York: Oxford University Press.

Lusthaus, Dan (2004). "Yogācāra School." In *Encyclopedia of Buddhism*, 2 vols., ed. Robert E. Buswell, Jr., vol. 1, pp. 914–21. New York: Macmillan Reference USA/Thomson/Gale.

MacDonald, Anne (2009). "Knowing Nothing: Candrakīrti and Yogic Perception." In *Yogic Perception, Meditation and Altered States of Consciousness*, ed. Eli Franco and Dagmar Einar, pp. 133–68. Vienna: Österreichische Akademie der Wissenschaften.

Oman, John Campbell (1908). *Cults, Customs & Superstitions of India*. London: T. Fisher Unwin.

Pinch, William (2006). *Warrior Ascetics and Indian Empires*. Cambridge: Cambridge University Press.

Qvarnström, Olle (2003). "Losing One's Mind and Becoming Enlightened." In *Yoga, The Indian Tradition*, ed. Ian Whicher and David Carpenter, pp. 130–42. London: RoutledgeCurzon.

Rastelli, Marion (2009). "Perceiving God and Becoming Like Him: Yogic Perception and Its Implications in the Viṣṇuitic Tradition of Pāñcarātra." In *Yogic Perception, Meditation and Altered States of Consciousness*, ed. Eli Franco and Dagmar Einar, pp. 299–317. Vienna: Österreichische Akademie der Wissenschaften.

Sanderson, Alexis (2006). "The Lākulas: New Evidence of a System Intermediate Between Pāñcārthika Pāśupatism and Āgamic Śaivism." *Indian Philosophical Annual* 24: 143–217.

Sarbacker, Stuart Ray (2005). *Samādhi. The Numinous and Cessative in Indo-Tibetan Yoga.* Albany: State University of New York Press.

Singleton, Mark (2010). *Yoga Body: the Origins of Modern Posture Practice.* London and New York: Oxford University Press.

Sjoman, N. E. (1996). *The Yoga Tradition of the Mysore Palace.* New Delhi: Abhinav Publications.

Syman, Stefanie (2010). *The Subtle Body: The Story of Yoga in America.* New York. Farrar, Strauss and Giroux.

Van der Veer, Peter (2001). *Imperial Encounters: Religion and Modernity in India and Britain.* Princeton, NJ: Princeton University Press.

Vasudeva, Somadeva (2004). *The Yoga of the Mālinīvijayottaratantra.* Pondicherry: l'Institut Français de Pondichéry.

White, David Gordon (1996). *The Alchemical Body: Siddha Traditions in Medieval India.* Chicago: University of Chicago Press.

——— (2003). *Kiss of the Yoginī. "Tantric Sex" in its South Asian Contexts.* Chicago: University of Chicago Press.

——— (2009). *Sinister Yogis.* Chicago: University of Chicago Press.

Note for Instructors

David Gordon White

As Jonathan Z. Smith has famously written, the task of the religious studies scholar is not only to make the strange seem familiar, but also to make the familiar seem strange. Put another way, our goal is both to reorient and to disorient. Of course, orientation is about finding one's bearings, and in the South Asian contexts out of which most of the world's yoga traditions arose, the east (*pūrva*) was always the direction of reference, because it was there that the sun rose and the day began. For this reason, the Sanskrit term *pūrva* has also had a temporal referent, in the sense of "prior to," "before." Accordingly, the chapters in this volume are, with a few exceptions, arranged chronologically, beginning at the beginning. Following the editor's introduction, which itself provides a chronological account of the origins and development of the many yogas that have come down to us, the contributions to this volume may be read as a historical narrative, from the Buddhist sources of Yoga philosophy as found in an early medical text down to the modern-day Jain system of *prekṣa* meditation.

This is where the process of reorientation and disorientation may begin in the classroom. Given the fact that the people who "do" yoga number in the tens of millions in the West alone, many students will come to a course on yoga with a number of preconceptions received from their teachers and trainers. Primary among these will be the received notion that all yogas are one, and that that one Yoga tradition has remained unchanged since its origins in the mists of antiquity. An alternative assumption is that yoga has evolved in a straight line and following some sort of historical determinism from the teachings of the *Bhagavad Gītā* and the *Yoga Sūtra* down through the classical works of *haṭha yoga* and into modern-day Vinyāsa, Aṣṭāṅga, Kriyā Yoga, and so forth. What a chronological reading of the outstanding translations and introductions of this volume makes abundantly clear is that there are as many discontinuities as there are continuities in the history of yoga, and that there are nearly as many yoga systems as there are texts on yoga. Furthermore, even within a single genre of yoga literature, such as the Yoga Upaniṣads, one finds a sharp divergence between the respective philosophies of northern and southern traditions, with both varying significantly from the (in fact very limited) yoga content of the "classical" Upaniṣads from which they take their name. The term yoga has itself been interpreted in widely variant ways, with both the *Bhagavad Gīta* and commentaries on the *Yoga Sūtra* asserting that the true sense of the term yoga is *viyoga*, "non-yoga." As for the *rāja yoga* that the great Swami Vivekananda championed as the "royal" yoga and "essence" of the *Yoga Sūtra*, commentators from earlier centuries employed the same term to denote a yogi's consumption of his female consort's sexual emissions (*rajas*)! Guiding students through the twists and turns of these multiple readings of yoga and the practices and theories in which they are embedded should serve to disabuse them of many of their prior assumptions.

This work of disorientation will, of necessity, be complemented by one of reorientation, of making the strange seem familiar. There *are* continuities—historical, philosophical, ritual, and so forth—between and among the various yoga traditions; however they are rarely found where one expects to find them. This being said, one cannot help but notice that even when they are seeking to refute one another, the authors of these works were clearly engaged in some sort of conversation. So, while there are distinctively Hindu, Buddhist, Jain, Tantric, non-sectarian, and even Islamic yoga traditions, there are a number of pervasive themes that recur across texts and time. In their introductions, the contributors to this volume (who also harbor differing opinions concerning yoga) have taken great pains to describe both the distinctiveness of and the continuities between the texts and traditions they are interpreting. So, for example, Dundas's introduction is an excellent guide to the specificities of Jain yoga traditions, while those of Chapple and Qvarnström/Birch link Jain formulations to those of the *Yoga Sūtra*, *Bhagavad Gītā*, hathayogic texts and so forth. Wujastyk, Larson, and Malinar discuss Buddhist influences on the *Yoga Sūtra* and *Bhagavad Gītā*, while Ernst delineates the hathayogic sources of Islamic treatises on breath control. As the six contributions on yoga in South and Inner Asian Tantric traditions make clear, sectarian differences among Hindus, Buddhists, and Jains paled in comparison to the commonalities of their shared Tantric worldview, metaphysics, goals, and techniques.

Another aspect of reorientation involves finding continuities in practice. When one reads the term yoga in one of its most general senses, as "discipline," another common feature of the various yoga traditions emerges. This is the notion that through the many disciplines called yoga, the practitioner seeks to stop, still, or immobilize one or more of four essential components of his person: his thought, breath, seed, and body. This common goal, of immobilization, flows from a shared assumption that suffering existence is a "flow" (*saṃsāra* literally means "con-fluence"), and that salvation is to be realized, precisely, by removing oneself from that flow. What distinguishes the principal types of yogic practice from one another are the components of the self that are the objects of one's discipline. So it is that in meditative traditions, the principal focus will be on immobilizing thought, usually in conjunction with breath control, the inner repetition of mantras, and so on. In most forms of Tantric yoga, thought, semen, and the body are highlighted to varying degrees. In *haṭha yoga*, the focus can be on all four components, as immortalized in a medieval vernacular poem attributed to the Nāth Yogī Gopīcand: "Steady goes the breath, and the mind is steady, steady goes the mind, the semen. Steady the semen, and the body is steady, that's what Gopıcand is sayin'." Drawing students' attention to these various combinations of the four principal objects of yogic discipline may serve as an interactive pedagogical technique in the classroom.

As this volume goes to press, culture warriors from worlds apart are staking the nearly identical claim that yoga is fundamentally Hindu. In the United States, a number of Christian evangelists are taking this position for the expressed purpose of controlling the bodies of Christian women, while in India, Hindu fundamentalists are doing the same in the service of their ongoing campaign of identity politics. In a word, each is instrumentalizing a simplified idea of yoga for ulterior motives of social, cultural, or political domination.

As for their shared claim, that yoga is fundamentally Hindu, this can only stand if one allows that there has only ever been one "yoga," and that that yoga has remained unaltered since its inception, i.e., that the yoga being taught today in yoga studios across the globe is identical to the yoga of the Upaniṣads or that taught by Kṛṣṇa in the *Bhagavad Gītā*, the two earliest treatments of "yoga" in the Hindu canon. However, upon inspection, these two original Hindu teachings on yoga are found to diverge on several points, and so one must conclude that from the very outset there have been at least two Hindu systems of yoga. And, as the contributions to this volume make plain, the past 2,500 years have seen the emergence of many, many systems of yoga—the earliest of which may not have been Hindu at all, and many of which arose outside of India—whose theories and practices have often been diametrically opposed to one another. To cite but one example from this volume, the author of the eighteenth-century *Haṃsavilāsa* held the teachings of the *Yoga Sūtra* up for ridicule, calling them "nonsense."

More than any other text, it was this work, the *Yoga Sūtra* of Patañjali, that Swami Vivekananda—the late-nineteenth-century reformer, nationalist, and father of modern yoga—championed as the theoretical foundation for all authentic yoga practice. But, as Peter van der Veer has recently shown, Vivekananda, too, was instrumentalizing this ancient yoga tradition in his own way. Vivekananda preached that the *Yoga Sūtra* was not only "scientific" and "spiritual," but also emphatically anti-sectarian—and that it was precisely because it transcended all religious and sectarian boundaries that yoga could be placed in the service of fostering Indian unity. Following in Vivekananda's wake, T. Krishnamacharya, the father of the postural yoga practiced by millions today, did not, in spite of his own orthodox Hindu identity, emphasize the "Hindu" content of yoga training. In his earliest published work on yoga, the circa 1935 *Yoga Makaranda,* Krishnamacharya took a position similar to Vivekananda's, arguing for the spirituality of the "science of yoga" (*yoga-vidyā*) as a corrective for India's flirtations with Western ways, and concluding that "Yoga will bring back honor and respect to Mother India."

As important as they are for twenty-first century understandings of yoga, Vivekananda and Krishnamacharya stand near the end of a long line of innovators who created something entirely new even as they harked back to the ancient foundations of yoga. Gorakhnāth, the medieval founder of the Nāth Yogīs and purported author of the earliest Sanskrit-language guides to *haṭha yoga*—a revolutionary form of practice involving "locks" and "seals" and the inner transformation of semen into the nectar of immortality—was also the author of a collection of mystic poems. Known as the *Gorakh Bāṇī,* these verses glorified the yogi as a person who could reduce the gods of the Hindu male trinity (Brahmā, Viṣṇu, and Śiva) to slavery—hardly a "Hindu" position! Many of the yogas of history have never been Hindu at all, but rather Jain, Buddhist, perhaps even Islamic in their sectarian identities.

Now, it is the case that many modern-day yoga gurus have collapsed the rich and varied histories of the many yogas of India, greater Asia, and now the West, into a simplistic vision of yoga as an unchanging tradition grounded in the religion of the Vedas. However, the simple fact that some contemporary teachers and practitioners of yoga hold to such an untenable hypothesis does not make yoga Hindu, any more than the presence of a plastic Jesus on some dashboards would make all automobile drivers Christian.

Foundational Yoga Texts

—1—

The Path to Liberation through Yogic Mindfulness in Early Āyurveda

Dominik Wujastyk

It can come as a surprise to discover that buried in one of the earliest medical treatises in Sanskrit is a short tract on the yogic path to liberation. This tract—a mere thirty-nine verses—occurs in the Chapter on the Embodied Person (*Śārīrasthāna*) in the *Compendium of Caraka* (*Carakasaṃhitā*). The *Compendium* is a medical encyclopedia and perhaps the earliest surviving complete treatise on classical Indian medicine. It is even more surprising to find that this yogic tract contains several references to Buddhist meditation and a previously unknown eightfold path leading to the recollection or mindfulness that is the key to liberation. Finally, Caraka's yoga tract almost certainly predates the famous classical yoga system of Patañjali. Let us explore these points in turn.

Classical Indian medicine, *āyurveda* ("the knowledge for long life"), is based on the body of medical theory and practice that was first collected and synthesized in several great medical encyclopedias, including especially the *The Compendium of Caraka* and *The Compendium of Suśruta* (*Suśrutasaṃhitā*). However, there are traces of the formation of this medical system to be found in earlier Sanskrit and Pāli literature. The first occurrence of the Sanskrit word *āyurveda* in Indian history is in the *Mahābhārata* epic. The epic also refers to medicine as having eight components, a term that is so standard in later literature that the science "with eight components" (*aṣṭāṅga*) becomes a synonym for medicine. These components include topics such as therapeutics, pediatrics, possession, surgery, and toxicology.

But the very earliest reference in Indian literature to a form of medicine that is unmistakably a forerunner of āyurveda is found in the teachings of the Buddha (probably fl. ca. 480–400 BCE, but these dates are still debated). As far as we know, it was not yet called āyurveda, but the basic concepts were the same as those that later formed the foundations of āyurveda. The Pali

Buddhist Canon as we have it today probably dates from about 250 BCE, and records a fairly trustworthy account of what the Buddha said. In the collection of Buddhist sermons called the "Connected Sayings" (*Saṃyutta Nikāya*), there is a story that tells how the Buddha was approached by a monk called Sīvako who asked him whether disease is caused by bad actions performed in the past, in other words by bad karma. The Buddha said no, that bad karma is only part of the picture and that diseases may be caused by any of eight factors. The factors he listed were bile, phlegm, wind, and their pathological combination, changes of the seasons, the stress of unusual activities, external agency, as well as the ripening of bad karma. This is the first moment in documented Indian history that these medical categories and explanations are combined in a clearly systematic manner. The term "pathological combination" (Pāli *sannipāta*) is particularly telling: this is a technical term from āyurveda that is as specific as a modern establishment doctor saying something like "hemoglobin levels." This term signals clearly that the Buddha's list of disease-causes emanates from a milieu in which a body of systematic technical medical knowledge existed. And it is these very factors that later became the cornerstone of classical Indian medical theory, or āyurveda. The historical connection between the ascetic traditions—such as Buddhism and āyurveda—is an important one.

What is the date of the *Compendium of Caraka*? The chronology of this work is complex. The text already declares itself to be the work of three people. An early text by Agniveśa was edited (*pratisaṃskṛta*) by Caraka. Caraka's work was later completed by Dṛḍhabala. Jan Meulenbeld has surveyed the key historical issues with great care in his *History of Indian Medical Literature*. After assessing the Nyāya, Vaiśeṣika, and Buddhist materials that appear in Caraka's *Compendium*, Meulenbeld concludes that, "Caraka cannot have lived later than about AD 150–200 and not much earlier than 100 BC."

How does this dating relate to the early history of classical yoga? Is the yoga tract in Caraka's *Compendium* to be dated before or after the classical yoga of Patañjali? In his authoritative new edition of the "Samādhi" chapter of Patañjali's work on yoga, Philipp Maas (2006) has provided a compelling reassessment of the authorship, title, and date of the texts commonly known as the *Yoga Sūtra* and the *Vyāsabhāṣya*, but which call themselves collectively the *Pātañjalayogaśāstra*, or *Patañjali's Teaching on Yoga*. Based on careful arguments and evidence, Maas makes three main assertions:

1. The text of the *Pātañjalayogaśāstra*, i.e., the undivided *Sūtra* and its commentary the *Bhāṣya*, is a single composition that can be traced back to a single author.

2. That author can be called Patañjali.
3. This unified text can be plausibly dated to about 400 CE.

Maas shows that the earliest references to "Vedavyāsa" as the author of a *Bhāṣya* occur at the end of the first millennium, in the works of Vācaspatimiśra (fl. ca. 975–1000), in his *Tattvavaiśāradī*; and Kṣemarāja (fl. ca. 950–1050), in his *Svacchandatantroddyota*. From the eleventh century onward, authors such as Mādhava (fifteenth-century *Sarvadarśanasaṃgraha*) routinely refer to Patañjali's *Yogaśāstra*, his *Sāṃkhyapravacana* or his *Yoga Sūtra*, and to Vyāsa as the author of the *Bhāṣya*.

However, the earliest of these revisionist authors, Vācaspati, also refers elsewhere to Patañjali as the author of a part of the *Bhāṣya*. Vācaspati was apparently uncertain as to whether *sūtra* and *bhāṣya* were by the same author or not. In fact, this view was reasonably widespread amongst early authors such as Śrīdhara in his ca. 991 CE *Nyāyakandalī*, Abhinavagupta in his ca. 950 CE *Abhinavabhāratī*, and many others. Maas also shows that the earliest form of the work's title in manuscript chapter colophons was probably *Pātañjala-yogaśāstra-sāṃkhyapravacana*, "Patañjali's Sāṃkhya Teaching that is the Treatise on Yoga." Working from this as well as internal textual arguments, Maas concludes that Patañjali took materials about yoga from older sources, and added his own explanatory passages to create the unified work that, since about 1100 CE, has been considered the work of two people. The extracts were designated as *sūtra*s and ascribed to Patañjali, while the explanations and additional remarks were regarded as a *bhāṣya* and ascribed to Vyāsa (meaning "the editor" in Sanskrit).

As for the all-important issue of the date of the *Pātañjalayogaśāstra*, Maas notes that it is partly a matter of guesswork, but refers to the plausible citations by Māgha (in his 600–800 CE *Śiṣupālavadha*), Vṛṣabhadeva (fl. ca. 650 CE), and Gauḍapāda (in his ca. 500 CE commentary on Īśvarakṛṣṇa's *Sāṃkhyakārikā*s). Maas therefore argues that the *Pātañjalayogaśāstra* was, by the beginning of the sixth century, regarded as an authoritative representation of yoga philosophy. Such a reputation would have taken at least some time to become established. The earliest possible date for the *Pātañjalayogaśāstra* is Patañjali's apparent engagement with the Vijñānavāda teaching of Vasubandhu in the fourth century, as already proposed long ago by Woods (1914). Maas's final opinion is that the composition of the *Pātañjalayogaśāstra* can be placed in the period between 325 and 425 CE.

Whatever the nuances of the arguments, it is beyond reasonable doubt that the *Compendium* of Caraka precedes the *Pātañjalayogaśāstra*, that the yoga tract in the *Compendium* is older than Patañjali's yoga system, and that it propounds a yoga system that has closer links to Vaiśeṣika philosophy than to the Sāṃkhya of Patañjali's system.

Caraka's Yoga Tract

In the yoga tract in his chapter on the origin and structure of the human being, the *Śārīrasthāna*, Caraka first frames yoga as both spiritual liberation and the means of attaining it. Verses 138–39 are a direct citation from the *Vaiśeṣikasūtra*. Caraka continues with a description of the supernatural powers that accrue to the practitioner of yoga as a result of his self-discipline and the power of his concentration. This is very much in line with Patañjali's teaching on *siddhi*s, and indeed with common ideas of the result of yoga practice across Indian literature.

Among the earliest sources of the idea that supernatural powers result from meditation are the descriptions in the Buddhist canonical text, the *Sāmañña-phalasutta* of the *Dīgha Nikāya*, when characterizing the monk who has completed the four meditations (Pāli *jhāna*). The powers arise from being integrated (*samāhita*), and are as follows:

1. body-power (*kāyavasa*), or the power to self-multiply, vanish, fly through walls, even touch the sun or moon
2. knowledge from divine hearing (*dibbasotañāṇa*)
3. mind-reading (*cetopariyañāṇa*)
4. the recollection of past lives (*pubbenivāsānussatiñāṇa*)
5. divine seeing (*dibbacakkhu*)
6. knowledge of the destruction of the bad influences (*āsavakkhaya*)

Many of the key terms used in this list of six powers are the same as those used in Caraka's yoga tract when he describes the eight powers that yoga practice can produce.

Most interesting of all, Caraka frames a new eightfold practice leading to recollection (Skt. *smṛti*), and places recollection at the very center of yogic practice. For Caraka, it is recollection that leads to yoga, and yoga that leads to the acquisition of supernatural powers and to ultimate liberation.

The language and conceptualization of this passage in the medical literature places it squarely within the tradition of the Buddhist mindfulness meditation (Pāli *satipaṭṭhāna*), often practiced today under the name *vipassanā*. As Gyatso (1992) has shown, in the Buddhist tradition, the Pāli term *sati* (Sanskrit *smṛti*) can denote memory in two quite distinct senses. First, it denotes memory as the simple bringing-to-mind of events that happened at an earlier period in time, the mental act required to answer such questions as, "what did I have for breakfast?" In a second sense, it means the deepening of one's consciousness, of one's experiential awareness of the present moment. This is the alert self-recollection that people experience at special or shocking moments in life, or as a result of deliberate forms of meditation practice. Sometimes, such moments of recollection or mindfulness generate long-term memories of the first type, which are referred to as "flashbulb memories."

The Pāli compound word *satī-paṭṭhāna*, the meditational practice leading to recollection or mindfulness, corresponds to the Sanskrit *smṛti-upasthāna*. And in verse 146, Caraka's text uses these very words to describe the one practice that leads to all the other moral and spiritual practices he has listed. They arise from "abiding in the memory of reality," or in Sanskrit *tattva-smṛter upasthānāt*. In the following verse, 147, Caraka inverts the cause-effect relation: it is the practice of the virtues listed in 143–44 that leads to recollection. Finally, verse 147 also identifies the final goal of recollection with freedom from suffering, Sanskrit *duḥkha*, again the central doctrine of Buddhism. This theme of suffering and impermanence is picked up again in verses 152 and 153 in completely Buddhist terms. Caraka's use of these keywords taken directly from the Buddhist meditational and doctrinal milieu shows unambiguously that his yoga tract is an adaptation of extremely old ascetic material known to us mainly from Buddhism.

Given all this, it is all the more surprising that the comment at the end of verse 149 identifies recollection with the ordinary-language meaning of memory, i.e., calling to mind previous experience. It is tempting to see this comment as an addition by an author who was not familiar with the Buddhist understanding of recollection or mindfulness that underlies this tract.

Since recollection is at the center of Caraka's method of yoga, the eightfold path to recollection that he outlines in verses 148 and 149 is of special interest. This appears to be a very early "eightfold path" whose origins and detailed meaning are obscure and require further study. It bears no apparent relation to other early forms of yogic path, such as the sixfold path of the *Maitrāyaṇīya Upaniṣad*, or the eightfold path of Patañjali's *Pātañjalayogaśāstra*. The first four of Caraka's eight steps to mindfulness concern the deepening of perception and discrimination. The fifth step could mean an attachment to *sattva* in the sense of the Sāṃkhya *guṇa* of purity, although at the end of verse 141 the same word means, as it often does, "mind." The sixth step, practice, could refer to practicing mindfulness, but it could also point to memorization in the ordinary sense. The seventh step, the yoga of knowledge, brings to mind the famous teachings of the *Bhagavadgītā* on this subject, where liberation is attainable through true gnosis. But Caraka's *Compendium* elsewhere shows no awareness of the *Gītā*. The last step, "what is heard again," is syntactically a little odd, since it is not exactly a procedural step in a path. But it was clearly intended as the eighth "step." It again suggests memorization, rather than mindfulness in the Buddhist sense.

The last part of verse 151 raises new questions. The philosophers of the Sāṃkhya school have normally been presumed to be those who "count" or "reckon" (*saṃkhyā-*) the twenty-five *tattva*s or evolutes of the universe's creation. However, in verse 151, Caraka has the Sāṃkhyas counting not *tattva*s, but *dharma*s. This strongly suggests the use of the word *dharma*, or Pāli *dhamma*, in the sense of "entity," "fundamental phenomenon," or even more neutrally "thing," and might even suggest the enumerative and descriptive characteristics of the Buddhist Abhidharma literature. The connection with Sāṃkhya continues with verse 153, which is a direct parallel of *Sāṃkhyakārikā* 64.

Caraka's yoga tract is an early and profoundly syncretic text about the path of yoga. Its citations from Vaiśeṣika and Sāṃkhya treatises show its willingness to synthesize across philosophical divides. But it is the Buddhist technical vocabulary and the text's focus on mindfulness as the most important yogic practice leading to liberation that strikes us most strongly. This suggests that Caraka integrated into his medical treatise an archaic yoga method that owed its origins to Buddhist traditions of cultivating *smṛti*.

Caraka's yoga tract did not go unnoticed within the Sanskrit literary tradition itself. In the fourth or fifth century it was copied by the author the *Yājñavalkyasmṛti*, and from there again into yet another work, the *Viṣṇusmṛti*. In this way, its ideas gained a readership far beyond physicians.

The passage below is translated from the *Carakasaṃhitā*, Śārīrasthāna 1, verses 137–55. The Sanskrit edition used is the standard vulgate edition: Jadavji Trikamji Acarya, ed., *Maharṣiṇā Punarvasunopadiṣṭā, tacchiṣyeṇāgniveśena praṇītā, Caraka Dṛḍhabalābhyāṃ pratisaṃskṛtā Carakasaṃhitā, śrī Cakrapāṇidattaviracitayā āyurvedadīpikāvyākhyayā saṃvalitā*, 3rd ed. (Bombay: Nirnaya Sagara Press, 1941). Earlier translations of this passage, none of which develop its wider significance, include Priya Vrat Sharma, *Caraka-Saṃhitā: Agniveśa's Treatise Refined and Annotated by Caraka and Redacted by Dṛḍhabala (text with English translation)*, 4 vols. Varanasi: Chaukhambha Orientalia 1981–1994), vol. 1, pp. 409–11; and Ram Karan Sharma and Vaidya Bhagwan Dash, *Agniveśa's Caraka Saṃhitā* (*Text with English Translation and Critical Exposition Based on Cakrapāṇi Datta's Āyurveda Dīpikā*), 7 vols. (Varanasi: Chowkhamba Sanskrit Series Office, 1976–2002), vol. 2, pp. 345–50.

Suggestions for Further Reading

The formation and early history of the Ayurvedic medical system outlined above is discussed in more detail by Kenneth G. Zysk, *Asceticism and Healing in Ancient India: Medicine in the Buddhist Monastery* (New York and Bombay: Oxford University Press, 1991; reprinted Delhi 1998, 2000); and by Dominik Wujastyk, "Indian Medicine," in W. F. Bynum and Roy Porter (eds.), *Companion Encyclopedia of the History of Medicine*, 2 vols. (London: Routledge, 1993), vol. 1, pp. 755–78; Dominik Wujastyk, "The Science of Medicine," in Gavin Flood (ed.), *The Blackwell Companion to Hinduism* (Oxford: Blackwell, 2003), pp. 393–409; and Dominik Wujastyk, *The Roots of Āyurveda: Selections from Sanskrit Medical Writings*, 3rd ed. (London and New York: Penguin, 2003). The most authoritative discussion of the dates of Ayurvedic texts is Gerrit Jan Meulenbeld, *A History of Indian Medical Literature*, 5 vols. (Groningen: E. Forsten, 1999–2002), Meulenbeld's discussion of the *Carakasaṃhitā*'s date is in vol. IA, pp. 105–15. The original Pāli text of the *Saṃyuttanikāya* discussed above appears in Leon Feer (ed.), *Saṃyutta-Nikāya. Part IV: Saḷāyatana-Vagga*, 3rd ed. (London: Pali Text Society, 1973), pp. 230–31. It has been translated by Bhikkhu Bodhi, *The Connected Discourses of the Buddha: A Translation from the Pāli* (Somerville, MA: Wisdom Publications, 2000), pp. 1278–79.

The question of whether the Buddhist Canon records the direct teaching of the Buddha or is a later construction by the monastic community is much debated. The topic is surveyed by Alexander Wynn, "The Historical Authenticity of Early Buddhist Literature: A Critical Evaluation," *Wiener Zeitschrift für die Kunde Südasiens* 49 (2005): 35–70, who defends a conservative view of the authenticity of the Canon as a record of the Buddha's words. A discussion of how recent manuscript discoveries affect our view of the *Saṃyuttanikāya*'s formation can be found in Andrew Glass and Mark Allon, *Four Gāndhārī Saṃyuktāgama sūtras: Senior Kharoṣṭhī fragment 5* (Seattle: University of Washington Press, 2007).

I have translated the Sanskrit word *smṛti* as "memory," "mindfulness," and "recollection" according to context. It has been called "one of the most difficult words . . . in the whole Buddhist system ethical psychology to translate" (Davids 1890–1894). Even in the early literature of the Veda, words from the verbal root *smṛ-* can denote memory of past events as well as the present awareness of objects of consciousness, as was noted by Konrad Klaus, "On the Meaning of the Root *smṛ* in Vedic Literature," *Wiener Zeitschrift für die Kunde Südasiens*, 36 (Supplementband) (1993): 77–86. Several relevant papers on the concept of memory in Buddhism are gathered in Janet Gyatso (ed.), *In the Mirror of Memory: Reflections on Mindfulness and Remembrance in Indian and Tibetan Buddhism*, SUNY Series in Buddhist Studies (Albany: State University of New York Press, 1992). The following important study stays very close to the original sources: Tse-fu Kuan, *Mindfulness in Early Buddhism: New Approaches Through Psychology and Textual Analysis of Pali, Chinese, and Sanskrit Sources* (London and New York: Routledge/Taylor & Francis, 2008). The issues of memory, Buddhism, and the *Carakasaṃhitā* are briefly touched upon by Johannes Bronkhorst, "A Note on the Caraka Saṃhitā and Buddhism," in *Early Buddhism and Abhidharma Thought: In Honor of Doctor Hajime Sakurabe on His Seventy-seventh Birthday, 2002.20. May* (Kyoto: Heirakuji Shoten, 2002), pp. 115–21. Gerhard Oberhammer, *Strukturen yogischer Meditation* (Vienna: Verl. d. Österr. Akad. d. Wiss., 1977), discusses mindfulness in the context of the *Pātañjalayogaśāstra* and with reference to the parallels in the *Questions of King Milinda* (Pali *Milindapañha*). See Thomas William Rhys Davids, *The Questions of King Milinda*, 2 vols. (Oxford: Clarendon Press, 1890–1894), vol. 1, pp. 58–59; and more recently Thera Nyanaponika and Bhikkhu Nyanatiloka, *Milindapañha: ein historisches Gipfeltreffen im religiösen Weltgespräch* (Bern: O.W. Barth [bei] Scherz, 1998), pp. 62–63.

The critical reassessment of the yoga teaching of Patañjali is that of Philipp André Maas, *Samādhipāda: das erste Kapitel des Pātañjalayogaśāstra zum ersten Mal kritisch ediert = The First Chapter of the Pātañjalayogaśāstra for the first time critically edited* (Aachen: Shaker, 2006). His key conclusions about the unified nature of the *sūtra* and *bhāṣya* are on p. xiv, and his arguments about the date of the *Pātañjalayogaśāstra* are on pp. xv–xvi. The evidence for Patañjali's knowledge of Vasubandhu's works was given by James Haughton Woods, *The Yoga-system of Patañjali: or, the ancient Hindu doctrine of Concentration of Mind Embracing the Mnemonic Rules, called Yoga-sūtras, of Patañjali and the Comment, called Yoga-bhāshya, attributed to Veda-Vyāsa and the Explanation, called Tattvavaiçāradī, of Vāchaspati-miçra, Harvard Oriental Series*, vol. 17 (Cambridge, MA: Harvard University Press, 1914), pp. xvii–xviii.

Amongst the earliest descriptions of a structured path of yoga, having a series of *aṅgas* or "components" is that of the sixth *prapāṭhaka* of the relatively late *Maitrāyaṇīya Upaniṣad*. For the Sanskrit text, see V. P. Limaye and R. D. Vadekar (eds.), *Eighteen principal Upaniṣads: Upaniṣadic text with parallels from extant Vedic literature, exegetical and grammatical notes* (Poona: Vaidika Samsodhana Mandala, 1958), pp. 325–57. The *Maitrāyaṇīya*'s six-component yoga and some of its successors were usefully discussed by Anton Zigmund-Cerbu,

"The Ṣaḍaṅgayoga," *History of Religions* 3:1 (1963): 128–34. Van Buitenen characterized the text as containing some interpolations: J.A.B. van Buitenen, *The Maitrāyaṇīya Upaniṣad. A Critical Essay, With Text, Translation and Commentary, Disputationes Rheno-Trajectinae*, vol. 6 (The Hague: Mouton & Co., 1962), pp. 84–87. This point was taken up by Somadeva Vasudeva, *The Yoga of the Malinivijayottaratantra, Critical edition, Translation and Notes*, (Pondicherry: IFP-EFEO, 2004), p. 375, note 18, where it is asserted that this section of the *Maitrāyaṇīya*'s text may be an interpolation later than *Jayākhyasaṃhitā* and other early Śaiva sources.

Tsutomu Yamashita, "On the Nature of the Medical Passages in the *Yājñavalkyasmṛti*," *Zinbun*, 36:2 (2001/2002): 87–129, establishes that the *Yājñavalkyasmṛti*'s "*ātman* treatise" is later than Caraka's *Compendium* and that it derived almost all of its concepts in this section from the *Carakasaṃhitā*. For the *Yājñavalkyasmṛti* passage parallel to verse 146 in Caraka's yoga tract, see Samarao Narasimha Naraharayya and Rai Bahadur Srisa Chandra Vasu, *The Sacred Laws of The Aryas as Taught in the School of Yajnavalkya and Explained by Vijnanesvara in his Well-known Commentary Named the Mitaksara Vol. III: The Prayaschitta Adhyaya* (Allahabad: The Pāṇini Office, 1913), p. 148. The text edition is Narayan Ram Acharya (ed.), *Yājñavalkyasmṛti of Yogīśvara Yajñavalkya with the Commentary Mitākṣarā of Vijñāneśvara, Notes, Variant Readings, etc.* (Bombay: Nirnayasagara Press, 1949), p. 390, verse 3.160.

Verse 137 of the translation talks about "pains." The Sanskrit term *vedanā*, sometimes translated as "feelings," is one of the key terms in the Buddhist philosophy of dependent origination (Pāli *paṭiccasamuppāda*) and one of the five *khandha*s or experiential aggregates of Buddhist theory. These Buddhist concepts are discussed especially insightfully by Sue Hamilton, *Identity and Experience: the Constitution of the Human Being According to Early Buddhism* (London: Luzac Oriental, 1996).

Verses 138–139 contain a passage parallel to *Vaiśeṣikasūtra*s 5.2.16–17. These have been discussed by Antonella Comba, "Carakasaṃhitā, Śārīrasthāna I and Vaiśeṣika Philosophy," in Gerrit Jan Meulenbeld and Dominik Wujastyk (eds.), *Studies on Indian Medical History* (Groningen: Egbert Forsten, 1987), pp. 43–61; and by Masanobu Nozawa, "Concept of Yoga in *Vaiśeṣikasūtra*," in *Indian Thought and Buddhist Culture. Essays in Honour of Professor Junkichi Imanishi on His Sixtieth Birthday* (Tokyo: Shunjū-Sha, 1996), pp. 17–30. The discussion by Albrecht Wezler, "Remarks on the Definition of 'Yoga' in the Vaiśeṣikasūtra," in Luise A. Hercus et al. (eds.), *Indological and Buddhist Studies: Volume in Honour of Professor J. W. de Jong on his Sixtieth Birthday* (Canberra: Australian National University. Faculty of Asian Studies, 1982), is relevant, although it does not mention the *Carakasaṃhitā* passage. Meulenbeld 1999–2002, vol. IB, p. 200, note 213, gives references for the dating of the *Vaiśeṣikasūtra*. The original *Vaiśeṣikasūtra* text in question can be found in the edition of Muni Jambuvijayaji (ed.), *Vaiśeṣikasūtra of Kaṇāda, with the commentary of Candrānanda*, *Gaekwad's Oriental Series*, vol. 136 (Baroda: Oriental Institute, 1961), p. 42.

Translation of the *Carakasaṃhitā*, śārīrasthāna 1, verses 137–155

137

In yoga and liberation, all pains are transient. In liberation, the cessation is complete; yoga promotes liberation.

138–139

Happiness and pain result from the close proximity of the self, the senses, the mind, and their objects. By not commencing, while the mind is steady and focused on the self, that pair stops and an embodied person becomes powerful. Sages who understand yoga know that that is yoga.

140–141

Entering someone's mind, knowledge of objects, free action, vision, hearing, recollection, beauty, and invisibility at will: these are called the eightfold lordly power that yogins have. All that arises from meditation (*samādhāna*) with a purified mind.

142

Liberation comes from the absence of passion (*rajas*) and lethargy (*tamas*), due to the disappearance of potent karma. The disjunction from all conjunctions is called non-rebirth.

143–146

Constant attendance on good people, and the avoidance of those who are not good; performing vows and fasting as well as each of the separate restraints (*niyama*); steady concentration (*dhāraṇā*), knowledge (*vijñāna*) of the teachings about dharma, a penchant for solitude, an aversion to the objects of sense, striving towards liberation, and supreme willpower. Not initiating deeds (*karma*), destruction of past deeds, unworldliness, freedom from ego, seeing the danger in attachment, concentration (*samādhāna*) of mind and intellect, investigating the true state of things. All this develops from abiding in the mindfulness of reality (*tattvasmṛter upasthānāt*).

147

Attendance on good people, etc., through to willpower (i.e., vv. 143–44): these make mindfulness (*smṛti*) arise. After having become mindful of the essential nature of existing things, being mindful, one is released from suffering (*duḥkha*).

148–149

The eight causes that are said to bring mindfulness about are:

(a) perception of the cause (*nimitta-grahaṇa*)
(b) perception of the form (*rūpa-grahaṇa*)
(c) similarity (*sādṛśya*)
(d) contrast (*saviparyaya*)
(e) attachment to *sattva* (*sattvānubandha*)
(f) practice (*abhyāsa*)
(g) the yoga of knowledge (*jñānayoga*), and
(h) what is heard again (*punaḥśruta*)

Recollection is said to come from recollecting what has been seen, heard, and experienced.

150–151

The power of recollecting the truth (*tattva*) is the one path of liberation, the one that is revealed by liberated people. Those who have gone by it have not returned again. Yogins call this the way of yoga. Those sāṃkhyas who have reckoned the dharmas and those who are liberated call it the way of liberation.

152–153

Everything that has a cause is pain, not the self, and impermanent. For that is not manufactured by the self. And in that arises ownership, as long as the true realization has not arisen by which the knower, having known "I am not this, this is not mine," transcends everything.

154–155

When this final renunciation exists, all pains and their causes, with consciousness, knowledge, and understanding, stop completely. After that, the corporeal self that has become *brahman* is not perceived. Having departed from all conditions, not a sign can be found. But an ignorant person cannot know this knowledge of those who understand *brahman*.

—2—

A Prescription for *Yoga* and Power in the *Mahābhārata*

James L. Fitzgerald

The translated text that follows—a small treatise labeled "Prescription for *yoga*" *(yogavidhi)* in many of its original manuscript sources (chapter 289 of Book 12 of the *Mahābhārata*, thus "*Mahābhārata* 12.289)—is a remarkable presentation of *yoga* taken from among the many philosophical and religious texts found in the vast Indian epic *Mahābhārata*. This introduction to it will proceed by describing the immediate context of this text—the two speakers in it and a neighboring treatise that helps us understand better the point of this "Prescription for *yoga*"—and the broad trends of ancient Indian intellectual history that define its teaching generally.

The Immediate Setting

BHĪṢMA'S INSTRUCTIONS OF YUDHIṢṬHIRA

In this text, the fading, soon to die, warrior-sage Bhīṣma, the patriarch ("grandfather") of the Kuru Bharatas, is instructing his young kinsman, Yudhiṣṭhira ("son of the Bharata King Pāṇḍu," who is addressed sometimes as Bhārata and as "bull of the Bharatas"; Yudhiṣṭhira is also occasionally addressed with two names based on two of his mother's names, "son of Kuntī"—at stanzas 16, 34, and 56—and "son of Pṛthā"—at stanzas 24 and 27). Yudhiṣṭhira has recently won a horrific and tremendous war that should usher in a new era through his rule across the entire known world. Bhīṣma's instructions to the new king all deal with problems that troubled the new king, problems of knowing and understanding "right action" (*dharma*) in relation to some of the critical issues of the times—problems such as "How can kingship itself, with its inherent violence and opportunism, be understood to be right action?" Or, "How can the ancient forms of religion (ritual worship of the various Gods, the killing of animals in some of these rites, the pursuit of life in heaven after a single, unique life) be reconciled with new religious ideas that presume that people live in chains of rebirths determined mechanically by the aggregation of all a person's past deeds, good and bad alike, and among which any and all deeds of violence and injury are the very worst?" The time when the various instructions collected here were composed is roughly between 200 BCE and 300 CE. The selection translated here, 12.289, likely dates from near the end of this long stretch of time.

THE *MAHĀBHĀRATA'S* RELIGIOUS AND PHILOSOPHICAL TEACHINGS AMIDST THE CURRENTS OF THE ERA: *DHARMA, MOKṢA, YOGA*

The particular portion of Bhīṣma's instructions from which our selection comes is called the "Section on *mokṣadharma*s" (read further for explanations of both of these words). This section is a collection of various texts from the brahminic tradition that present sermons and treatises on the various forms of behavior that are both normatively good (prescribed as laws or duties) and also supposedly good for a person's welfare after death (that is, they are *dharma*s, the right things for a person to do; the word *dharma* embraces both those senses of "good action," being obligatory and being beneficial in the next life). These texts also present different important teachings that pertain to a person's ultimate welfare in life and beyond death (in this part of the *Mahābhārata* the word *dharma* may also, at times, refer to an "important truth or teaching" that entails some particular form of ultimately beneficial behavior). All of these sermons and treatises on various *dharma*s are presented against the backdrop of new teachings that became very prominent in northern India after 400 BCE in the mouths of various teachers such as the Buddha, teachings that argued that human beings were plagued or "bound" in various ways and needed to free themselves—from the general suffering of life (*duḥkha*), from the mechanical action of the aggregation of past deeds (*karman*, Anglicized as karma), and from the possibly endless chain of personal rebirths (*saṃsāra*) that is powered by the energy of one's karma. These new doctrines came frequently to use the word *mokṣa* (a word that comes from a verb-root that signifies to "let loose," like an arrow from the string of a bow, or "get loose," as in escape from danger or a bad situation) and related words like *mukti* and *mukta* to describe the various forms and degrees of these liberations.

These teachings regarding the fundamental misery of the human condition, the mechanical bondage of karma, and the chain of rebirths seem likely to have arisen from social and cultural milieus that were not Aryan and brahminic (see Bronkhorst 2007). The fundamental Vedic religious ideas of the

Aryan brahmins were predicated upon the idea that people might engage in various rituals (worshipping the Gods) and other forms of good action (*dharma-karman*) that would make the world reasonably comfortable and secure—the world was not a locus only of suffering in their eyes. And while they understood human actions to have ethical qualities and corresponding good or bad consequences for their agents, they did not envision their deeds as a life-long accumulation that mechanically determined their futures, nor did they think that persons were incarnated in a succession of bodies. In ancient times, brahmins did develop ethical themes by which some individual persons conceived of "immortality" and the "beatitude" (blessedness, perpetual perfect bliss) of union with the impersonal source-reality of the universe (*brahman*), but these ideas are fundamentally different from the ideas of liberation from suffering, karma, and *saṃsāra*. In a slow process that took several centuries, the two different worldviews intermingled, and the differing notions of the highest good (gaining immortality or the beatitude of union with *brahman*, on the one hand, and Escape or Absolute Freedom, on the other) came ultimately to be regarded as more or less synonymous. Once the non-brahminic ideas of *mokṣa* started to circulate and gain prominence, brahminic thinkers began appropriating parts of them into brahminic religious themes, especially in the centuries after 300 BCE, in some of the younger *Upaniṣad* texts and passages. Many of the texts of the *Mahābhārata*'s "Section on *mokṣadharma*s" are likewise appropriations of these ideas to greater or lesser degrees, and they represent attempts to fit these alien ideas together with continuing brahmin respect for the Gods, the Vedas, and ritual action.

Exactly where the ideas and practices that came to be labeled "*yoga*" fit into these developments is obscure (see Bronkhorst 1986, 1993; White 2009; and Eliade 2009). Those ideas and practices focus emphatically upon individual persons, particularly the human body and the mental structures that operate within the body, and especially upon the breathing that obviously powers both the body and its conscious structures. This focus makes those practices seem quite distinct from the early Vedic forms of brahminic religion which are centered upon the many Gods that control the world surrounding human beings, who live in various kinds of corporate groupings, as do the Gods. But whatever sociocultural background these practices had when eventually they made their entrance upon the stage of Indian religions in historically visible times, they served both the brahminic quest for beatific union and non-brahminic quests for liberation equally well. These practices typically called for withdrawal from the world of everyday life (renunciation, *saṃnyāsa*), affiliation with a preceptor, emphasis upon control of the body and the breath, and control of the mind by withdrawing consciousness from sensory objects and focusing it tightly for long periods of time on a single point of support (different phases or degrees of meditation: *dhāraṇā*, *dhyāna*, *samādhi*). The changes such regimes of "psycho-somatic technology" would effect in persons lent themselves to different metaphysical interpretations, a fact that made this a "psycho-somatic technology" that seems to have been regarded as effective by many different schools of thought across more than two millennia of Indian intellectual history.

It is also important to understand that these practices were not always nor everywhere labeled "*yoga*." *Yoga* is a Sanskrit word that came to be applied—primarily in the Hindu brahminic traditions—to some parts of this broad tradition of asceticism and praxis at some indeterminable point in time, and the word *yoga* applies some interesting ideas to it. *Yoga* is an ancient word signifying "hitch up" or "harness" draught animals to a wheeled vehicle or the blade of a plow, and the like, or "yoke" a pair of such animals together for such work. It would be interesting to ponder the ways in which this idea might fit, and in turn, be modified through its referring to and describing the various alterations of behavior, manipulations of the body, regulations of breathing, and arresting of mental activities that are characteristic of "*yoga*" (see the metaphor of the chariot at *Kaṭha Upaniṣad* 3.3–8). We cannot launch such an exploration here, but I will mention that central themes of the "harnessing" metaphor involve a graded continuum between different kinds of entities: lower-level, powerful entities or creatures (often the senses and/or parts of the body) that must be conquered, tamed, directed, regulated, or controlled by the higher-level entities (layers of the Mind). The higher-level entities are regarded as naturally closer to the ideal state of reality, however that is conceived. The harnessing theme is apt for the project of bringing the higher strata of a person into control over his or her lower strata, for this metaphor imports the notions of "traces," "reins," "lines of control" running from the higher entity to the lower (ideas such as *yama*s ["reins; restraints"] and *raśmi*s ["traces, lines, reins"]). The work of David White has shown the wide applicability of these motives (White 2009).

Another relevant theme implied in "harnessing" is that the person in control harnesses the lower-order being or entity for some purpose, for some enterprise or work. This aspect of *yoga* is highly relevant to a number of discussions of *yoga* in the *Mahābhārata*, especially those involving a divine *yogin*, such as Kṛṣṇa presents himself to be in the *Bhagavad Gītā* and as Nārāyaṇa is more implicitly presented at the end of 12.289, as you will soon see. Again, this is a theme of *yoga* that has been illuminated by David White's recent work. As he has shown, this theme of *yoga* stands in some tension with the theme of seeking *mokṣa*, and the practice of *yoga* described in our text here does face in both directions—toward the active use of *yoga* powers in the world even though Absolute Liberation is within reach, and, too, toward Absolute Liberation, *mokṣa*. Having described broadly the power and strength the *yogin* acquires and the way in which the *yogin* can make use of any and every entity in the known universe (in stanzas 58–62), the text remarks (actually earlier, in stanza 41) that the *yogin* may, at will, take up the "highest, or final, *yoga*" and gain *mokṣa* straightaway.

THE "PRESCRIPTION FOR *YOGA*:" CHAPTER 12.289 OF THE *MAHĀBHĀRATA*

The text at hand represents a relatively late and highly developed stage in this history. It offers a glimpse of a well-developed tradition of reflection and praxis on body and mind that on its face is directed toward freeing a person in different ways—Absolute Liberation, *mokṣa*, and, by merging with the Supreme God Nārāyaṇa in the end, beatitude. At the same time, its *yoga*-harnessing can be, and is, directed toward the development of very high degrees of power and control within the phenomenal world for as long as the *yogin* may wish. And finally, this text presents all of this as a self-conscious "School" of thought (a *darśana*, a "View" of important matters of reality and knowledge) to be known as the "Yoga" School, which I render here with the deliberately verbose "The School of Mastery by means of *yoga* harnessing." (I write "Yoga" when I believe the text refers to this school, and "*yoga*" when the word refers to generic forms of *yoga*.)

THE HIGHLIGHTS OF THE "PRESCRIPTION FOR *YOGA*"

As is so often the case with the instructional texts in the *Mahābhārata*'s "Section on *mokṣadharma*s," there are a number of currents running through this text. It is worth emphasizing that it is a teaching on liberation—liberation from the bondage of karma, which entails ultimately liberation from rebirth in the created world and liberation from all that is not the highest God Nārāyaṇa. But what is highly distinctive about this text is its emphasis that the *yogin* breaks these bonds with the strength (*bala*) he accumulates through *yoga* praxis. Through *yoga* he becomes as powerful as a God, and the text applies to him the word for God, *īśvara* ("powerful, mighty, one who has the ability to control entities that are below him"), that came to replace the older Vedic word for God, *deva* ("a bright, shining being" of "the bright realm," the *div/dyu*, the sky). Of course the successful *yogin* who becomes an *īśvara* is not *the* Supreme God, the Supreme Powerful One, the *parama-īśvara*, who was *never* bound by karma, who has been the original source and final end of the entire universe from time without beginning (either Viṣṇu or Śiva, eventually). As pointed out above, the successful *yogin* who becomes an *īśvara* according to 12.289 is said to merge into such a *parameśvara*, Nārāyaṇa, finally (stanza 62). (At the time 12.289 was composed, the theology of Viṣṇu had not developed fully; ultimately Nārāyaṇa came to be understood as one particular way of conceiving of the *parameśvara* Viṣṇu.)

The presentation of *yoga* between stanzas 11 and 56 is dominated by the idea of strength, *bala*, and fortitude of will. (The following paragraph, ending with the quotations of stanzas 28 and 39–41, is a quotation and adaptation of a close description of the teachings of 12.289 from a paper of mine that discusses this text in a more technical way. See Fitzgerald 2011: 194–97.) This *bala* is the power to break out of all forms of bondage (stanzas 11–23); it is the ability to enter at will into all other beings (including the Vedic Gods and the ancient seers of the Veda), the ability to withstand the power even of an angry Yamadeva, the Lord of the Dead, to make many thousands of clones of oneself and act in diverse ways in each and every one of them, and to have complete control over all forms of bondage (stanzas 24–28); it is the fortitude to hold the mind fixed in difficult "Holding Meditations" (*dhāraṇā*s, stanzas 29–41 and 54–55); it is the might to overcome various internal temptations and infirmities (such as lust and laziness) (stanzas 47–49); and it is the perseverance to adhere to the path of *yoga*, which is never easy (stanzas 50–53). Besides the great powers mentioned above, what one is said to gain through *yoga* is to "get back to 'That Place' (a general reference to Absolute Reality, in stanza 10) when those afflictions (the five afflictions of passion, error, affection, desire, and anger, stanza 11) are all gone" (stanza 12)—"spotless, [they] go the propitious way that goes farthest" (stanza 14)—and, of course, *mokṣa* (at stanzas 13, 18 28, 31, 35, and others). At one point (stanza 42), Yudhiṣṭhira interrupts to ask what foods the *yogin* eats to gain strength and Bhīṣma discusses foods and fasting for several stanzas (43–49). In stanzas 50–53, Bhīṣma offers an extended statement regarding how terribly difficult and challenging the path of *yoga* actually is.

An apt summation of this Yoga exposition is contained in *ślokas* 28 and 39-41 (which I present in slightly simplified translations):

> Certainly the powerful yogin, who has complete control over the bonds that hold him, has at his disposal the absolute power to escape them at will. [289.28]
>
> A yogin who concentrates intently in great formal observances focused on his navel, head, heart, etc., perfectly harnesses his subtle self with the Self. [289.39–40] Having burned off his past deeds good and bad, his wisdom spotless, he may, if he wishes, take up the highest yoga harnessing and quickly get Absolutely Free. [289.41]

Yoga Paired with Sāṃkhya

As happens frequently with presentations of *yoga* in the *Mahābhārata* (see Fitzgerald 2011: 185, n. 2), the presentation in 12.289 is paired with the presentation of another developing *darśana* tradition, called "Sāṃkhya," which I gloss as "The School of Total Knowledge." (The paired description of Sāṃkhya occurs in the immediately following chapter of Bhīṣma's instructions of Yudhiṣṭhira, 12.290.) In the texts of the *Mahābhārata,* at least, the school of Sāṃkhya and the school of Yoga appear to share the same vision of what exists in the world and how persons are constructed: both are committed to understanding the world and persons in terms of a "stack" or "ladder" of levels of being that all descend from some common source entity, often by each lower entity emerging from the prior one through a process of progressive coarsening or thickening, until the densest and most opaque of the material elements [earth] is reached. Though there is not unanimity about the dating of all relevant textual passages, I believe "Sāṃkhya," as the name of an intellectual theme or method, was unknown in India until about the turn of the Common Era, when it appears in a number of places in the *Mahābhārata,* in the *Śvetāśvatara Upaniṣad*, and in Aśvaghoṣa's account of the life of the Buddha. The term appears on the scene rather suddenly, and it represents a newly conceived and articulated version of the method of liberation that had been developing up until then in connection with the traditions of *yoga* praxis and reflection (see Schreiner 1999). The goal of Sāṃkhya is to achieve a radical (and "*mokṣa*-conferring") disaffection from the world, a radical purging of egocentrism and desire from one's taken for granted understanding of the world with oneself in it. This disaffection, called *vairāgya* (a dissociation from life's motivating stimuli at the visceral level of a person's being), is effected by the *systematic, enumerative contemplation of the entire system of the world.* The word Sāṃkhya signifies "comprehensive intuition," or "all-gnosis," and its cognates signify "enumerate, know the whole of some complex entity by itemizing and totaling every component of it." The connection between the ideas of enumeration and summing up and taking a complete grasp of a thing is obvious. It seems that in the "Sāṃkhya revolution," different intellectual motives emerged and converged within old traditions of reflection upon the makeup of the world and persons and the effecting of Escape or beatitude by means of *yoga*-control. And I would suggest that basic Buddhist ideas—of freeing oneself from suffering, karma, and rebirth that embrace both intellectual "re-visioning" of the world and oneself; the cultivation of wisdom, *prajñā*, through "Insight meditation"; and the psycho-somatic quieting of the entire body-mind organism (the cultivation of *śamatha* through trance-meditation)—played an important role in this "Sāṃkhya revolution." This convergence of motives and themes prompted some thinkers to argue for a "gnostic" approach to *mokṣa*, one that de-emphasized those aspects of *yoga* that were concerned with mastering and using entities in the world by exercising acquired yogic power in the fashion of a God, a Lord, an *īśvara*. That is to say, 12.289 here would seem to represent exactly what the new Sāṃkhya was turning away from.

The issue of precisely what prompted the separation of an emphatically gnostic tradition from the older tradition of *yoga* is complex and we cannot go into it any further now. It is also true that this separation made some teachers, or members of their audiences, nervous, for a frequent theme of the joint presentations of Sāṃkhya and Yoga in the *Mahābhārata* is that they are both equally effective and both lead to the highest good. Such an argument seems highly understandable in the case of a splintering development that wishes to carry away with it as many of the advantages of its origin as may prove possible. Such an argument is also highly plausible in this particular case, for, as the offspring of the *yoga* tradition, the epic forms of "Sāṃkhya" very much resemble the basic teachings of *yoga*. It is precisely over the issues of power and lordship (being an *īśvara*) that they part company from *yoga*. I would end by suggesting that the Sāṃkhya emphasis upon intellection does not rule out Sāṃkhya "knowers" making use of *yoga* harnessing as a component of their exhaustive, enumerating, intellectual apprehension of the universe, as described in 12.290. In that text they do not suggest that they make use of *yoga*, but they do attribute the teachings of their school to a powerful "master" (*īśvara*) of *yoga* harnessing, Kapila.

I will close my discussion of this pair of texts, in which our "Prescription for *yoga*," is set, and thus of my introduction to 12.289, by returning to the theme of the Supreme God Nārāyaṇa, with whom the *yogin* merges when he chooses to exit the universe definitively (stanza 289.62). The Sāṃkhya presentation too emphasizes that Nārāyaṇa is the highest principle of the universe, and the successful Sāṃkhya knower too enters Nārāyaṇa, in the end. Each of these presentations concludes with a series of stanzas in a more ornate poetic form than is typical in the *Mahābhārata*, and these concluding series of stanzas develop the connection of each school of thought to the theology of Nārāyaṇa. The successful *yogin-īśvara* ultimately assimilates himself to the God Nārāyaṇa and becomes a controlling agent of *yoga* harnessing identical with God Himself. In the case of Sāṃkhya, these concluding stanzas claim that the Sāṃkhya system of thought is an embodiment of the God Nārāyaṇa Himself, an embodiment he manifests at the beginning of each cycle of creation and reabsorbs at the end of each cycle.

A final practical note: My translation of 12.289 rests upon two alterations of the printed Sanskrit text of the Critical Edition of the *Mahābhārata*. First, the editor of the Critical Edition pointed out a typographical error in his printed text at 12.289.17a, where the text was corrected to *sūkṣmāḥ*, which I have rendered here as "puny." The text as printed did not connect the word *sūkṣma* with the "birds trapped in a net." Second, as may be seen from the stanza numbers printed in my translation, I have rearranged the order of a verse or two between 289.58 and 62, moving 61cd to the head of the sentence, immediately following 57. I did this for the sake of the clarity of the English translation.

The selection translated here is from pages 1583–91 of *The Śāntiparvan [Part III: Mokṣadharma, Being the Twelfth Book of the Mahābhārata, the Great Epic of India*, edited by S. K. Belvalkar (Poona: Bhandarkar Oriental Research Institute, 1954). This book is volume 15 of *The Mahābhārata for the First Time Critically Edited*, 19 vols., edited by V. S. Sukthankar, S. K. Belvalkar, and P. L. Vaidya (Poona: Bhandarkar Oriental Research Institute, 1933–66). The present introduction and translation have been excerpted from *The Mahābhārata*, vol. 8 (The Book of the Peace, Part Two), translated, edited, and annotated by James L. Fitzgerald (University of Chicago Press)

Suggestions for Further Reading

There is a small core of English-language scholarship that has investigated *yoga* in the *Mahābhārata* (*MBh*) firsthand and in a way that stays close to the often less than clear texts. Progress in charting all the details has been slow, so older works are still of use, though they have been superseded in some of their details over time. I proceed through this small set in chronological order. Edward Washburn Hopkins, "Yoga-technique in the Great Epic," *Journal of the American Oriental Society* 22 (1901): 333–79, is still worth study. A revisionist work in its day is the now classic piece by Franklin Edgerton from 1924 that lays out some of the fundamental "theological" ideas of Yoga and Sāṃkhya (by "theological" I refer to any absolutely fundamental claims, whether involving anthropomorphic beings or not): "The Meaning of Sāṃkhya and Yoga," *American Journal of Philology* 45:1 (1924): 1–46. Next is V. M. Bedekar's survey, "Yoga in the Mokṣadharmaparvan of the Mahābhārata," contained in a volume celebrating the philosophical investigations of the great German expert Erich Frauwallner, *Beiträge zur Geistesgeschichte Indiens: Festschrift für Erich Frauwallner, aus Anlass seines 70. Geburtstages*, ed. Gerard Oberhammer (=*Wiener Zeitschrift für die Kunde Sud- und Ostasiens und Archiv für Indische Philosophie* 12–13 [1968], 43–52). In 1999, Peter Schreiner asked, "What Comes First (in the Mahābhārata): Sāṃkhya or Yoga?" (*Asiatische Studien: Études Asiatiques* 53:3, pp. 755–77) and, after a systematic investigation, concluded that *yoga* is anterior to Sāṃkhya in the *MBh* by every important measure. Next is John Brockington's comprehensive survey, "Yoga in the Mahābhārata," in *Yoga: The Indian Tradition,* ed. David Carpenter and Ian Whicher (London: Routledge-Curzon, 2003), 13–24. Last, another work that is not a survey: my own forthcoming examination and discussion of the important pair 12.289 (translated above) and its Sāṃkhya companion 12.290 in "The Sāṃkhya-Yoga 'Manifesto' at MBh 12.289–290" (in *Battles, Bards, Brahmins.* Papers from the Epics Section of the 13th World Sanskrit Conference, ed. John Brockington and Peter Bisschop [Delhi: Motilal Banarsidass, 2011], 185–212).

Two important discussions of the "philosophy" or "theology" of the *MBh* generally treat *yoga* as well. Angelika Malinar's comprehensive examination of the *Bhagavad Gītā* (*The Bhagavad Gītā: Doctrines and Contexts*) Cambridge: Cambridge University Press, 2008) ranges across the entire *MBh* and treats various questions of *yoga* in the *MBh* at length, since *yoga* is such a centrally important concept in the *Bhagavad Gītā.* Produced a century earlier was chapter 3 ("Philosophy in the Epic") of E. W. Hopkins's often splendid *Great Epic of India* (New York: Charles Scribner's Sons, 1901). Unfortunately, Hopkins's comprehensive listing of doctrines found in the epic has as one of its purposes to argue that the text is disjointed, a point which he exaggerates here in an objectionable way.

The above works are confined to the *Mahābhārata.* There are some important works that deal with *yoga* in the *MBh* against the background of the broader development of *yoga* in India. First among these is the now classic work of Mircea Eliade, *Yoga: Immortality and Freedom* (Princeton, NJ: Princeton University Press). Originally published in French in 1954 and in English translation in 1958, it was re-issued in 2009 with an introduction by David White, the general editor of the current volume. David White's *Sinister Yogis* (Chicago: University of Chicago Press, 2009) addresses the development of *yoga*, including *yoga* in the *MBh*, from the important, too long neglected perspective of *yoga*'s concerns with bodies and powers that control bodies in the material world.

Finally, while there are many accounts of the development of the non-brahminic traditions of India and of the asceticism and meditation that are important within them, three of the works of the prolific historian of Indian philosophy Johannes Bronkhorst are directly germane to what we find in the *MBh.* Two detailed examinations of texts he produced were his study, *The Two Sources of Meditation in Ancient India* (Stuttgart: Franz Steiner Verlag Wiesbaden, 1986) and his 1993 book, *The Two Sources of Indian Asceticism* (Bern: Peter Lang). Growing out these two works and other arguments in the history of Indian philosophy which he has developed is an argument put forward in his recent book that the religious history of ancient India must be understood in terms of the mixture of the brahminic Vedic tradition with a quite different religious culture most evident in the Magadha region of eastern India: *Greater Magadha: Studies in the Culture of Early India* (Leiden: Brill, 2007).

A Prescription for yoga and Power in the Mahābhārata *Mahābhārata* 12.289.1–62

Yudhiṣṭhira said:

As you know everything, grandfather, please tell me the difference between the School of Total Knowledge and the School of Mastery through *yoga* harnessing. Truly, all is known to you, most excellent of the Kurus. [289.1]

Bhīṣma said:

Brahmins of the School of Total Knowledge praise total knowledge, and those of the School of Mastery through Yoga Harnessing praise yoga harnessing. They each proclaim the superiority of their own position with reasons that advance their own side. [289.2]

> O enemy-withering King, the consummate experts of yoga harnessing declare the excellence of their side with arguments such as "How can anyone who is not a powerful Lord become Absolutely Free?" [289.3]
>
> On the other hand, perfect brahmins of the School of Total Knowledge all make this argument: "Obviously, there is one and only one way to become Absolutely Free upon leaving the body: One becomes thoroughly detached upon coming to know *all* the pathways through the experiential realms of this world." Men of profound wisdom declare this School of Total Knowledge to be "The Theory of Absolute Freedom." [289.4–5]

Each of them countenances the reasoning on his own side as an apt and beneficial statement, and surely men like yourself, who assent to men of learning generally, must countenance the thinking of the learned here. [289.6] Those in the School of Yoga Harnessing rely upon reasons that are directly evident to the senses, while those of the School of Total Knowledge teach the conclusions of a tradition of systematic inquiry and instruction. Yudhiṣṭhira, my son, both of these are doctrines regarding fundamental reality, [289.7] and both are doctrines regarding knowledge, and both are esteemed by men of great learning. When they are carried out according to their prescribed teachings, either one ought to lead one on the course that goes to the farthest place. [289.8] The degree of cleanliness involved in each of them is the same, and so too their kindliness toward other beings, and their adherence to special vows. But, blameless one, their theories are different. [289.9]

Yudhiṣṭhira said:

If their vows, cleanliness, and kindliness are the same, grandfather, how are their theories different? Tell me this. [289.10]

Bhīṣma said:

Using yoga harnessing initially to eradicate absolutely the five afflictions of passion, error, affection, desire, and anger, they reach That, the highest reality. [289.11] Just as big fish break through a net and get back to the water again, those who use yoga harnessing get back to That Place, the highest reality, when those afflictions are all gone. [289.12] In the same way, just as strong animals break a snare and get free of all their bonds and make a clean getaway, [289.13] so, king, strong men using yoga harnessing cut through the bonds that come from greed and, now spotless, travel the propitious way that goes to the farthest place. [289.14] But other animals that are weak perish in those snares, king, no doubt of it; and men perish too unless they use the power of yoga harnessing. [289.15] O son of Kuntī, when feeble fish are caught in a net they perish, and so do men practicing yoga harnessing when they are weak. [289.16] O tamer of your enemies, puny birds trapped in a net perish, while the strong ones get out; [289.17] so it is with men held by the bonds of their past deeds who practice yoga harnessing: The weak perish and the strong get free. [289.18]

O mighty one, a weak man practicing yoga harnessing is like a faint, weak fire that goes out when heavy logs are laid upon it. [289.19] But after a wind blows upon that fire and makes it powerful again, it might quickly burn up the entire earth. [289.20] In the same way, when a man practicing yoga harnessing has become powerful, his Fiery Energy blazes mightily and he can scorch the entire world like the sun at the time of the world's end. [289.21]

Just as a feeble man gets swept away by a river's current, so a weak man practicing yoga harnessing is helplessly swept away by the objects of sense. [289.22] And just as an elephant stands firm against the current of a river, so too he who has acquired the power of yoga harnessing forces the many objects of his senses to part and flow around him. [289.23]

Men practicing yoga harnessing who are mighty Lords filled with power from the harnessing enter at will into Progenitors, Seers, Gods, and the elements, son of Pṛthā. [289.24] Neither Yama, the Lord of the Dead, nor the End-Maker, Time, when he is enraged, nor ferociously aggressive Death—none of these, king, exercises power over the man who practices yoga harnessing—that man has unlimited energy. [289.25] O Bull of the Bharatas, a man practicing yoga harnessing might, after he has acquired power, take on many thousands of identities and wander the earth in all of them. [289.26] With one, O son of Pṛthā, he might betake himself to the sense objects, while he might perform severe asceticism with another; or he might draw them back into himself again, as the sun does the rays of its energy. [289.27] Certainly, king, the powerful man practicing yoga harnessing, who has control over the bonds that hold him, has at his disposal the absolute power to escape them at will. [289.28]

So, lord of peoples, I have told you the powers there are in yoga harnessing. Now I shall tell you some of its finer points to illustrate it to you further. [289.29]

Lord, bull of the Bharatas, hear, as illustrations, some of the finer points regarding the holding of one's mind in concentration. [289.30]

As a careful bowman hits his target when he concentrates, so a man practicing yoga harnessing who is perfectly under control reaches Absolute Freedom, no doubt of it. [289.31]

As a man carefully carrying a pot full of oil can mount a stairs with it, if he puts his mind unwaveringly on that pot and keeps his mind under control; [289.32] so, king, a man practicing yoga harnessing, who has lashed himself tightly, holding himself motionless, makes himself so spotless he looks like the sun. [289.33]

O son of Kuntī, as a pilot who concentrates intently guides his ocean-going ship swiftly into port,[289.34] so, king, he who knows the fundamental principles of the world and has engaged in concentration of his Self by means of yoga harnessing, reaches a position that is very hard to get to, once he leaves this body behind. [289.35]

> O bull among men, as a charioteer who has harnessed fine horses and concentrates intently takes his bowman directly to the intended spot, [289.36] so, king, a man practicing yoga harnessing who concentrates in the Holding-Meditations reaches the highest place directly—just as an arrow that goes straight to its target when released. [289.37]

A man practicing yoga harnessing who stands without moving after making himself enter into his Self, gains the place that never decays—just as a man who stands without moving in order to spear fish gains an evil place. [289.38] O warrior of immeasurable courage, a man practicing yoga harnessing who concentrates intently in great formal observances focused on these spots—his navel, his neck, his head, his heart, or his chest, or his two sides, or his sight, touch, or smell—perfectly harnesses his subtle self with the Self. [289.39–40] Having burned off his past deeds good and bad, his wisdom spotless, he may, if he wishes, take up the final yoga harnessing and quickly get Absolutely Free. [289.41]

Yudhiṣṭhira said:

What sorts of things does a man practicing yoga harnessing take for his foods—and which ones does he remove—in order to gain strength, Bhārata? Please tell me this. [289.42]

Bhīṣma said:

> A man practicing yoga harnessing who is committed to eating seeds and the mash left after pressing oil-seeds, and who is also committed to avoiding oils, gains strength. [289.43]
>
> O tamer of your foes, a man practicing yoga harnessing who eats rough barley and is pleased with that food alone over long periods of time cleanses himself and gains strength. [289.44]
>
> A man practicing yoga harnessing who, for periods of fortnights, months, or across the varied seasons of the year, wanders about from cave to cave, drinking nothing but water mixed with some milk, gains strength. [289.45]
>
> O lord of men, a man practicing yoga harnessing who fasts continuously for an entire month is completely cleansed and gains strength. [289.46]

King, these exalted men overcome cold, heat, and rain; and desire, anger, and fear as well; also sleep, shortness of breath, and the penis, the objects of the senses, [289.47] apathy—so difficult to conquer!—and terrible craving, all the sensations of touch, and laziness—so difficult to conquer!—O most excellent of kings. [289.48] Then, their passions gone, those very wise exalted men illuminate the subtle self with the Self by way of the sublimity of their meditations and recitations. [289.49]

This path of brahmin sages is held to be very difficult to traverse; no one travels on it comfortably, O bull of the Bharatas. [289.50] Only a youngster could easily fly down a path dotted with robbers through a terrible forest abounding in snakes and lizards, where there is very little water and it is hard to move about because there are pits and many bramble-thickets, and most of it is dense, unbroken woods or stands of trees burned up in forest fires. [289.51–52] So if a brahmin gets onto the path of yoga harnessing and finds it comfortable, then he should get off of that path, for tradition teaches that he must have many faults. [289.53]

O lord of earth, a man practicing yoga harnessing finds it very easy to stand on the sharpened razors' edges of Holding-Meditations, but those whose minds are not properly formed find it very difficult to stand on them. [289.54] And, son, Holding-Meditations that have been disrupted lead men along a course that is no good, like ships at sea without captains. [289.55] But, O son of Kuntī, one who stays in the Holding-Meditations as prescribed, gets Absolutely Free of death and birth, and pleasure and suffering too. [289.56]

Arisen in diverse learned traditions, this has been declared among those of the School of Mastery through Yoga Harnessing—but it was among brahmins that the whole of the supreme method of control through harnessing was definitively fixed. [289.57]

> The fact is, exalted one, a man practicing yoga harnessing should enter into and then fuse with [289.61cd] That, the Highest, The Mighty All, *brahman*; then the Lord Brahmā, then the favor-granting Viṣṇu, Bhava (Śiva), the God Dharma, the six-faced God (Skanda), the six majestic sons of Brahmā, [289.58] the Attribute that is noxious Darkness, the Attribute that is tremendous Energy, the Attribute that is pure Lightness, the highest Originary Matrix, Complete Attainment, the Goddess who is the wife of Varuṇa (that is, the element water), all of Fiery Energy (the element fire), the vast and mighty firmness (the element earth), [289.59] the spotless moon amidst the stars, the All-Gods, the serpents, the ancestors, all the mountain peaks, the terrific oceans, all rivers, clouds, forests, [289.60] elephants, mountains, the throngs of Yakṣas, the quarters of the sky, the throngs of Gandharvas, and men and women. [289.61ab] Thus vast and tremendous, his body that Mighty All, he gains Absolute Freedom shortly afterward. [289.61d]

King, this account focused upon this God of tremendous power and thought (that is, the successful yogi) is splendid! Transcending all mortal practitioners of yoga harnessing, this one acts, his body that Mighty All, his soul the supreme Lord Nārāyaṇa. [289.62]

—3—

Yoga Practices in the *Bhagavadgītā*

Angelika Malinar

The *Bhagavadgītā* (BhG) is a dialogue between the epic hero Arjuna and his charioteer and comrade Vāsudeva-Kṛṣṇa, which was composed and transmitted as part of the *Mahābhārata* epic. The epic tells the tale of a conflict between two branches of a royal lineage, the Pāṇḍavas and the Kauravas. This conflict culminates in a battle between the two opposing, yet related parties, which lasts eighteen days and brings about the destruction of most of the lineage and many other warrior clans. Immediately before the account of battle begins in the sixth book of the epic, the Pāṇḍava hero Arjuna raises serious doubts about the legitimacy of this war between relatives and dreads the painful outcome. Kṛṣṇa replies with a long teaching which criticizes any egotistical perspective on the performance of duties or results of one's actions. Instead, detachment and determination to fight for the maintenance of the cosmic order and the welfare of all beings should be one's guide. This general direction of the argument is presented in different doctrines, uses of terminology, and practical recommendations. One of the most important doctrinal frameworks of the text is yoga in theory and practice, the other being the ideal of *bhakti* (devotion) which demands dedicating one's life to the one and only highest self, the god Kṛṣṇa. This latter framework is grounded in the revelation that the human hero is indeed a god embodied on earth to fight against the enemies of the cosmic order (*dharma*). The text consists of seven hundred stanzas in eighteen chapters and was most probably composed in different steps between the second century BCE and the beginning of the Common Era.

The BhG includes not only a variety of ideas about yoga as doctrine and practice, but also notions of yoga peculiar to this text, such as the doctrine of *karmayoga* (yoga of action), which has been widely discussed in the subsequent history of its reception. Broadly speaking, the term yoga is used in the BhG to refer to: (1) methods of controlling one's activities with the aim of obstructing the production of *karman* (the consequences of actions); (2) doctrines and practices of meditation and the acquisition of liberating insight; (3) states of self-control and strength in the hour of death; and (4) extraordinary powers that allow one to control other agents in the world, including the cosmic cause of creation itself (*brahman*, *prakṛti*). This last notion is usually presented as a characteristic feature of the divinity of Kṛṣṇa as the "Lord of Yoga" (*yogeśvara*), who uses his yogic powers for the welfare of all beings and thereby embodies *yoga aiśvara*, the yoga of sovereignty (BhG 9.5). This serves to explain the paradoxical nature of the god's way of being, for on the one hand he is present in the world as creator and cosmic sovereign, while on the other he resides as the "highest self" (*paramātman*) in a transcendent, invisible realm. In the chapters on the idea of *bhakti*, attachment and exclusive devotion to God (BhG 9–12), the god's yoga is turned into an object of devotional activity and serves as a model of desireless action to be emulated by the devotee. Such devotional practices are said to substitute for and even surpass ascetic and liberation-oriented forms of yoga and are clearly distinguished from what can be regarded as "yoga in practice" in a more technical sense.

The spectrum of ideas of yoga presented in the BhG is also reflected in different concepts of practice, which range from the ability of the divine yogin Kṛṣṇa to be present in apparitional bodies, to breath control, to sitting upright. Despite such differences a common denominator is discernible, a kind of consensus about the general structure of yoga practice. In many instances throughout the text, yoga practice is depicted as a fight, struggle, or conquest of one's own nature (*svaprakṛti*), that is, the agency of one's physical and mental apparatus (BhG 3.5). This connects yoga in the BhG with nontechnical uses of the word *yoga* elsewhere in the epic in the sense of harnessing, yoking, deploying, and so on, which is used in many passages in the MBh in the context of warfare and the deployment of weapons and armies. This points to a key notion of many of the yoga teachings in the BhG: yoga is all about taming and gaining control over oneself (*ātman*), that is, over the ongoing mental, emotional, and physical activities that dominate much of one's corporeal existence. Practice thus consists of all the efforts a yogin undertakes to bring these many "natural" activities under control. Therefore, the yogin is often described as the one "whose self is restrained" (*yuktātman*) or "purified" (*viśuddhātman*), who is able to restrain and tame both mind (*manas*, *citta*) and senses. This is summarized in the injunction to practice yoga by wielding "the sword of knowledge" (*jñānāsi*) against the inner enemies of desire and passion, the characteristic features of the ego-oriented life, which is also regarded to be the cause of Arjuna's crisis (4.41–42). Yoga is thus first of all a confrontation with one's natural disposition (*svaprakṛti*), which needs to be calmed, fixed, and redirected according to the purposes of the yogin. Therefore, the yogin is enjoined to seat himself on a well-prepared seat and stabilize his body, concentrate on the tip of the nose, and exercise breath control (6.11–13). Elsewhere, the stabilization of one's concentration is depicted as a gradual effacement of all sense objects, and a drying out of the streams of thoughts, emotions, and bodily fluids, which includes fasting to the point of foregoing even drink (2.59). If one does not manage to control the mind, the senses will again turn to the outer world and will lead the practitioner astray. Then he will end up either as a hypocrite indulging in sensuality in the guise of practicing ascetic meditation (3.6), or else as a "fallen yogin" who cannot control his senses and who is therefore fated to fall apart like a "shredded cloud" (6.48). These descriptions are to be distinguished from practices that are associated with the various levels of yogic accomplishments and the states of yogic meditation and of union with the object of meditation. BhG 6 provides not only the most detailed information, but also an evaluation of different practices. It is pointed out (6.3) that the most important practice is pacification (*śama*), which obviously requires a certain level of self-control, such that the yogin may effectively proceed to efface all thoughts and mental activities. At such higher levels of practice only one object or realm remains, upon which yogic meditation should rest, called "the highest," beyond which there is nothing else.

The BhG includes different realms and thus ultimate goals of yogins, such as *brahman* (the cause of creation) or the immortal self, as well as the god Kṛṣṇa, who is depicted as being beyond both *brahman* and the immortal self. No special type of yoga is taught that would allow one to reach the god; rather, Kṛṣṇa is either superimposed on well-established pathways of yoga or his yoga is depicted as the object of devotional practices that culminate in a vision of him. More information about yogic practice may be garnered from the passages that deal with the connection between yoga and certain types of actions on the one hand (BhG 2.39–53; chapters 3 and 4), and with yoga as a pathway to liberation on the other (2.54–72; chapters 5 and 6).

However, the BhG not only presents a variety of practices, but also offers, through its discourse on the nature and deployment of *karman* (activity, action, duty), a reflection on the conditions of any practice. Any recommended practice should ideally be based on an analysis of the basic conditions on which it depends. Practice is not viewed as "becoming active" after having been inactive, but primarily means confronting the constant activities that each and every living being manifests. The idea that there exists something like inactivity is a delusion, and delusion is an obstacle to any practice. As is stated in BhG 3.5, there is not a single moment when a living being is inactive. This means that practice of any kind implies consciously and purposefully curbing, employing, and redirecting these activities to obtain the projected goals. In the BhG, this notion is developed on the basis of a specific concept of physical existence and "nature" (*prakṛti*, *brahman*) taught in Sāṃkhya philosophy. This is also the basis for what is perhaps the most renowned doctrine of the BhG—the doctrine of *karmayoga*, the so-called yoga of action, that is, the detached performance of all activities. The text thus offers one of the most influential accounts of yogic detachment as the basis for all practice to be found in early Indian literature. This idea refers primarily to the way in which daily ritual and social duties should be performed and is then extended to a merely physical, yet purposeful, performance of all actions (4.21). In BhG 2, this notion is first presented as flowing from a determination whose starting point is a clear recognition of one's duties and aims and of the purpose of action. This is depicted as *buddhiyoga*, the self-control brought about by the correct application of *buddhi*, the faculty of insight and discrimination and the highest of all cognitive faculties. The terminology used here and in many other passages of the text is based, once again, on ideas developed in the Sāṃkhya school of philosophy. The notion of yogic determination is offered as a critique of ritual specialists who follow the doctrines of the Vedas and claim that actions (*karman*) are instruments for fulfilling the desires and intentions of the acting individual (2.43–48). Contrary to their position, it is argued here that all activities should be carried out without any desire for personal benefit. One is to abandon the quest for fruits and thus distance oneself from the traditional Vedic view, which is depicted as a "thicket of delusion" (2.52–53). As a consequence, yoga in terms of *buddhiyoga* is presented as both a cognitive state and a method for maintaining it. This results in an attitude of "determination" (*vyavasāya*; 2.41), which is based on right decisions and correct understanding that need to be employed in each and every situation. This determination allows the ties of *karman* to be severed and guarantees success in all undertakings. It is a state of "skilfulness in action" (2.50) that is primarily obtained not through practices of yogic meditation, but by (1) being determined and rigorous with regard to one's tasks (*adhikāra*; 2.47); (2) giving up all personal attachment to the results of one's acts (2.48); and (3) developing an aversion (*nirveda*) to the traditional views launched by followers of the Veda (2.52). All of this means disciplining one's emotions by being yoked to or armed with a yogic determination.

This line of thought is extended in BhG 3 in a discussion of *karmayoga* proper, which is again offered by way of criticizing other doctrines, especially those demanding the relinquishing of one's social existence. The idea of *karmayoga* is presented in BhG 3.4 in opposition first to the idea that one has to stop acting completely (*akarmya*), and second to the notion of renouncing one's social duties (*saṃnyāsa*) and taking up an ascetic or mendicant life. However, the idea of *karmayoga* is also directed against the "wrong" yogic practice of "hypocrites" who outwardly appear to practice yoga while actually craving the objects of their meditation (3.6). This is a reference to the topic of the "false ascetic"—well attested in Sanskrit literature—that is, a yogin who uses the trappings of practice and the ascetic lifestyle as a disguise for pursuing quite different interests. In opposition to such abuse of yoga practice, the author of BhG 3 proposes that ascetic accomplishment must be proven through practice (3.7); that is, in the demonstrated ability actually to act ascetically, to be a *karmayogin*. Karmayoga is thus not only a type of yoga practice, but also a criterion for evaluating the quality of other forms of practice.

Yoga is seen here as a way of acting that denies all personal interests and emphasizes that everything should be done out of a sense of obligation and for the sake of "holding the world together" (*lokasaṃgraha*; 3.20), that is, for the welfare of all beings. The term *karmayoga* has been interpreted as "disinterested action" or "detached action," which is appropriate if one bears in mind that such detachment only concerns individual interest and does not imply indifference toward the purpose of the actions that are undertaken. More precisely, the purpose of action is diverted away from the individual to a desire to care for the maintenance of the cosmic order since it provides the basis for the life and prosperity of all beings. This idea of upholding the cosmic order is explained by referring to the cycle of ritual and social reciprocity, the "wheel of sacrifice" (3.14–16). It is argued that a sacrificer turns into a yogin and does not accumulate *karman* when he sacrifices *karman*. This means that he offers up his activities (*karman*) in the service of maintaining the sacrificial cycle of reciprocity and consumption upon which all living beings depend. In this way a deed is turned into "fuel" and consumed in activities that are carried out for "the welfare of all beings." "Yoga of action" thus means sacrificing one's deeds in the consuming fires of ritual and social reciprocity. The ability to act in this way is depicted not only as an ideal of social life, but also as a criterion for assessing ascetic accomplishments and the general value of ascetic practices. *Karmayoga* is thus a method for sacrificing skillfully; that is, of avoiding karmic consequences. This allows for the claim that desireless sacrificers are yogins and, conversely, that "true" yogins are indeed sacrificers. What is commonly understood as the "renunciation" (*saṃnyāsa*) of ritual and social activity is no longer required. The text thus documents the mediation of the values of sacrifice and of yoga which, as Madeleine Biardeau has shown, is also a concern found in other texts of the period. This realignment is also demonstrated in the identification of such yogic practices as breath control with sacrificial activities in 4.25–29.

Although the concept of *karmayoga* is presented as "true" yoga and as something that yogins actually do, in the BhG it stands in contrast to yoga as a practice of meditation and a doctrine of liberation, the topics of BhG 2.54–72, and chapters 5 and 6. Even as these passages provide the most elaborate descriptions of yoga practice in the BhG, they also display a concern to mediate these ideas with the new concept of *karmayoga*. While BhG 5 deals with the mechanism of *karmayoga* from the perspective of yoga, BhG 6 presents yoga as a path to salvation culminating in *brahmanirvāṇa* (effacement of all differences in the cause of creation), a path in which disinterested action (*karmayoga*) plays only a preparatory role, a field of training for the adept who would continue on to "true" yoga practice.

BhG 5 offers an explanation for the way in which a yogin is liberated from *karman* even if he continues acting. Therefore, the chapter may be regarded as a critique of the previous (and probably) original sacrificial understanding of *karmayoga*, from the perspective of yoga. It is argued that the consequences of action can be avoided when the yogin "conquers creation" (5.19) and has thereby become identical with the cause of creation, meaning that his physical, mental, personal self is identified with the cosmic principles that comprise it (5.7). As a consequence he sees "the same" in everything and realizes that it is not "he," but rather only the powers of nature (*guṇa*) or the cosmic cause of all actions (*brahman*; *prakṛti*) that are active (5.8–9). This state is described as a yogin's accomplishment, which consists in his being the same as *brahman* without being liberated in(to) it. This serves to explain why a yogin can indeed be *brahman* while remaining alive and why he continues to be active prior to reaching *brahmanirvāṇa*, the effacement of all differences in the cause of creation. Moreover, it establishes the referential framework for understanding why it is possible to act without karmic consequences: the yogin does not produce *karman* because he acts like the cosmic cause of all actions (*brahman*; *prakṛti*), which is also forever free from any karmic consequence (5.19). Actions only produce karmic baggage if they are appropriated by an egotistic agent.

The presentation of yoga as a doctrine of liberation in BhG 6 is not only linked to ideas of yoga discussed elsewhere in the epic, but also points to parallels with Buddhist notions, and may reflect a widespread practice accepted in different scholastic frameworks. In BhG 6 two different paths of yoga, the one theistic, and the other non-theistic, are juxtaposed. While the former culminates in the vision of the god Kṛṣṇa as the "one" (*eka*) who is the "all" (*sarva*), the latter ends in ultimate happiness (*sukha*) upon reaching *brahmanirvāṇa*, the "effacement [of all differences] in the cause of creation." Since the presentation of yoga as a doctrine of liberation is inserted following the exposition of *karmayoga*, it becomes necessary to address it at the beginning of BhG 6. In doing so, *karmayoga* is turned into a preparatory practice for those who wish to become (true) yogins (6.3). While *karman* is a method at this lower level of practice, "cessation" (*śama*) is declared to be the method of the one "who has climbed the path of yoga" (*yogārūḍha*; 6.4) and thus is already a yogin. For this practice, the yogin sits down in a lonely, well-prepared place and concentrates his gaze on the tip of his nose (6.12–13). The yogin must keep himself upright in order to remain in that stable concentration, which, according to BhG 6.14–15, allows him to concentrate on the god Kṛṣṇa alone. After this reference to Kṛṣṇa alone, the description of practice continues by stressing that yoga practice is based on a moderate lifestyle, with a balanced diet and appropriate amounts of sleep and rest (6.16–17). Persistence and relentless efforts result in taming the natural activities of body, mind, and senses, which then allows the yogin to cease all thoughts and to realize that his being is the same as all other beings in the world. He then becomes *brahman*, identical with the cause of the world and of all beings. In this manner a yogin eventually obtains a state of happiness (*sukha*) and peace (*śānti*), which is called *brahmanirvāṇa* (5.24). The state of *brahmanirvāṇa* is defined as the complete cessation of mental activity (*nirodha*). This aligns with a well-established concept of yogic meditation as a liberating practice that emphatically requires the stoppage of all thought processes. This is to be distinguished from the yoga that results in the vision of the self, or of God as this self (as is the case when Kṛṣṇa is declared to be the object and goal of yoga). In this way the BhG includes not only what may be distinguished as "theistic" and "non-theistic" yoga, but also two types of yoga and meditation found in Buddhist texts as well: first, yoga as a practice that aims at *nirodha*, complete cessation of mental activity followed by ultimate happiness; and second, as a practice of meditation that culminates in insight (*prajñā*; BhG 2.54ff.) or vision (of the self, god, etc.). Indicative of the emphasis on *nirodha* and on the experience of happiness is the fact that the yogin is described as *brahmabhūta*, one who has become *brahman*. The yogin enjoys "the touch of *brahman*" (*brahmasaṃsparśa*), which means the experience of unsurpassed happiness (6.28). This emphasis on "touch" allows the complex structure of yogic practice to be described in quite concrete terms. Touch and touching play a role in descriptions of yoga wherein yogins are asked to avoid both the touching and the "touch of outer objects" (BhG 5.21). Many descriptions of yogins depict them as indifferent to and immune from (but not unaware of) whatever circumstances, words, or deeds they are exposed to. This is also the point of the well-known comparison of the yogin to a tortoise (BhG 2.58): just as the tortoise reacts to an unwelcome touch by withdrawing its limbs into its shell, so the successful yogin reacts to the outer world. Thus, when the yogin is no longer "touchable" by others, he is ready for the touch of *brahman*. Only then may he experience the extraordinary, transsensual happiness that awaits him at the end of a path that has required the abandonment of all pleasure. The "touch of *brahman*" permits a new vision of the cosmos as a universe of sameness (*samatva*), in which a cow and brahmin are just the same (5.18); that is, they all consist of the same material constituents and in the end they all merge into one and the same cosmic cause of creation (6.29). According to BhG 6, Yoga is that practice which brings about "the disjunction (*viyoga*) from one's conjunction (*saṃyoga*) with suffering" (6.23), which not only means the end of suffering, but also the dawning of incomparable happiness.

Since the text of the BhG is a conversation, the dialogue-partners address each other with epithets referring either to their pedigree (Arjuna being the son of his mother Kuntī or Pṛthā and descendent of mythical king Bharata) or to their heroism (Arjuna as the "Winner of Wealth").

The following translations from the *Bhagavadgītā* are based on the text as constituted in the critical edition of the *Mahābhārata* (MBh 6.23–41) edited by V. S. Sukthankar et al., 21 vols. (Poona: Bhandarkar Oriental Institute, 1933–59). For a full translation of the text, see J.A.B. van Buitenen, *The Bhagavadgītā in the Mahābhārata. Text and Translation* (Chicago: Chicago University Press, 1981); a translation with a running commentary is offered by R. C. Zaehner, *The Bhagavad-Gītā with a Commentary based on the Original Sources* (Oxford: Oxford University Press, 1969). For a comprehensive analysis of the doctrines of the BhG, see Angelika Malinar, *The Bhagavadgītā: Doctrines and Contexts* (Cambridge: Cambridge University Press, 2007); for more on yoga in the BhG, see Angelika Malinar, "Yoga and Yogin in the Bhagavadgītā," in *Proceedings of the Fifth Dubrovnik Conference on the Sanskrit Epics and Purāṇas, August 2008*, ed. M. Jezic and P. Koskikallio (Zagreb: Croatian Academy of Science), forthcoming. On sacrifice and yoga, see Madeleine Biardeau and Charles Malamoud, *Le sacrifice dans l'Inde ancienne* (Paris: Presses Universitaires de France, 1976).

Bhagavad Gītā 2–6

1. Teachings on Yoga as the Basis for All Practice and as a Method for Avoiding the Consequences of Action (karman)

BHG 2: YOGIC DETERMINATION (BUDDHIYOGA)

Hear now about the faculty of discrimination (*buddhi*), which is known to you with regard to Sāṃkhya [and] with regard to Yoga. When yoked through the faculty of discrimination, O son of Pṛthā, you will get rid of the bond of *karman*. (2.39)

There is no loss of effort here, nor a reversal [of what has been achieved]. Even a little of this practice (*dharma*) saves from great danger! (2.40)

That faculty of discrimination (*buddhi*), which is completely determined, is unified, O Kuru hero, while the faculties of discrimination of those who lack determination are countless and many-branched. (2.41)

Ignorant followers of Vedic doctrines declaim with flowery speech when they assert that "there is no alternative [to ritual action]." (2.42)

For those who consist of desire, heaven is the highest [goal]. They are keen on gaining pleasure and power, which are found in many different rituals and brought about in [the next] birth by the fruits of ritual acts. (2.43)

Your entitlement (*adhikāra*) is only to the ordained act, never to its fruits. Be neither motivated by the fruits of [ordained] acts nor indulge in inactivity! (2.47)

Perform the [ordained] acts as one who abides in yogic determination (*yoga-stha*), give up [your] attachment (*saṅga*), O Winner of Wealth, and be indifferent toward success and failure. Yoga is called indifference (2.48)

For [mere] action is far less valuable than self-control through determination. Seek refuge in determination! Despicable are those who are motivated by the fruits [of their deeds]. (2.49)

The person who is restrained by his determination gets rid of both good and bad deeds. Therefore: Yoke yourself to yoga (self-control)! Yoga means skillfulness in [ordained] acts. (2.50)

For wise men, restrained through determination, shun the fruits that arise from their deeds. They are free from the bonds of birth and reach a state of non-affliction. (2.51)

When your determination has escaped the thicket of delusion, you will feel an aversion (*nirveda*) toward what you had to learn and have learned. (2.52)

When your determination abides in stable concentration and remains unshaken [even] when it departs from traditional Vedic knowledge, you have obtained the state of yogic self-control. (2.53)

BHG 3: THE YOGA OF SACRIFICAL ACTION (KARMAYOGA)

A man does not obtain freedom from [the consequences of] action by refraining from action completely, nor is this goal achieved through renunciation (*saṃnyāsa*) alone. (3.4)

For not even a single moment does a living being exist without being active since everyone is helplessly propelled to action through the powers (*guṇa*) that arise from nature (*prakṛti* [the cosmic cause of all activity]). (3.5)

He who curbs the faculties of action, yet who in his mind imagines the sense objects, is full of delusion: he is called a hypocrite. (3.6)

But he who curbs the senses with his mind and then practices self-control in action using his faculties of action without any attachment stands out [from the rest]. (3.7)

Carry out the ordained acts, since action is better than non-action. Even your journey in the body (*śarīrayātra*) will not succeed without action. (3.8)

This world is bound by acts, except those [undertaken] for the sake of sacrifice (*yajñārtham*). For this purpose, you must perform your duty, O son of Kuntī, as one who is free from attachment (*muktasaṅga*). (3.9)

Creatures arise from food, food arises from rain, rain arises from sacrifice, sacrifice arises from [ordained] action (*karman*). You must know that [ordained] action arises from *brahman* [the ritual knowledge and formulations contained in Veda], and *brahman* arises from the "indestructible" [*akṣara*, the syllable *Oṃ*, the essence of Vedic knowledge]. Therefore the ubiquitous *brahman* is forever grounded in the sacrifice (*yajña*). (3.14–15)

He who does not keep this moving wheel rolling accordingly lives in vain, O son of Pṛthā, since he indulges his senses, living a life that is sin. (3.16)

Therefore, you must perform the ordained act without attachment, for the man who fulfills [his] duty obtains the highest [realm]. (3.19)

For through deeds alone King Janaka and others obtained complete success. You too must act while only looking to what holds the world together (*lokasaṃgraha*). (3.20)

BHG 4: YOGIC SACRIFICE

Because he has given up attachment to the fruits of his deeds, being always satisfied and independent, he does not do anything, even though he is engaged in activity. (4.20)

Because he hopes for nothing, has himself and his mind under control and gives up all possessions, he is not beset with defilement, since he simply performs the act physically. (4.21)

In the case of the liberated man whose attachment has vanished and whose mind is steadied by knowledge, *karman* [the accumultated consequences of deeds] dissolves completely when he lives for the sake of sacrifice (*yajñāya*). (4.23)

Offering is *brahman*; the oblation that is poured with *brahman* into the fire of *brahman* is *brahman*. He who [thus] meditates on the ritual acts as *brahman* will certainly reach *brahman*. (4.24)

Some yogins offer sacrifices directed at deities alone, others offer the sacrifice through sacrifice into the sacrificial fire that is *brahman*. (4.25)

Some (yogins) sacrifice the senses, such as hearing and so forth, into the fires of complete restraint; others offer up the sense objects in the "sacrificial fire of the senses" (*indriya-agni*). (4.26)

Still others offer up all the activities of the senses and the activities of the breaths (*prāṇa*) into the sacrificial fire of the yoga practices of self-control (*ātma-saṃyama-yoga-agni*), which is kindled by knowledge. (4.27)

Some are dedicated to breath control (*prāṇāyāma*) and offer in-breathing in out-breathing and out-breathing in in-breathing when they stop the [natural] flow of out-breathing and in-breathing. (4.28)

Others offer up the breath into the breath when they reduce the consumption of food. Yet, all of them are sacrificial experts, since their stains have been extirpated through sacrifice. (4.29)

Acts do not tie down the person who controls himself because he has cast away his deeds through yoga and his doubts have been dispelled through knowledge, O Winner of Wealth. (4.41)

This doubt, which arises from ignorance and has taken hold of your heart: cut it away from yourself with the sword of knowledge and practice this yoga. Take up your arms and prepare [for battle], O Son of Bharata! (4.42)

2. Teachings on Practices of Liberation

BHG 2: FIRM INSIGHT

Arjuna said:

What is the language of a man whose insight is firm, who abides in concentration? What does a man whose thought is clear say? Does he stay [in one place or] does he move about? (2.54)

Kṛṣṇa said:

When a man gives up all the desires that occupy his heart and is satisfied with himself in himself, he is called "a man whose insight is firm." (2.55)

He whose mind remains unimpressed when faced with hardships, who has no desire when faced with pleasures, and is free from passion, fear and scorn, is called a "sage whose insight is firm." (2.56)

He who is without emotion with regard to whatever good or evil he may obtain and who neither rejoices nor shows hatred possesses insight that is firmly established. (2.57)

When he entirely withdraws his senses from their objects as a tortoise withdraws its limbs, his insight is firmly established. (2.58)

The sense-objects vanish for the embodied self, who no longer imbibes them, with the exception of drink; but drink also disappears for him who has seen the highest. (2.59)

The man who abides in yogic control is awake in what is night for all creatures; likewise it is night for the envisioning ascetic when the other creatures are awake. (2.69)

As the rivers flow into the ocean, which remains unmoved even when it is filled up, so do all desires enter into the one who has gained peace—as opposed to the one who desires desire (*kāmakāmin*). (2.70)

BHG 5: YOGA AS SUBSTITUTING AGENCY

The person who has purified himself, conquered himself and (conquered) his senses is accomplished in yoga. Although he is active, he is not defiled because his self is identical with the self of all beings (*sarvabhūtātmabhūtātmā*). (5.7)

"I do nothing at all." This is what the accomplished one, the knower of reality shall think when he sees, hears, feels, smells, eats, walks, dreams, breathes, talks, excretes, grasps, [or] opens his eyes and closes them, because he bears in mind that "the senses are occupied with the sense-objects." (5.8–9)

Having cast all activities onto *brahman* [the cosmic cause of all actions] and given up attachment, he acts but is not defiled by demerit, just as a lotus petal is not [defiled] by water. (5.10)

Yogins perform their duty with their body, mind, faculty of discrimination or even only with their senses, because they have given up all attachment through self-purification. (5.11)

The learned ones see a knowledgeable, well-mannered brahmin, a cow, an elephant, a dog and an eater of dogs as one and the same. (5.18)

Here in this world they indeed have conquered creation, since their minds rest in [the recognition of] sameness (*sāmya*). For the indifferent cause of creation and action (*brahman*) is devoid of flaws, and therefore they abide in that cause (*brahman*). (5.19)

Because he is no longer attached to touching outer objects, he indeed finds happiness in himself. He whose self is controlled through union with *brahman* (*brahmayogayuktātmā*) finds permanent happiness. (5.21)

The pleasures that arise from touching are breeding grounds for suffering simply because they have a beginning and an end, O son of Kuntī. The wise ones do not indulge in them. (5.22)

He who here on earth is capable of resisting the overflow of desire and anger [setting in] before discarding his body, is an accomplished yogin [and] a happy man. (5.23)

He who finds happiness, bliss and light within himself is a yogin, who, being *brahman*, realizes the effacement of all differences in the cause of creation. (5.24)

The wise one who is dedicated to liberation and whose senses, mind and faculty of discrimination are under control, keeps the afflictions from the outer world outside, fixes his gaze between the eyebrows, and equalizes the [rhythm] of both the in-breathing and out-breathing that flow within the nostrils. Only he whose desire, fear and wrath are gone is always liberated. (5.25–26)

BHG 6: OBTAINING THE TOUCH OF BRAHMAN

He is a renouncer as well as a yogin who performs the prescribed task without craving its fruits—not he who is without fires and rites. (6.1)

What is generally called "renunciation" (*saṃnyāsa*) you should understand to be "yoga," O son of Pāṇḍu, because no one becomes a yogin who has not cast away his intentions [of gaining the fruits of his acts]. (6.2)

For a wise man who wishes to climb the yoga path, "action" (*karman*) is said to be the method. For the one who has already climbed the yoga path, "cessation" (*śama*) is said to be the method. (6.3)

Indeed, when the renouncer of all intentions [concerning the fruits of his acts] neither clings to the sense objects nor to his deeds, he is said to be the one "who has climbed the yoga path." (6.4)

One should raise oneself by oneself and not degrade oneself, for oneself alone is one's kinsman [and] oneself alone is one's enemy. (6.5)

The self is a kinsman to the person who has conquered himself by himself, but to him who has no self [i.e., a self that is under control], his self will simply turn out to be his enemy. (6.6)

For he who has mastered himself and has become peaceful, the higher self [i.e., the faculty of discrimination; *buddhi*] is completely stable in cold and heat, in joy and pain, in honor and abuse. (6.7)

The yogin should constantly harness himself while he abides in concealment [i.e., in solitude]. He lives on his own, having his mind and himself under control. He is without expectations or social ties. (6.10)

On a clean spot he builds for himself a firm seat, neither too high nor too low, covered with cloth, deer-skin or *kuśa* grass. (6.11)

While sitting on this seat he concentrates his mind, with its mental and sensual activities under control; he should practice yoga for self-purification. (6.12)

While holding his body, head and neck upright he is immobile [and] stable; without taking notice of his surroundings he gazes intently at the tip of his nose. (6.13)

At peace with himself and fearless, he is firm in the observance of chastity. With his mind subdued, the accomplished yogin sits [on his seat] directing his thoughts to me [Kṛṣṇa] as he holds me to be the highest. (6.14)

When the yogi whose mind is controlled constantly harnesses himself in this way, he will reach the peace that lies in me, and which thereby surpasses *nirvāṇa*. (6.15)

However, yoga is not for one who eats too much or who eats nothing at all; nor [is it] for one who sleeps too much or is always awake. (6.16)

Yoga becomes a destroyer of pain for the person who eats and fasts in right measure, who has his movements under control in all activities and whose [periods of] sleeping and waking are in balance. (6.17)

When he has fixed his completely subdued mind in himself and is without desire for pleasures, then he is called an accomplished yogin. (6.18)

Like a flame does not flicker when placed in a windless spot: this is a well-known metaphor for the yogin whose mind is controlled when he applies yogic practice to himself [literally, "who yokes himself to yoga"]. (6.19)

When the mind comes to rest as it is stilled through the practice of yoga, then he sees the self in himself through himself. (6.20)

He then experiences that exceptional happiness which surpasses the senses because it can only be experienced through the faculty of discrimination (*buddhi*); and when he remains therein and does not depart from it, when he has obtained it and cannot imagine anything else worth obtaining, he firmly remains therein and is not shaken by suffering, however profound it may be. (6.21–22)

He will then understand the definition of yoga as "disjunction (*viyoga*) from the conjunction (*saṃyoga*) with suffering." This yoga must be practiced with determination and with a mind that is free from sorrow. (6.23)

A yogin who constantly yokes himself in this way is free from defilement; he easily enjoys the touch of *brahman*, which is infinite happiness. (6.28)

He sees himself in all beings and all beings in himself. Having controlled himself through yoga, everywhere he sees the same. (6.29)

—4—

Pātañjala Yoga in Practice

Gerald James Larson

History and Texts of Pātañjala Yoga

There are all sorts of traditions of yoga in India and elsewhere, both sectarian and non-sectarian, but there are primarily two systematic forms of South Asian yoga that are especially salient for understanding Yoga in its many permutations. These are a philosophical system of yoga known as Pātañjala Yoga (yoga in the lineage of Patañjali; hereafter PY), focusing largely on meditation training relating to the functioning of ordinary awareness (*citta-vṛtti*); and *haṭha yoga* ("Exertion Yoga"), focusing largely on meditation training relating to the functioning of the body, its postures, breathing, and general health. Both systems, of course, interact with one another, since the functioning of ordinary awareness is always contingent on the states of the body, and similarly, the exercises that a yogin performs regarding posture, breath, muscle control, bodily fluids, and so forth, always impinge on the functioning of awareness.

As systematic forms of yoga, PY appears to be considerably older than *haṭha yoga* and is likely the source from which much of later *haṭha yoga* is derived, although it must be admitted that the precise historical development of yoga traditions in India is still being debated in contemporary scholarship. In any case, PY is the focus of this chapter. The later *haṭha yoga*, usually associated with the names Gorakṣanātha and Matsyendranātha, will be treated elsewhere.

PY itself is usually referred to as *Pātañjala-yoga-śāstra*, that is, the learned tradition (*śāstra*) of Yoga in the lineage belonging to Patañjali, or *Pātañjala-yoga-darśana*, the philosophical school of Yoga in the lineage of Patañjali. This learned tradition or school of philosophy is set forth systematically in a Sanskrit text entitled *Yoga Sūtra* (hereafter YS) or sometimes *Pātañjala-yoga-sūtra*, compiled or attributed to a certain Patañjali in the early centuries of the Common Era (roughly 350–450 CE). The sūtra collection itself is a compilation of 195 brief sūtras or aphorisms in four sections or chapters (called "Pādas") containing 51, 55, 55, and 34 sūtras respectively. Some of the aphorisms may be considerably older than the fourth century CE when they were compiled into the present extant collection. The collection itself is accompanied by a commentary (*Bhāṣya*), attributed to a certain Vyāsa (hereafter VB), and to be dated approximately to the same time as the sūtra collection itself. Indeed, it has been maintained with some plausibility that the commentary was composed by the compiler of the sūtra collection, thereby making the commentary what is known in Sanskrit as a "self-composed" commentary (*svopajña*).

PY is said to be a "common tradition" (*samāna-tantra*) with one of the oldest systems of Indian philosophy known as Sāṃkhya, a system of thought that proceeds by "enumerating" (*saṃkhyā*) a set of twenty-five basic principles. The old Sāṃkhya philosophy takes shape in the last centuries BCE and attains its classical or systematic formulation in the first centuries of the Common Era in the work of a certain Vārṣagaṇya and a younger contemporary, Vindhyavāsa. Unfortunately only fragments of the teachings of these two teachers remain. The system, however, is given an elementary summary explication in an extant text entitled *Sāṃkhyakārikā* ("Verses on Sāṃkhya") composed by Īśvarakṛṣṇa in about 350–450 CE. As such, this text is roughly contemporary with the composition of the YS and its commentary, the VB. The *Sāṃkhyakārikā* is said by Īśvarakṛṣṇa to be a summary of a so-called *Śaṣṭi-tantra*, the "System of Sixty," referring either to an old name of the Sāṃkhya system or one or more texts by that name. Moreover, the YS together with its commentary is said to be an "explanation of Sāṃkhya" (*sāṃkhya-pravacana*). It would appear to be the case, then, that PY is a system of thought and practice combining an ancient philosophical system (Sāṃkhya) with a systematic compilation of older traditions of disciplined meditation (Yoga) practices.

As mentioned above, it has been suggested that the commentary (the VB) that accompanies the YS is a "self-composed" (*svopajña*) commentary. If such is the case, the obvious question to be answered is why two distinct names are connected with the sūtra collection and the commentary, Patañjali and Vyāsa. Sufficient evidence to resolve the issue of the names is not yet available, but it is possible to offer a few comments. The name Vyāsa, a legendary name ascribed to all sorts of texts in Sanskrit literary history, is obviously incorrect. There is, however, the old Sāṃkhya-yoga teacher, mentioned previously, named Vindhyavāsa, who was working at about the same time as the compilation of the YS and who may well be the author of the commentary. The specific reasons for such a suggestion need not detain us other than to say that there are some enticing clues to suggest that Vindhyavāsa is a plausible hypothesis. Perhaps the most important clue is that Vindhyavāsa was in polemical interaction with Buddhist thinkers in the first centuries CE, especially with the great Buddhist author, Vasubandhu, and was influenced by many Buddhist ideas. Many aspects of the YS and its basic commentary appear to reflect such polemical interactions. Thus, even if Vindhyavāsa was not himself the author of the commentary on the YS, the author must surely have been a Sāṃkhya-yoga teacher very much like Vindhyavāsa.

The name Patañjali is the same as that of the famous grammarian Patañjali, who lived in the first or second century BCE, and some have suggested that they are the same person. While it is unlikely that the grammarian could have been the compiler of the entire extant YS, since the dates of the grammarian's work and the compilation of the YS are clearly divergent, a case can be made that a portion of the sūtra collection may be traceable to the famous grammarian, namely, the *yogāṅga*-section, YS 2:28 through about 3:5, that is, the portion of the sūtra collection that deals with the eight "limbs" (*aṅgas*) of Yoga practice. There is some evidence to suggest that the famous grammarian may have been interested in some of the older forms of yoga practice. Thus, when the Yoga system of philosophy was compiled in the first centuries CE, the compiler—for example, Vindhyavāsa or one of his colleagues in the same period—may have attributed the system as a whole to one of Yoga's first and most famous adherents, thereby legitimating the value of the new learned system (*śāstra*) of Yoga and linking it to another of the great learned systems of Indian scientific work, the grammar of Patañjali.

This is admittedly only speculation based on some suggestive clues, and it should be frankly admitted that the name of the compiler of the *Yogasūtra*s may have been some other Patañjali and not the famous grammarian. Likewise, this other Patañjali could have been the author of the "self-composed" (*svopajña*) commentary. It could, of course, also be the case that there may have been some other author of the commentary, different not only from Vyāsa but from Vindhyavāsa as well. These matters are not settled in current scholarship but are important issues to be pursued in any attempt to write a cogent history of the development of Yoga as a systematic system of thought and practice in India.

Many commentaries have been written on both the *Sāṃkhyakārikā* and the YS with the VB. Only two authors of commentaries are especially important for our purposes, however. These are Vācaspatimiśra, who lived and wrote in the tenth century CE, and the sixteenth-century Vijñānabhikṣu. Vācaspatimiśra has written important commentaries on both Sāṃkhya and PY. His Sāṃkhya commentary is entitled *Sāṃkhya-tattva-kaumudī* ("Moonlight on the Truth of the Sāṃkhya"), and his massive commentary on the YS and the

VB is entitled *Tattva-vaiśāradī* ("Expertise on the Truth [of Sāṃkhya-yoga]"). Vijñānabhikṣu's commentary on Sāṃkhya is entitled *Sāṃkhya-pravacana-bhāṣya* ("Commentary on the Explanation of Sāṃkhya"), and his commentary on PY is *Yoga-vārttika* ("Critical Annotations on Yoga"). Both Vācaspatimiśra and Vijñānabhikṣu were adherents of Vedānta philosophy, a system of philosophy that differs from both Sāṃkhya and Yoga. It is generally recognized, however, that Vācaspatimiśra's commentaries on the various systems of Indian philosophy are exhaustive, reliable, and balanced. The same is not the case with Vijñānabhikṣu. He was a vigorous polemicist against all traditions that diverged from his own Vedānta, and, hence, his commentaries are not nearly as reliable as Vācaspatimiśra's. Also, of course, his work comes nearly a thousand years after the YS and the VB, long after Sāṃkhya and Yoga were vigorous living traditions of thought and practice in their original forms. In what follows, therefore, we will obviously be relying more on Vācaspatimiśra's interpretations of the YS and the VB.

Before proceeding to the discussion of PY practice, one other introductory matter must be addressed, and that is a brief characterization of the essentials of Sāṃkhya philosophy, since it is essential for understanding the meaning of the basic ideas underlying PY. Sāṃkhya philosophy consists in the "enumeration" (*saṃkhyā*) of twenty-five basic principles (*tattva*s), or, more precisely, two ontologically distinct realities, that is, "consciousness" (*puruṣa*) and "materiality" (*prakṛti*), the latter of which has twenty-three internal components in addition to itself, thereby making a total of twenty-four principles. In other words, consciousness is ontologically distinct from materiality and represents a unique principle separate from the twenty-four-fold structure of materiality. Sāṃkhya is in this sense a rigorous dualism, although it is an unusual form of dualism. Consciousness is said to be content-less (or, in modern terms, non-intentional). It is simply a witnessing translucent presence. Materiality itself is made up of three constituent processes or dynamic strands (*guṇa*s) that are always present together and always operating mutually in various permutations; *sattva*, the intelligibility or thinking process (symbolized by the color white); *rajas*, the energizing process (symbolized by the color red); and *tamas*, the objectifying or objectification process (symbolized by the color black or blue). These constituent processes are not qualities of materiality, but rather actually constitute materiality. Consciousness and materiality are in proximity to one another and without beginning (or, put somewhat differently, each dimension of reality is all-pervasive). This beginning-less proximity brings about a continuous process of unfolding structures or components within materiality that include intellect (*buddhi* or *mahat*), ego (*ahaṃkāra* or *asmitā*), mind (*manas*), and the five sense capacities (*buddhīndriya*s), five motor capacities (*karmendriyas*), five subtle elements (*tanmātras*), and five gross elements (*mahābhūtas*). Intellect, ego, mind, the sense capacities, and the motor capacities are largely governed by the constituent process *sattva*, while the subtle elements and gross elements are largely governed by the constituent process *tamas*. The constituent process *rajas* energizes the ongoing overall transformations of materiality (*prakṛti*).

At this point, it is crucial to grasp several remarkably counterintuitive but important twists or reversals that are fundamental to the Sāṃkhya and PY positions, not only philosophically but also for understanding the underlying nature of the practice involved.

First, given the number of twenty-five principles, one might be inclined to think that the consciousness principle is one and the materiality principle is twenty-four. In fact, however, the situation is reversed. Consciousness, although a unique singularity in its essence, is, rather, plural in its manifestations. Materiality, on the other hand, although apparently plural in its manifest components, is singular in number. In other words, in Sāṃkhya and PY the distinction between one and the many is the opposite of what one usually thinks. Materiality, although having many internal components, is really a single, rationally intelligible (*sattva*), dynamic (*rajas*), and objective world (*tamas*). Consciousness, to the contrary, manifests itself pluralistically, even though in its essence it is a unique singularity, that is, content-less or non-intentional, and totally distinct from the *guṇa*-realm of materiality.

Second, although one might think that consciousness (*puruṣa*) includes our usual understanding of the self in terms of mental life, ego, and mind in all of its operations, in fact, for Sāṃkhya and PY, intellect, ego, and mind and our usual notions of selfhood are included within materiality (or, in modern terms, are construed in a physicalist manner). The intellect, ego, and mind, along with sense capacities and motor capacities, are all part of our physical or material makeup. Any and all of these may become, in other words, "objects" for meditation and, in fact, are material objects for meditation. In this regard, there is a somewhat different vocabulary in Sāṃkhya and PY for these various objects. For Sāṃkhya, intellect, ego, and mind along with sense capacities and motor capacities are all separate subtle "objects" abiding in gross physical forms (the brain, ear, eye, and so forth). For PY, intellect, ego, and mind are combined into one single composite notion of "ordinary awareness" (*citta*), which is a subtle object known as the "subject" (*grahītṛ*). Sensing and motor capacities are subtle objects known as "sensing" or apprehending capacities (*grahaṇa*), and the manifest world of ideas and empirical objects are known as subtle and gross objects (*grāhya*). All three dimensions of ordinary experience or awareness (*citta*)—that is, subject, object, and the sensing that links subject and object together—are functions of materiality and are ontologically distinct or "isolated" (*kevala*, *kaivalyam*) from consciousness (*puruṣa*). Put directly, for Sāṃkhya and for PY, a crucial intuition that grows out of ongoing meditation or yogic practice is that "awareness" is fundamentally distinct or separate or isolated from "consciousness."

Third, this then leads to the most important insight of Sāṃkhya and PY. Because consciousness is a content-less (non-intentional) translucent witness or presence, it can only appear as what it is NOT: that is, it appears as if it were the same as the manifest material world. Similarly, materiality in turn, which is lacking in consciousness, by virtue of having been witnessed or reflected in non-intentional consciousness, appears as what it is NOT: that is, it appears as if it were conscious. In other words, there is a double negation at the heart of sentient existence in all its forms, a profoundly mistaken confusion, a fundamental mixing up or "union" of "awareness" and "consciousness" that triggers the profound suffering characteristic of the manner in which one experiences the gods, the experience of one's involvement in social life and the experience of one's own personal life. The meditational goal of Sāṃkhya and PY, then, is to bring about the "disunion" (*vi-yoga*) of "awareness" and "consciousness," or what PY refers to as the realization of the absolute "otherness" of the *guṇa*-realm of materiality from the *guṇa*-less realm of consciousness. What the yogin seeks to accomplish in meditation is the "cessation of the functioning of ordinary awareness" (*citta-vṛtti-nirodha*) (YS I.2) so that the "witnessing" presence of consciousness (*draṣṭṛ*) may show itself in its sheer translucent excellence (YS I.3). There is nothing otherworldly or mysterious about this realization. The un-doing of the confusion between "awareness" and "consciousness" simply allows for the yogin to attain an experiential realization of the presence of a radical freedom at the heart of sentient existence, an experiential clarity that radically transforms self-understanding, thereby providing relief from the suffering that has been brought about by the afflictions attendant upon mistaken or muddled awareness.

Pātañjala Yoga in Practice

According to the commentaries on the YS, chapter 1 (or the first Pāda) of the text has to do with gaining a correct understanding of "concentration" (*samādhi*). Chapter 2 (second Pāda) has to do with the meditative practices (*sādhana*) needed to prepare the yogin for the cultivation of "concentration." Chapter 3 (third Pāda) has to do with the "extraordinary cognitive capacities" (*vibhūtis*) that arise from pursuing the higher levels of yogic concentration.

Chapter 4 (the final Pāda) provides an overall summary of what has gone before, focusing on the nature of individual awareness (*citta*), different sorts of karma, the reality of a single existing world, and some concluding comments about liberation, ending in the final affirmation that "spiritual liberation (*kaivalyam*) is the standing forth of pure consciousness in its own inherent nature."

The overall focus of the entire YS is the proper cultivation of "concentration" (*samādhi*) in all of its modalities, and, thus, the proper place to begin by way of discussing specific practice is chapter 2, the chapter that addresses concrete practice (*sādhana*). Chapter 2 begins by stressing the need to perform ascetic exercises (*tapas*), recitation and study (*svādhyāya*), and devotion to God (Īśvara) in order to overcome the basic afflictions that derive from the failure to distinguish "ordinary awareness" (*citta*) from consciousness (*puruṣa*). These afflictions include the basic ignorance or the mistaken confusion of not distinguishing awareness from consciousness, and the resulting problems of improper self-understanding, counterproductive attachment, dysfunctional anger, and clinging to the illusions of conventional life (YS 2:1–14). Then, the text provides a summary of Sāṃkhya philosophy, culminating in the description of the "sevenfold insight" (*prajñā*), the first four components of which are roughly parallel to the Four Noble Truths of the Buddhists (suffering, its cause, its alleviation, and the path to be followed), and the final three components of which are the achievement of the cessation of conventional awareness, the cessation of the functioning of the constituent processes (*guṇas*), and the achievement of the realization that *puruṣa* is different from the *guṇas* (YS 2:15–27).

Chapter 2 then proceeds to set forth the famous eight "limbs" (or the eightfold path) of Yoga practice (*yoga-aṅgas*) (YS 2:28–55 and YS 3:1–8). The first five stages of Yoga practice are described in YS 2:30–55 and include behavioral restraints (*yama*), purificatory ritual observances (*niyama*), correct meditation postures (*āsana*), appropriate breathing practices (*prāṇāyāma*), and sense-withdrawal exercises (*pratyāhāra*). The final three "limbs" are set forth in YS 3:1–8 and include spatial fixation on the object of meditation (*dhāraṇā*), even temporal flow regarding the object of meditation (*dhyāna*), and cultivation of one-pointed "concentration" (*samādhi*).

The first five "limbs" are largely practical, preparatory exercises that have little to do with the cultivation of concentration. They are described as "external limbs" (*bahir-aṅga*) (YS 3:7–8), that is, outer preliminary, preparatory meditative exercises. The first limb, behavioral restraint (*yama*), includes a conventional list of behaviors widely valued in all traditions of Indian religion and philosophy, including non-violence, speaking the truth, not taking what belongs to others, sexual continence, and non-covetousness (YS 2:30 and 35–

39). The second limb, purificatory ritual practice (*niyama*), includes cleansing the body, suppressing desire for the sake of contentment, ascetic practice, study and recitation, and meditation on (or deep longing for) the yogic God (*īśvara-praṇidhāna*). Both the VB and Vācaspatimiśra construe devotion to God in the sense of devoting all one's actions to God without becoming attached to the fruits of action (YS 2:1, 32, and 40–45). The third limb, correct meditation posture (*āsana*), means simply any posture of the body that is "comfortably steady" for the sake of meditation practice (YS 2:46). These postures enable the practicing yogin to remain comfortably in the same position for a long period in a relaxed fashion (YS 2:47) and without being troubled by cold or heat, and so forth (2:48). The fourth limb, appropriate breath exercise (*prāṇāyāma*), has to do with cutting off or lessening the processes of inhalation and exhalation (YS 2:49) so that the practicing yogin can increase the periods of the retention of breath (either after inhalation or exhalation) (YS 2:50). Moreover, breath exercise involves focusing the breath on a particular place (*deśa*) in the body, measuring the length of time (*kāla*) of each inhalation and exhalation and retention, and counting the number of breaths (*saṃkhyā*) (YS 2:50). Eventually a level of breathing arises that transcends the ordinary awareness of inhalation, exhalation, and retention (YS 2:51), enabling the practicing yogin to move to higher levels of meditation (YS 2:52–53). The fifth and final "external" limb (*bahir-aṅga*), sense-withdrawal exercise (*pratyāhāra*), involves detaching one's attention from the objects of the various sense capacities (YS 2:54–55).

When all of these preparatory practices have been properly cultivated under the guidance of an appropriate teacher, the practicing yogin is ready to move on to the final three "internal" (*antar-aṅga*) limbs of the practice of Yoga. These three "limbs" are to be practiced simultaneously and are referred to as "comprehensive reflection" (*saṃyama*).

The sixth limb of the eightfold limbs of Yoga, and the first of the "internal" limbs, is "fixation" (*dhāraṇā*) of the *citta* on a specific location in space (YS 3:1). The VB indicates that such fixation may be based on certain parts of the yogin's body. These include the vital center of the navel, the lotus of the heart, the light in the head, the tip of the nose, the tip of the tongue, and so forth. Or, the focus can be on any external object.

The seventh limb of the eightfold limbs of Yoga, and the second of the "internal" limbs, is "meditating" or "contemplating" (*dhyāna*) or attaining an even (temporal) "tone" of awareness in regard to the object in the particular place attained by fixation (YS 3.2). This means a "like" or "similar" flow, from moment to moment, of the notion of the object so fixed in the yogin's awareness with no apprehension of any other object.

The eighth and final limb of the eightfold limbs of Yoga, and the third of the "internal" limbs, is "one-pointed" (*ekāgra*) concentration (*samādhi*) (YS 3:3). The text reads as follows: "That same [meditative state] in which only the object shines forth as if devoid of the inherent cognizing presence of the practitioner is the one-pointed awareness (*samādhi*)." When the yogin has mastered the threefold "comprehensive reflection," then the light of insight (*prajñā-āloka*) shines forth (YS 3:5).

Concentrations (*samādhi*) and Coalescences (*samāpatti*)

In order to understand what happens at the higher levels of practice in PY, it is essential to be clear about the meaning of two crucial notions, namely, "concentration" (*samādhi*) and the closely related notion, "coalescence" (*samāpatti*). With regard to the former, the VB states at the outset that "Yoga is concentration (*samādhi*), and this [concentration] pertains to all the levels of ordinary awareness." To some degree, this is an etymological comment, in the sense that the word "*yoga*" in PY is said to mean "concentration" as distinct from another possible meaning along the lines of "yoking" or "union." More than this, however, the comment also suggests that "concentration" relates to a wide variety of states of awareness. Five such states are then enunciated: distracted, torpid, partially distracted, one-pointed, and restricted. Among these five, only the final two, one-pointed and restricted, are considered to be relevant for the practice of PY. The first three states of awareness are dominated largely by *rajas* (the distracted state) or *tamas* (the torpid state) or have only small amounts of *sattva* (the partially distracted). Only the "one-pointed" and "restricted" are states of awareness with dominant amounts of *sattva*, the "one-pointed" having also a trace of *rajas*, the "restricted" being a pure *sattva* state. Since *sattva* states have to do primarily with intelligibility or the constituent process of thinking clearly and correctly, what "concentration" or *samādhi* means in PY is the manner in which a yogin correctly knows or apprehends the manifest world. "One-pointed" (*ekāgra*) concentration refers to a correct awareness that has an object or content of some sort, and such awareness is known as "correct awareness with some sort of object or content" (*saṃprajñāta-samādhi*). "Restricted" (*niruddha*) concentration refers to a correct awareness that has no object or content, a state of awareness that is pre-reflective, content-less, or non-intentional. Such awareness or concentration is known as "correct awareness that is seed-less" (*nir-bīja-samādhi*) or "correct awareness that is non-intentional or without an object or content" (*a-saṃprajñāta-samādhi*).

Regarding "one-pointed" concentrations, according to YS 1:17, there are basically four varieties, namely, empirical awareness (*vitarka*), rational awareness (*vicāra*), aesthetic or sensorial awareness (*ānanda*), and self-awareness (*asmitā*). The terms "aesthetic" and "sensorial" mean mere sensing or what is referred to in modern philosophy as a "quale" or the "qualia" experiences, that is, raw "feels" without intellectual elaboration. The VB on YS 1:17 characterizes these awarenesses as follows.

> Empirical awareness has to do with the experience of gross objects or contents. Rational awareness has to do with subtle objects or contents. Aesthetic (or sensorial) awareness has to do with the joy of sensuous awareness or the sheer sensing (or the act of cognizing) of objects or contents. Self-awareness has to do with the feeling of being one with one's self. The first, that is, empirical awareness, encompasses all four levels of awareness. The second, that is, rational awareness is without empirical awareness. The third, that is, aesthetic awareness is without empirical or rational awareness. The fourth, that is, self-awareness, is just self-awareness alone without the other three. All these states of awareness (*samādhis*) have objects or contents.

There is an additional, optional sort of "one-pointed" awareness, and that is what might be called "theological awareness," or, if you will, "divine awareness" (*īśvara-praṇidhāna*, or literally, a "deep longing for God") (YS 1:23). That is to say, in addition to meditating on an empirical object, a rational object, an aesthetic object, or simply on oneself, one may also meditate on the yogic notion of God.

As previously mentioned, all of these one-pointed concentrations (*samādhi*s) are intentional in the sense that they are "about" something, or, in other words, have some sort of specific content (*saṃprajñāta*). The first two varieties of one-pointed awareness are concerned respectively with gross and subtle objects or contents (*grāhya*). Empirical awareness concerns the everyday realm of ordinary or gross experience. Rational awareness concerns the subtle realm of ideas and conceptualizations that inform ordinary experience, or what Gaspar Koelman has aptly called the "objective universals" within experience—that is, ideations, fantasies, images, concepts, and so forth, that inform the empirical world of experience but are clearly on a different level of apprehension. The third variety of one-pointed awareness has to do with the processes or instrumentalities of sensing, including mental functioning, hearing, touching (feeling), seeing, tasting, and smelling (*grahaṇa*). Finally, the fourth variety of one-pointed awareness has to do with self-awareness or the ordinary subject of awareness (*grahītṛ*).

The four varieties of one-pointed awareness encompass three distinct levels of experience. First, there is the level of objects or contents (*grāhya*), which itself breaks into two sub-levels—gross-empirical and subtle-rational. Second, there is the level of processes or instrumentalities of cognizing and sensing (*ānanda* or *grahaṇa*). Finally, there is the level of self-awareness or subjective awareness (*asmitā* or *grahītṛ*). It is important to recognize in this sort of analysis the overlapping of notions due to the peculiar physicalist or materialist orientation of PY (and Sāṃkhya). That is, all three levels of experience (*grāhya, grahaṇa*, and *grahītṛ*) are objects or contents in ordinary awareness or "mind-stuff" (*citta*) and are, therefore, material processes within materiality. The term "*grāhya*" in this context means "object," and includes gross empirical objects and subtle "objective universal" or rational objects. The term "*grahaṇa*" in this context means the processes or instrumentalities of "sensing" and "cognizing," but these instrumentalities are themselves "objects" (*grāhya*) as well. That is, they too are types of subtle objects (or, perhaps better, action nouns) and can be the focus for meditation. Finally, the term "*grahītṛ*" in this context means ordinary self-awareness or subjective apprehension, but it, too, is also a type of subtle object (*grāhya*) and can be a focus for meditation. Altogether, then, the three levels of experience give rise to four separate types of objects, or perhaps better, "contents" (*grāhya*).

1. Gross empirical objects: *vitarka*.
2. Subtle rational ("objective universal"): *vicāra*.
3. Processes or instrumentalities of sensing: *ānanda*.
4. Ordinary self-awareness or subjective apprehension: *asmitā*.

Ordinary self-awareness or what would ordinarily be called "subjective awareness" is, according to this analysis, a type of "object" or "content." It is illumined by consciousness (*puruṣa* or *citi-śakti*), but ordinary subjectivity or self-awareness is a material process distinct from non-intentional consciousness. The same must be said about the processes of sensing, that is to say, ordinary mental functioning, hearing, touching, seeing, tasting, and smelling. Each of these, of course, has a gross objective base, as brain (or, in this ancient context, the heart region, since in ancient Indic thought, the seat of cognition is the "heart" region), ear, skin, eye, tongue, and nose, but the actual functioning or "sensing" capacity must be distinguished from the gross organ and is itself a subtle object. As is perhaps obvious, dementia, deafness, paralysis, blindness, and the inability to taste or smell provide clear evidence that the sensing capacity must be clearly distinguished from the gross organ. What the yogin must come to understand in ongoing meditation is that sensing and cognizing as well as subjective awareness are themselves subtle objects or material entities within the framework of ordinary awareness or "mind-stuff" and are to be clearly distinguished from consciousness. When the yogin achieves such a realization, he has attained "truth-bearing insight" (YS 1:48), and this insight is a special cognitive experience that transcends both scriptural knowledge and inferential knowledge (YS 1:49). This insight is also called the "dharma-cloud meditation" and the "supreme" or "ultimate" "reflection" (YS 4:29). When this special cognitive experience occurs, there arises, then, a strong predisposition (*saṃskāra*) that leads toward spiritual liberation (*nirodha*, *kaivalyam*) and that counteracts all other predispositions (YS 1:50).

Finally, when the yogin turns away even from that predisposition, or, in other words, even from that special cognitive experience—inasmuch as all ordinary awareness has been overcome—the yogin passes into "object-less" or "seed-less" (*nir-bīja*) *samādhi*. The yogin's non-intentional "perfect *sattva*" rests in the presence of pure, content-less consciousness, which is identical with the achievement of "isolation" or spiritual liberation, that is, the quiescent co-presence of "perfect *sattva*" and *puruṣa*" (YS I.51).

In addition to the understanding of concentration (*samādhi*), it is also important to understand the relation of concentration to the notion of "coalescence" (*samāpatti*). Furthermore, it is important to offer an interpretation of the various levels of concentration and coalescence. Commentaries differ from one another somewhat on the various levels of concentration and coalescence, and in what follows the interpretation of Vācaspatimiśra will be examined, since his work is without question the most authoritative, prior to the medieval period, in the intellectual history of Indic thought.

Regarding the issue of the relation between concentration and coalescence, the two terms are often used synonymously in the texts, but there is a distinction implied between concentration and the content exhibited in the state of concentration. The term "*samādhi*" is from the root, "*dhā*," together with the adverbial particles "*sam*" plus "*ā*" meaning "to put, place or hold together" (not unlike the English term, "con-centrate," from Latin, "cum" plus "centrum, "meaning "to center along with"). The term "*samāpatti*" is from the root, "*pad*," together with the adverbial particles "*sam*" plus "*ā*," meaning "to come together, to meet or to encounter." The terms are obviously close but not identical. The difference between them is the difference between "concentration" and that upon which the concentration is directed or focused. One-pointed awareness (*samādhi*), unlike the largely multiple, distracted, and confused awarenesses of everyday life, is a highly concentrated or focused awareness, and that "one point" upon which the awareness is focused becomes, then, the unique and single object "encountered" (the *samāpatti*). "Objectless" or "seedless" (*nir-bīja*) awareness, in contrast, is a highly concentrated or focused awareness without a determinate object or content. The "objectless" awareness, in other words, is a non-intentional awareness.

The possible varieties of one-pointed concentrations that bring about coalescences with certain contents are set forth in YS I.41.

> (When the ordinary awareness [of the yogin] has been sufficiently cleansed of its dysfunctional functioning [and become] like a transparent jewel, there arises an encounter or coalescence with [gross and subtle objects], the processes of sensing, and the subject of cognizing. [The cleansed ordinary awareness] then shows forth or highlights the true nature of those contents.

Just as black pigment or collyrium highlights the eyes, so the yogin's cleansed awareness shows forth the true nature of the contents exhibited in the one-pointed awareness, and, as has been discussed, there are four types or levels of awareness to be exhibited: empirical, ideational/rational, sensorial, and subjective (YS I.17).

Each type of "one-pointed" awareness may be accompanied by "verbal characterization or construction" (*sa-vikalpa*), and, hence, accessible to linguistic description, inferential reasoning, and so forth. Or, it may be free from such constructions (*nir-vikalpa*), hence permitting an immediate or direct apprehension of an object or content. Altogether, then, there are eight levels of *samādhi* and/or eight types of cognitive one-pointed objects or contents (*samāpatti*s). Vācaspatimiśra comments as follows (under YS 1:46) about these eight levels.

> The first four *samāpatti*s, referring to gross and subtle objects or contents, are clearly or obviously determinate by reason of having a specific "seed" (content). But, the condition of having a specific "seed" or content also applies to the *samāpatti*s pertaining to "sensing" and/or "cognizing" and subjective apprehension inasmuch as the distinction between "verbally constructed" or "verbally unconstructed" equally applies to them. Thus, there are four *samāpatti*s that pertain to gross and subtle objects and four that pertain to the contents related to "sensing" and subjective apprehension—(altogether, then) eight (*samādhi*s and *samāpatti*s) are recognized as established.

The first type of "one-pointed" awareness, namely, empirical awareness, encompassing the everyday world of ordinary experience, thus has two subdivisions. There is a lower level of empirical awareness in which objects (*artha*), language (*śabda*), and meanings or ideas (*pratyaya*s) are mixed together in single constructed or verbalized cognitions. This, of course, is the level of ordinary, everyday experience (YS 1:42). Since it is a one-pointed awareness, of course, it is a highly focused or disciplined empirical awareness. Perhaps, to use some modern examples, it is not unlike the focused excellence of a competent engineer, a highly trained athlete, or a professional musician whose objects of meditation might be respectively a specific project design, a particular game strategy, or the performance of a piece of music. In this regard, in both the popular and scholarly literature of Yoga, there is a tendency to write about *samādhi*s in terms of obscure mystical states. The original intent of the classical texts, however, is to speak about levels of awareness that are clear, distinct, and precise characterizations of what is truly real!

On this first level of empirical concentration, there is also, however, a higher level of empirical awareness in which memory no longer operates and, hence, a level in which the constructed or verbalized cognitions of everyday experience, involving language, learning, and inferential reasoning, are no longer intended. This is a level in which the yogin experiences the empirical object in and of itself "as if" (*iva*) separate from the constructions of verbal cognition (*vikalpa*) and self-awareness (YS 1.43). To remain with our earlier metaphor, this is a level of awareness in which the engineer becomes totally engrossed in the design qua design. Or, the highly trained athlete becomes totally engrossed in a game-move (for example, a specific play in a soccer match). Or, the musician becomes totally engrossed in the music itself. The one who is meditating becomes detached from everything except the meditation-object itself.

The second type of "one-pointed" awareness, namely, ideational/rational awareness (*vicāra*), likewise has two subdivisions, a lower "constructed or verbalized" awareness and a higher "unconstructed" awareness, that is, a direct awareness of the abstract object or content. The lower form of this awareness involves the "constructed" spatial (*deśa*), temporal (*kāla*), and causal (*nimitta*) contexts in which verbalized cognitions or constructions involving language, learning, and inferential reasoning are functioning. The higher form of this awareness arises when the spatial, temporal, causal, and linguistic/inferential framework is transcended and the pure "rational object" is apprehended in and of itself, "as if" devoid of the cognizing process and subjective presence. There is a total engrossment in the abstract subtle contents. Again, to use some modern illustrations, the "constructed" *samāpatti* would not be unlike the "objects" or contents experienced in the awareness of a mathematical physicist, a pure mathematician, a music theorist, or a professional philosopher, and the "unconstructed" or direct "coalescence" (*samāpatti*) would be a total engrossment in the subtle object contemplated "as if" the cognitive process itself and one's own subjective presence had been eliminated.

The lower and higher forms of the third and fourth types of "one-pointed" awareness, namely, aesthetic/sensorial and subjective awareness, are somewhat more difficult to characterize, since they go beyond what we usually mean by the term "object." For PY, however, it must be recognized that the sensing capacities as well as ordinary subjectivity itself are part of the material makeup of a sentient being and can, thus, become "objects" for meditation, albeit, of course, highly subtle material objects. Regarding the aesthetic/sensing awareness, there is a reflexive turning back whereby the cognizing processes themselves become the focus. It is likely that the terms "bliss" (*ānanda*) and "joy" (*hlāda*) (YS 1.17) are used for this level of awareness because there is no determinate object or content beyond the affective (aesthetic) feeling of sensing/cognizing itself. The lower level aesthetic/sensing "coalescence" is evidently a kind of sublime abiding in which the content or "seed" (*bīja*) is the blissful abiding itself, as sheer hearing, feeling, tasting, and so forth. The higher level or "unconstructed" awareness would then be something like an affect-less abiding in which only an indescribable intentional flow of awareness itself is the "seed." The only modern illustrations that come to mind are those from the highest levels of science and art. When a disciplined mathematician, for example, comes upon a new proof and describes it as "elegant," or when a disciplined connoisseur hears a great performance of music or sees a great painting and describes the experience as "noble" or "sublime," these could be possible examples of the lower level of aesthetic/sensing awareness. All such experiences involve objects, of course, but the true focus is the blissful apprehension of "elegance" or "nobility." More than that, however, there are also those moments of what might be called the sheer act of "sensing" or "cognizing" apart from any affect or feeling, a sheer "sensing" or "cognizing" that often follows as a kind of "after-taste" the apprehension of "elegance" or "nobility." Such awarenesses could possibly be illustrative of the higher level of aesthetic/sensing awareness.

The fourth and final type of "one-pointed" awareness has self-awareness or subjective apprehension as its "seed." Like the aesthetic/sensing awareness level, this level is a reflexive turning back in which, as it were, ordinary subjectivity shows itself as being a kind of "object" or content. The lower level of this awareness involves the discriminative realization that subjectivity or ego is a constituent process (*sattva*) within the *guṇa*-realm of materiality (*prakṛti*), and that there is a witnessing consciousness (*puruṣa*) that is beyond subjectivity itself. The higher level of the awareness of subjectivity, in which subjectivity itself dissolves, is described simply as "being itself" or "being alone" (*sattā-mātra*). It is the unmanifest presence of primordial materiality (*mūla-prakṛti*).

These, then, are the eight levels of "one-pointed" concentrations with their accompanying "coalescences." Beyond these is only the "seedless" presence of the witnessing consciousness.

The edition of the *Yoga Sūtra* used for this translation is Ram Shankar Bhattacharya, ed., *The Yogasutra of Patanjali together with the Bhasya of Vyasa and the Tattvavaisaradi of Vacaspatimisra* (Varanasi: Bharatiya Vidya Prakashan, 1963). The following translation is in two parts. Part I is an idiomatic interpretive translation in prose style of the first 40 *sūtras* of chapter 1 (Pāda I: Samādhi Pāda) for the sake of general background. Part II is a complete translation of *sūtras* 41–51 with the complete commentary attributed to Vyāsa. In Part II, the *sūtra*s themselves are presented in boldface. The commentary is in non-boldface type.

Suggestions for Further Reading

For an edition and translation of the portion of the *Yoga Sūtra* treated here, see Pandit Usharbudh Arya, ed. and trans., *Yoga-Sūtras of Patañjali*, vol. 1 (The Samādhi Pāda) (Honesdale, PA: Himalayan Institute, 1986). An edition and translation of the complete *Yoga Sūtra*, together with extensive commentary, is Edwin F. Bryant, *The Yoga Sūtras of Patañjali* (New York: North Point Press, 2009). Useful studies of the *Yoga Sūtra* are Georg Feuerstein, *The Yoga Sūtra: An Exercise in the Methodology of Textual Analysis* (New Delhi: Gulab Varzirani, 1979); Caspar M. Koelman, *Pātañjala Yoga* (Poona: Papal Atheneum, n.d.); and Ian Whicher, *The Integrity of the Yoga Darśana* (Albany: State University of New York Press, 1998). The entire sweep of the yoga tradition, from the *Yoga Sūtra* and its commentarial literature down through twentieth-century modern yoga, is treated encyclopedically in Gerald James Larson and Ram Shankar Bhattacharya, eds., *Yoga: India's Philosophy of Meditation* (Encyclopedia of Indian Philosophies, vol. 12) (Delhi: Motilal Banarsidass, 2008). Several Indic yoga traditions, including Jain yoga and Tantric yoga, are treated in Ian Whicher and David Carpenter, eds., *Yoga: the Indian Tradition* (London: Routledge Curzon, 2003).

Part I: Pātañjala Yoga Sūtra: Chapter 1, "On Concentration"

YS 1:1–40

This treatise has to do with the nature of disciplined meditation (*yoga*) and is based upon past teachings regarding the nature of meditation (1). Yoga or disciplined meditation involves the cessation (*nirodha*) of the functioning of ordinary awareness (*citta-vṛtti*) (2). When ordinary awareness has ceased to function, consciousness is experienced by the yogin for the first time (as a phenomenon distinct from awareness) (3). Prior to bringing about cessation or inhibition of ordinary awareness, consciousness conforms with ordinary awareness (or, in other words, does not reveal itself as something distinct from ordinary awareness) (4).

The notion of "ordinary awareness" is fivefold and may be afflicted or unafflicted (in the sense that everyday experience may be dysfunctional or purposeful in the functioning of a sentient being) (5). The five functions of ordinary awareness are correct cognitions, misleading or false cognitions, verbal discourse, sleeping (and other conditions such as waking, dreaming, and so forth), and memory (6–11).

The cessation (or inhibition) of these functions of ordinary awareness can be accomplished by the yogic (meditational) disciplines of continuing practice and renunciation and/or detachment (12). The expression "continuing practice" means training in meditation for the sake of attaining cognitive stability (13) in the sense of uninterrupted (repetitive) practice over extended periods of time (14). The expression "renunciation and/or detachment" means the complete control that the yogin achieves over any and all attachments either to the perceptible objects of the ordinary world or to the scriptural objects or contents set forth in the sacred texts (15). Moreover, there is a supreme "renunciation or detachment" that involves turning away from ordinary awareness altogether (and see above, sūtra 2) for the sake of experiencing the unique presence of consciousness that is absolutely distinct from awareness of any sort (see above sūtra 3) (16).

The cessation or inhibition of ordinary awareness by means of "continuing practice" and "renunciation or detachment" encompasses two sorts of yogic intense concentration (*samādhi*), that is, altered or "extra-ordinary" states of awareness, the first of which provides clear cognition of the nature of empirical (*vitarka*) objects, intellectual or ideational (*vicāra*) objects, aesthetic or sensing (*ānanda*) processes, and self-awareness or subjectivity (*asmitā*). These intense concentrations are known as "altered" or "extra-ordinary" states of concentration that involve an object or specific content (*saṃprajñāta*) (17). The second sort of yogic intense concentration is a state in which awareness itself, whether ordinary or extra-ordinary, has dissipated with only consciousness itself appearing (see above, sūtra 3), a state wherein only predispositions that are outside of awareness remain operative (18–22). [Sūtras 19 through 22 discuss various classifications of yogins and appear to be notations relating primarily to 17 and 18.]

In addition to the intense concentrations known as "altered" or "extra-ordinary" states of concentration that involve an object or specific content (*saṃprajñāta*)—for example, concentration on empirical objects, ideational objects, aesthetic or sensate processes, and self-awareness—there is the alternative possibility of making God (Īśvara) an intentional object of meditation (23–28).

When meditation has been successfully practiced, one then attains the realization of the presence of one's own consciousness, and the various distractions and obstacles are no longer present (29–32). Peace of mind (*citta-prasādana*) or stability of awareness arises, and the yogin's complete control (see above, sūtra 15) ranges throughout the entire range of reality from the smallest particle to the largest entity (33–40).

Part II: Pātañjala Yoga Sūtra 1: 41–51 with the Bhāsya attributed to Vyāsa

YS 1:41 [Preface by VB] The coalescence and/or engrossment of ordinary awareness when the condition of steadiness has been attained—What precisely is its nature or what sort of content does it have? Thus it is stated,

[When the ordinary awareness of the yogin] has been sufficiently cleansed of its dysfunctional operations (*kṣīṇa-vṛtti*) [and has become] like a transparent jewel, there arises a profound coalescence or engrossment (*samāpatti*) in regard to [gross and subtle] objects (*grāhya*), the process of cognizing (*grahaṇa*) and the subject of cognizing (*grahītṛ*). Ordinary awareness (*citta*) then takes on, or exhibits or highlights (*añjanatā*), the true nature of those contents.

[VB] The expression "dysfunctional operations" has the meaning "thrown out" or "cast aside." "Transparent jewel" is the mentioning of an "illustration." Just as a crystal, colored (or tinged) in a certain manner due to whatever form is proximate to it, shines forth or exhibits the shape (or color) of that particular form, so ordinary awareness, influenced by an object to be grasped (or influenced by an apprehended object) shines forth or exhibits (or coalesces with) the shape of the inherent form of that object. In a similar fashion, (ordinary awareness) shows forth the essential form of the subtle (dimension) of objects when in the presence of subtle objects and colored (or tinged) by those subtle objects. In a similar fashion, (ordinary awareness) shows forth the essential form of the gross (dimension) of objects when in the presence of gross objects and colored (or tinged) by those gross objects. In a similar fashion, (ordinary awareness) shows forth the essential form of the entire manifest world when in the presence of the determinate form of the world and colored (or tinged) by that world. It must also be understood that the situation is similar in regard to the various sensing capacities. (Ordinary awareness) appears or shines with the essential form of the sensing capacities when in the presence of the sensing capacities colored (or tinged) by the sensing capacities as themselves the objects of apprehension. (Ordinary awareness) appears or shines forth with the essential form of consciousness in terms of subjectivity when in the presence of consciousness as subjectivity colored (or tinged) by consciousness appearing as subjectivity that is itself an object. (Ordinary awareness) appears or shines with the essential form of the "released" (or, in other words, ontologically distinct) "consciousness" when in the presence of released consciousness colored (or tinged) by the released consciousness as itself an object. It is said, thus, that the condition of "profound coalescence" or "engrossment" of ordinary awareness like a transparent jewel exhibits (or takes on the appearance) of whatever forms appear in it including subjectivity, sensing, and subtle and gross objects, or, in other words, consciousness, the senses, and any and all conventional objects.

YS I:42 Therein (*tatra*) [with regard to the notion of *samāpatti*], the engrossment or coalescence having to do with empirical awareness (*savitarkā*) is accompanied by the [verbal] constructions (*vikalpa*), words (*śabda*), referents [objects] (*artha*), and the [resulting] cognitions (or cognitive awarenesses) (*jñāna*).

[VB] That is to say, there is the word "cow," the object referred to by "cow," and the cognition of "cow." These are perceived or apprehended as a single, undivided experience (of "cow"), even though they are quite distinct. Some aspects of words are being apprehended, some characteristics of referents (or objects) are being apprehended and some characteristics of cognitions are being apprehended. There is a distinct aspect (or functioning) for each of these. For the yogin who has attained this level of engrossment or coalescence and come upon the experience of a "cow" and so forth, in (his) intuitive level of concentration, if that experience includes the constructions of words, referents (or objects) and cognitions (in a single "mixed" apprehension), that "mixed" apprehension is known as an empirical engrossment or coalescense.

YS I.43 [Preface by VB] When, however, the referent (or object) stands forth in its own inherent form, when the insight arising from concentration no longer includes memory and the conventional understanding of words and is devoid of the constructs involving reliable teaching and inference, in other words, when the referent (or object) is distinguished in awareness solely in terms of its direct inherent nature, that (involves) the engrossment or coalescence known as "meta-empirical" or "unconstructed" engrossment or coalescence. That is a higher perception. And that is the seed (or basis) for both reliable teaching and inferential knowledge. Reliable teaching and inferential knowledge arise from this (direct perception). But that apprehension (or direct perception) is not dependent upon the cognitions relating to reliable teaching or inference. Thus, the yogin's direct perception arising from "meta-empirical concentration" is not mixed with any other means of knowing. The definition of the "meta-empirical" or "unconstructed" "engrossment or coalescence" (that is related to the "meta-empirical concentration") is set forth with this next *sūtra*.

The "meta-empirical" or "unconstructed" (*nirvitarkā*) engrossment or coalescence (*samāpatti*) that arises when the memory is purified [or eliminated], is the reflection [or shining forth] (*nirbhāsā*) solely of the object [referent] itself, as if it were devoid of the yogin's own cognizing presence (*svarūpa-śūnyā iva*).

[VB] That is (known as) the "meta-empirical" or "unconstructed" engrossment or coalescence, which (engrossment) is constituted by an insight, dependent on the inherent form of the (empirical) object (itself), purified (or, in other words, devoid or absent of) memory and the constructed cognitions (or memory of the constructed cognitions), inference, reliable teaching and the conventional meaning of verbal expressions—(an insight) so focused on the object itself that the very process of apprehension (of the cognizing yogin himself) is, as it were, abandoned (or disregarded) and in which only the meaning of the object itself is present. And so it (the explanation) has been fully given.

YS I.44 In the same manner is to be explained the engrossment (*samāpatti*) with subtle [intellectual or ideational] contents (*sūkṣma-viṣaya*), whether relating to specific intellectual notions (*sa-vicāra*) or pure intellectual contemplation (*nir-vicāra*).

[VB] Therein the subtle (intellectual or ideational) engrossment is said to be that which has to do with the manifest qualities relating to subtle elements characterized by the experience of such limitations as space, time, and causality. This subtle element (or subtle realm) that becomes an object for contemplation, when the appropriate intuitive concentration (is occurring), manifests itself (or exhibits itself) as determined by characteristics that can be apprehended in a single cognitive act. That "pure intellectual contemplation" engrossment is said to be that (cognitive condition) when the subtle element (or subtle realm), constituted and accompanied by all its essential characteristics, is nevertheless always and under all circumstances apprehended without the distinctions of what has past, what is present and what is yet to be. This is just the inherent form of the subtle element (or subtle realm). It has become an object by means of this inherent form. It provides the content of the intuitive concentration. And when there is just the intuition containing only the object itself, as if the presence of the cognizer is absent, then it is called "pure intellectual contemplation." In regard to this discussion overall, (the engrossments) whose contents are gross objects have to do with "empirical" engrossment and "meta-empirical" or "unconstructed" engrossment; and (the engrossments) whose contents are subtle (intellectual or ideational) objects have to do with "specific intellectual notions" engrossment and "pure intellectual contemplation" engrossment. The overcoming of cognitive or verbal projection as has been explained for "meta-empirical" engrossment applies as well for both the empirical as well as the ideational.

YS I.45 And subtle objectivity (*sūkṣma-viṣayatva*) [encompasses all the non-empirical contents of awareness] up through the unmanifest (*a-liṅga-paryavasāna*) [that is, up through unmanifest *prakṛti*].

[VB] The smell subtle element is the subtle objective base of the (gross) earth element; the taste subtle element of the (gross) water element; the form subtle element of the (gross) fire element; the touch subtle element of the (gross) wind element; and the sound subtle element of the (gross) space (or atmosphere) element. Ego (is the subtle objective base) of these (subtle elements). Furthermore, the discerning faculty (i.e., *buddhi*, *mahat*) (is the subtle objective base) of this (ego). Finally, the unmarked (or unmanifest) primordial base (i.e., *mūlaprakṛti*) (is the subtle objective base) of this (the discerning faculty). There is no subtle objective base higher or other than the unmarked (or unmanifest) primordial base. An objection is raised: Is not the consciousness (likewise) subtle? That would seem to be obvious!

In the case of the unmanifest, it is higher than the discerning faculty (in the sense that it provides the material base for the discerning faculty). This is not the case with consciousness, however. How is that? Consciousness is not the material cause of the discerning faculty, but only the reason (for its functioning). Hence, the subtlety (in terms of its material or objective base) has been explained as reaching its final limit in primordial materiality.

YS I.46 These [four engrossments] only represent concentration (*samādhi*) that has (specific) content (*sa-bīja*).

[VB] These four engrossments have contents that are external objects—hence, the concentration is also constituted as having an objective content. In this regard, the empirical and meta-empirical engrossments have to do with gross objects. The ideational and contemplative engrossments have to do with subtle objects. In the same manner, the accompanying intuitive concentration is explained as being fourfold.

YS I.47 When the yogin has gained skill (*vaiśāradya*) in cultivating the highest [of the four] concentrations (*nirvicāra*), there arises a tranquility pertaining to the presence of the self (*adhyātma*) [that is, *puruṣa* or "consciousness"].

[VB] "Skill" (means) that the *sattva*-awareness of the intellect (of the yogin), whose natural condition is luminous cognition, and which has separated itself from the coverings of impurity, has attained an independent even flow no longer influenced by *rajas* and *tamas* (or a state of awareness in which *rajas* and *tamas* are no longer operating). When this skill has reached to the highest (among the four) cognitive concentrations, then there is a tranquility pertaining to the presence of the Self in which all objects appear as they truly are, unfettered by the sequence of ordinary temporality, characterized by the clear light of intuitive insight. And as it has been said, "The wise (yogin) having attained the tranquility of intuitive insight, no longer grieving, reflects upon all suffering creatures, like someone standing on a mountaintop looks down upon those standing on the plains below."

YS I.48 Therein [when skill in achieving the highest levels of objective engrossment has been attained, the yogin attains] what is known as "truth-bearing insight."

[VB] The technical name of this insight, which arises when the ordinary awareness has been so trained or concentrated, is "truth-bearing." And that insight conforms to what truly is (i.e., to *prajñā*, the highest intuitive insight); it concerns only what is true. In regard to such insight, there is not the slightest hint or whiff of false knowledge. And so it has been said: "Practicing this sort of insight that utilizes the threefold modalities of verbal instruction, inference and the experiential realization of continuing meditation, a yogin attains the highest Yoga."

YS I.49 [Preface by VB:] That (intuitive insight), however, (of the preceding *sūtra*) is different from ordinary insight.

This highest intuitive insight (*prajñā*) has content [or concerns objects] that is [or are] different from the insights arising out of verbal instruction (*śruta*) or inference (*anumāna*), since it involves the direct awareness of specific aspects of objects (*viśeṣa-artha*).

[VB] Verbal knowledge, or the cognition arising from what is taught, has to do with the general aspects of what is being known. It is not possible to identify the particular aspect of a thing being described just by verbal knowledge. Why? A word is a conventional designation that is not involved in the specific apprehension of something. So likewise inference only deals with the general aspects of what is being known. Wherein something has attained a new position, therein one can infer that some sort of motion has occurred. Wherein no new position has been attained, it can be inferred that no movement has taken place. A conclusion is reached by means of inferring general features. There is no specific immediate knowledge of an object either through verbal instruction or inference. And there is no apprehension by ordinary perception of a thing that is subtle, obstructed or at a great distance. And the specific feature of a thing cannot be said to be non-existent because it cannot be established by an ordinary means of knowing. Such a specific feature is only to be apprehended through the insight of concentration—such features as subtle elements or consciousness. Therefore, this (highest level of *sa-bīja*) insight involves objects (or contents) that have specific features, which are other than the sorts of things known by verbal instruction and inference.

YS I.50 [Preface by VB] When the yogin attains the intuition that arises from concentration, the resulting residual effect leads to a repetitive sequence.

The resulting residual effect [or predisposition] (*saṃskāra*) arising from that [intuitive concentration, namely the "truth-bearing" intuition] counteracts or impedes the predispositions in ordinary awareness.

[VB] The predisposition that arises from intuitive concentration [literally "the insight or wisdom arising from concentration"] counteracts the predispositions of ordinary awareness. Since ordinary predispositions are overcome, the cognitions of ordinary awareness no longer arise. When there is cessation of ordinary cognitions, concentration becomes firmly established. The intuition or insight arises from concentration; because of this predispositions arise derived from this insight; and a repetitive sequence arises. First, there are insights; then, there are residual predispositions; and so on, and so forth. Is it not the case, then, that such a process will also activate a certain kind of correlative behavior in ordinary awareness? (To the contrary), the predispositions generated by the intuitive concentration, since the destruction of afflictions is brought about, do not bring about any kind of additional behavior in ordinary awareness. Ordinary awareness, rather, ceases from its ordinary activity. Ordinary awareness tends towards the final condition of (quiescent) discriminative realization.

YS I.51 [Preface by VB] And what happens (or what becomes) then of this residual effect or predispostion (*saṃskāra*)?

When there is cessation even of this (*saṃskāra*), since everything has ceased, there is [only] seedless [or objectless] concentration (*nirbījaḥ samādhiḥ*).

This (seedless or objectless concentration) not only counteracts the intuitive realization of concentration; it counteracts likewise the predispositions that arise out of the intuition. Why? The predisposition that arises out of the experience of cessation restricts the predispositions that arise out of correct awareness with some sort of object or content. The existence of (specific) predispositions brought about in ordinary awareness when in the condition of cessation can be inferred, since there is an experience of the passage of time when in the condition of cessation.

Ordinary awareness becomes dissolved in its own stable natural condition, accompanied by predispositions made up of the realization of isolation arising from the concentration of (or in) cessation. Therefore, these predispositions, counteracting or going against the ordinary functioning of ordinary awareness, are not the causes of the final realization, since ordinary awareness has desisted from its now-quieted ordinary functioning, accompanied as it now is by the predispositions made up of the realization of isolation. When such cessation has occurred, consciousness stands forth in its own inherent form [see above, *sūtra* 3] That is, it is said to be pure, contentless, and distinct (separate, "released"). This, then, is the first (portion or chapter), entitled "The Concentration Section" (*Samādhi-Pāda*) of the Commentary by the learned paṇḍit Vyāsa, of the Pātañjala Yogaśāstra, known as "The Explanation of Sāṃkhya" (*Sāmkhya-pravacana*).

— 5 —

Yoga in the *Yoga Upaniṣads*: Disciplines of the Mystical *OṂ* Sound

Jeffrey Clark Ruff

The *Yoga Upaniṣads* (YU) are a collection of twenty-one medieval Sanskrit texts. They are Hindu texts. No one knows who wrote them, and this is a common characteristic of medieval and early modern texts categorized as "*upaniṣads*." Whoever the authors were, they thought it was important to follow the style of the so-called classical *Upaniṣads*, which were written over a thousand years earlier in Northern India.

Most of the earliest YU (or parts of the texts) date roughly from the ninth to thirteenth centuries, while others date from as late as the eighteenth century. The earlier texts were written in North India, in the brahminic Hindu heartland of the Ganges and Yamuna rivers (possibly in or around the city of Varanasi, but no one knows for sure). The early modern texts in this genre were written in South India, most likely by Tamil- or Telugu-speaking brahmins.

Medieval and early modern Hindus authored hundreds of "minor" *Upaniṣads*, and these are often categorized into thematic collections that suggest to the reader something about their content: *Yoga Upaniṣads*, *Saṃnyāsa Upaniṣads*, *Vedānta Upaniṣads*, *Śiva Upaniṣads*, *Śākta Upaniṣads*, *Viṣṇu Upaniṣads*, and others. The *Yoga Upaniṣads* deal with our topic, "yoga," while the others focus on devotion to gods or goddesses (Śiva, various goddesses, Viṣṇu, and other divine beings), or on other aspects of Hindu life (such as giving up normal social life, or having a particular view of the world).

These divisions are worthwhile because they accurately label the different contents of these collections. Scholars have used these, or similar divisions, for over a century as genre conventions, thus providing the added usefulness of easily finding them in bibliographies and indexes. A drawback of these divisions is that they suggest a kind of intentional or purpose-driven voice behind the texts that is not always there. They are texts called *Upaniṣads* that happen to focus on yoga, yet many of them were written at different times and places. Thus, they do not really represent a single tradition or school of thought.

In brahminic Hinduism, "*upaniṣad*" is the category of texts that contain esoteric, mystical, and philosophical speculations. The primary meaning of *upaniṣad* is "true correspondence," "connection," or "mysterious equivalence." Since, according to the theories and beliefs of Hindus, sacred "connections" are hidden—difficult for human beings to see or understand—derivative meanings of *upaniṣad* are "secret," "mysterious," or "arcane." Because of this, the term *upaniṣad* usually means secret teaching, esoteric connection, mysterious knowledge, or arcane doctrine. If one were to draw a parallel in English language usage, it could be said that the *Upaniṣads* are the "sacred mysteries" of the ancient Hindu books of wisdom (the *Vedas*).

The word *upaniṣad* derives from the Sanskrit roots *upa* + *ni* + *sad*. The terms together have been long misunderstood rather literally to mean, "to sit close beside." Many understand this definition as a title describing the "educational" setting of the texts: i.e., that students "sit close beside their teachers" instead of the esoteric correspondences (things close to or connected to each other) between *all things*.

This characterization has been so widely disseminated since the nineteenth century that one will find it in almost every introduction to the texts, both Western and Indian. It is a misleading yet largely harmless interpretation. It is not an altogether useless definition since these texts were originally, and for a long time, oral-aural teachings learned by students (*śiṣyas*) at the feet of their teacher (*guru*): the tradition describes this as from "ear to ear." These "secret" (*rahasya*) teachings were passed down by word of mouth to the followers of a particular teacher. The students perfected their intuition through learning and meditative practice in order to perceive and recognize the hidden connections (*upaniṣad*) between different philosophical and mystical concepts and between the different levels of reality: individual, mundane, and cosmic.

The *Upaniṣads* overflow with examples of the "connections" between different aspects of reality: between the spiritual or true self and ultimate reality, between certain words (such as the sound of "*oṃ*" which appears repeatedly in the YU and absolute truth), between sounds and creation, and between vital breaths and sunbeams, to name but a few. In one application, the visualization or imagination of these "true connections" is viewed as an act of religious practice. In part, this is what the YU mean when they use various words that we often translate as "meditation, reflection, visualization, remembering, being mindful of, or concentration." For example, in the yoga of these texts, stars, the moon, the sun, ritual fires, various flowers, butter churns, fire drills, and actions such as religious pilgrimage or others are visualized as occurring inside the human mind or body (which we will see in the texts translated here). Therefore, a text called *Upaniṣad* is a *"secret teaching" revealing the "hidden connections" that energize the matrix of reality.*

Exploration of the nature of these correspondences is the science of *upaniṣad* (connection). Indic brahminic traditions constructed their ancient worldview by and from this starting point. This way of sense-making (its very sensibility) takes for granted that all things are connected: that reality is a kind of weave or matrix of interconnections. Everything connects to everything else in one way or another, and the order of existence that this produces is organized both vertically and horizontally. Cows, people, plants, rocks, the gods, powers, forces, and events exist in a pattern that is like that of woven cloth or piled bricks. Every object or concept relates to all others directly or indirectly and they all work together in a larger pattern. The traditions consider these direct or indirect connections to be discoverable through ritual, speculation, and meditation. Nevertheless, this larger weave or pattern is not visible to the average person, cow, or even god.

This weave of correspondences constitutes a theory of reality, and the *yoga* of sounds and visualizations are two of its practical methods. The concept of *ātman* (often translated as eternal self, true self, soul, etc.) demonstrates one example of this way of thinking. The body (*ātman*) is the true self (*ātman*)—this common form of wordplay in the *Upaniṣads* signals two different but connected concepts by using the very same word. One might describe this kind of sense-making as connection by homophony (this technique is seamlessly interwoven with other forms of wordplay: simile, metaphor, pun, rhyme, alliteration, and creative interpretations based on the root meanings of words). This essential connection (body and true self) has an additional connection: body has a subtle connection with self, and these together connect with the cosmos in its totality. The *ātman* is ultimately identified with the absolute reality, *brahman*. This is not simply an abstract theory or logical exploration: it relates *directly* to the methods developed by the sages.

True knowledge of the connections becomes a program for practical experimentation for *activating* (making real, "real-izing") the connections within the body and consciousness of individuals. Following this way of thinking, actions in an individual's life affect changes in the rest of the world—even the universe in its totality—and vice versa. These traditions maintain that some connections are stronger, more potent, and more concentrated than others. Thus, the Upanishadic traditions seek the most potent connections. They seek these connections intellectually but also through religious practices and disciplines. The strongest connections provide the most potent realizations of truth and reality. These most potent realizations of reality lead directly to superhuman power, ultimate freedom, and unconditional immortality. Accordingly, pure ignorance, these traditions tell us, leads inexorably to pain and suffering. A lesser secret truth (activated through practices such as ritual or repeating mantras without awareness) will lead to a desirable rebirth or sojourn in some god's paradise. A greater secret truth will lead the sage to liberated immortality, ultimate being, and genuine truth.

Hindu knowing (*veda*, *vidyā*, *jñāna*) and doing (*karma*) partake of the same dynamic of correspondence. Ignorance or confusion expresses itself in wasted, painful, or useless actions. Abstract knowledge without action is weak; in other words, it does not "do" or "make" anything. Knowledge with properly corresponding actions "makes" or empowers "reality." Important to the sages' knowledge and practice was a harnessing (*yoga*) of the creative energy hidden in the weave of correspondences that empower reality. The sages played this language game very deeply and in multiple dimensions. They did not merely see these correspondences as two-dimensional patterns of reality (only to be observed and analyzed), but they also performed and experimented, "activating" or "realizing" the creative power (*māyā*) inherent in these connections. In other words, they actively participated in manipulating the weave. In this usage, *māyā* has its earliest semantic range, extending to art, wisdom, poetry, and uncanny creative power. The term also has the derivative meaning of "illusion." This notion of illusion has at least two usages: impermanent expressions of reality (appearances that *change*) and somewhat later, as an extension of the concept of illusion, "*inferior* or *dangerously misleading* appearances." These pejorative meanings of *māyā* came to be employed by the world-rejecting forest traditions, such as those of some later classical *Upaniṣad*s and Buddhism. In the earliest tradition, illusion is a secondary meaning, yet from the time of the Buddha, it begins to replace the primary meaning such that, in contemporary Indic usage, *māyā* retains virtually no trace of its earlier positive meanings.

In this way, Vedic tradition presents a highly magical set of views and practices. Over many centuries, this magical worldview was supplemented by and in many ways replaced with more mystical, philosophical, and psychological viewpoints. This set of developments waxes and wanes in such a way that there is no linear "evolution" of (practical if magical) Vedic concepts toward the psychological and symbolic usages of contemporary cosmopolitan Hinduism. Once this trend was set in motion, traditions of symbolic wisdom and introspective meditation gradually replaced the more magically charged ritual tradition. These developments did not have any significant effect on the vast array of folk traditions within Hinduism; to this day, these folk traditions remain practical in their concerns for good health, fertility, wealth, and fortune, and pursue these goods of life through ritual, practical, holy, and magical means. It also did not profoundly affect every one of the various traditions of yoga, but it was crucial for the texts translated here.

Undergirding these conceptual frameworks is the recognition that by knowing the systems of connections, one could perceptually grasp the nature of reality and ultimate truth by a special kind of inference and mystical intuition. Connection, correspondence, and substitution provide a mystical algebraic vocabulary for knowing the fundamental structures, nature, and possibilities for reality, the cosmos, and the self. As an applied science of hidden connections, the *Upaniṣads* also afford almost limitless opportunities for developing original methods for discovering the "reality of reality" or the "truth of truth" (*satyasya satya*). These speculations and technologies shaped the fundamental beliefs of many of the later elite traditions of Hinduism, and were very influential on the YU.

Hindus consider the *Upaniṣads*, like all Vedic texts, to be the sages' direct aural cognitions (*śruti*) of absolute reality in contrast to "remembered" texts, or traditional wisdom (*smṛti*). *Śruti* is literally "that which is heard." The primordial seers (*ṛṣis*) are said to have "heard" and "seen" ultimate and absolute truth in visionary trance and later communicated in words their direct experiences of *Veda* (wisdom, true knowledge, the Word).

There are many kinds of texts in the body of Vedic knowledge. The *Veda Saṃhitās* (1500–800 BCE) are the earliest. There are several other genres, but the "classical" *Upaniṣads* (500 BCE to 300 CE), the last of these ancient texts, are the "culmination of Vedic lore" (or Vedānta). Texts of all of these genres are considered by Hindus to be revelations of eternal true knowledge (*veda*), eternal words and sounds (*veda*, *brahman*, *śabda*, *mantra*), and the worldly manifestation of the unchanging, unlimited matrix of reality (*brahman*). The YU, and all of the other medieval *Upaniṣads*, mostly date from after 800 CE, but they consciously continue the themes, approaches, and attitudes of these much older genres.

Many brahminical traditions classify *Upaniṣads* as the *jñāna* section of the Vedic lore. *Jñāna* and other related terms (*vijñāna*, *prajñā*) are cognates with the English word "knowledge" but they have a more specialized meaning than "knowledge" does in English. In the Hindu context, it is knowledge of ultimate truth, not simply general information, intellectual cleverness, or memorized data. As such, the term is more like its Greek cognate, *gnosis*, which has the deeper, transformative meaning of ultimate knowledge. In the translations, I have typically used the terms "deep knowledge" or "true knowledge" to translate *jñāna* and "true judgment" to translate the related word *vijñāna*.

Although varied and often contradictory, the *Upaniṣads* provide the foundation for the system of Vedānta that became influential in Hindu thought even down to the present day, especially in popular and devotional expression. This worldview distinguishes manifestations of reality in terms of volatility verses permanency. Change, fluctuation, and transformation characterize mundane reality. Stability, eternality, and unity characterize the ultimate source and being of all reality. The Upanishadic worldview turns upon the distinction between things that are ever changing and in flux and the underlying unchanging reality of *brahman*. The tradition considers the visible fluctuating manifestations of reality as insecure, undependable, and undesirable. Because of this, the tradition seeks knowledge (*jñāna*) and practical methods (*yoga*) for escaping the "turning water wheel" of changing reality. The hopes and the goals of the sages are to discover and realize (to make real in their own lives) the unchanging realm of ultimate being, the *brahman*.

This search for the unchanging ultimate in Vedānta led to the development of a series of important concepts. These explorations include the identity of genuine eternal being (*brahman*) and personal true self (*ātman*), the theory of reincarnation or transmigration of souls, the necessity of freedom from suffering, ignorance, and repeated births, and the practices and lifestyle that lead to this ultimate freedom—*yoga* and renunciation. Beyond these concepts, the *Upaniṣad*s contain a range of other concepts, ideals, and goals. These selected few become the foci of the later Vedānta that the YU and other minor *Upaniṣad*s explore.

First among these concepts, the sages declare that the absolute reality, *brahman*, is identical with the essential self, *ātman*, the true nature of each individual. The oldest of all texts in the genre, the *Bṛhadāraṇyaka Upaniṣad* (1.4.10) states that the whole universe was originally *brahman*, and that it only knew itself (*ātman*), thinking "I am eternal being" (*aham brahmāsmi*). It then goes on to say that if human beings can truly and genuinely realize the same thing, "I am *brahman*," then they become the universe; and, that not even the gods could prevent this occurrence, adding that if people think that they are different from a god or each other, then they do not understand "the truth." In other words, if a person does not understand the mysterious true nature of life, then he or she does not actually understand anything at all.

These characterizations of *brahman* are diverse, even including the concept that *brahman* is beyond classification. A fundamental speculation of the Upanishadic sages is that *brahman* always retains its oral and aural (sonic) character: *brahman* is *oṃ*, the "sound" of truth or reality. The individual sage must appreciate this notion and seek the experiential knowledge of it in order to know the "reality of reality." Thus, this speculative theme emphasizes both the model of reality and the model for knowledge and action. The term *brahman* originally meant something like "growth" or "creativity," but it came to mean the mystical source of everything. Since *brahman* is ultimately "everything," it is not surprising that these texts describe it in numerous ways: "a formulation of truth," the *Veda*, the life breath, speech, the origin, true being, "That" (*tat*)—for so it is referred to—is never-ending-being, the universal, the absolute, reality, genuine being, the ultimate, original being, ultimate being, truth, eternity, creativity, and never-ending growth. Scholars often simply leave the word untranslated, but in my translations I have tried to communicate the sense and intentions of the texts by picking terms from the preceding list to match with the content of the text.

This fundamental assumption, that the genuine truth of an individual is the absolute truth of all that exists, produces a fundamental problem: human beings may already be essentially perfect, but they are prevented from enjoying the bliss of this perfection because they are ignorant or confused, and the YU often communicate this insight through metaphor and simile: like a bird caught in a net or a bramble, the true self yearns to be free but cannot shake itself loose from the snare of confusion and folly. The *Yoga Upaniṣad*s often use the migratory goose as one of their primary similes: the true self is like a honking gander. Migration over the Himalayan mountains becomes a symbol of escape from bondage. The sources in the Further Reading section, particularly the books of André Padoux and David G. White, explain in detail the symbolism and the use of the term "gander" in Hindu religious thought, and its use as a sacred word.

Just as they sought the eternal unchanging *brahman*, the *Upaniṣad*s also searched for a permanent solution to the vicissitudes of activity in the world (*karma*), whether pleasant or painful. Although proper ritual actions and other religious observances (also denoted by the term *karma*) could win a good rebirth after a sojourn in the realm of the moon, the Upanishadic sages sought freedom from *all* rebirths. The liberating knowledge of the *Upaniṣad*s is that there is an eternally blissful existence beyond the vault of the heavens through which one must pass to attain liberation. The oldest idea was that the sun was like a lid or doorway to a different type of reality, and that escaping through that door led to immortality and ultimate freedom. Patrick Olivelle's and Paul Deussen's books on the *Upaniṣad*s, which are listed in the Further Reading section of this chapter, explain in good detail the idea of escaping the world as we know it, through the doorway of the sun. The *Īśa Upaniṣad* provides a concise presentation of this doctrine and its imagery.

The YU take this idea from the earlier tradition of the classical *Upaniṣad*s, and transpose it to the inner body of the practitioner of yoga. For them, it was not the actual sun that one sees up in the sky that was the material doorway to freedom, but rather a sun that was projected onto the inside of the human body through visualization meditations and singing the sacred sounds. The texts translated here will show how they imagined this. There are also other variations in the YU, but the escape of the true self through the top of the head by means of sacred sounds and visualizations is one of the primary practices.

The Canons of *Yoga Upaniṣads*

The texts of the YU draw their ideas and images from the heritage of classical Vedānta. They are medieval texts, but their imagery plays with the metaphors, symbols, and objects of ancient Vedic fire rites, Vedānta philosophy of the classical *Upaniṣad*s, classical yoga, medieval mythology, sectarian texts such as the *Āgama*s and *Tantra*s, and the *haṭha* ("forceful") *yoga* of the Nāth Siddhas, as well as other medieval *yoga* textual traditions. Their goals are ultimate freedom (*mokṣa*) and direct experience of the genuine being (*brahman*). The practices of the northern tradition are limited to forms of *mantra yoga*. Later, in South India they draw much from the practices and ideas of Tantra and *haṭha yoga*. Meditation on the most sacred brahmanical *oṃ* mantra is the cornerstone of the *yoga* of these texts, while the *haṃsa* mantra and its lore complete this *yoga's* foundation.

The two canons of the YU include twenty-one separate texts. Some of the texts have different titles in various manuscript collections, and so there are more than twenty-one different titles, but these only represent the same twenty-one texts. The North Indian texts were written between 800 CE and 1300 CE. The northern texts are generally very brief (usually fewer than 50 verses). The exact dates of their composition are unknown, but I will list them here in roughly chronological order: (800–1100) *Brahmavidyā*, *Kṣurika*, *Cūlikā*; (1100–1300) *Brahmabindu* (also titled *Amṛtabindu*), *Amṛtabindu* (not the same as the previous, and later re-titled as *Amṛtanāda*), *Dhyānabindu*, *Nādabindu*, *Tejobindu*, *Yogaśikhā*, *Yogatattva*; and (around 1200) *Haṃsa* (also titled *Haṃsanāda*).

All of the northern texts exist in expanded form in the southern collections (sometimes under different titles). The South Indian texts exist in various versions, some very similar to the older northern texts. Those texts that are similar to their northern counterparts generally appear in the south between 1300 and 1500. Southern texts that are greatly expanded versions of the northern titles appear after 1500, but before 1750. All other South Indian YU appear in the written record between 1600 and 1750. The South Indian collection includes:

Advayatāraka, *Amṛtabindu*, *Amṛtanāda* (also known as *Amṛtanādabindu*), *Brahmavidyā*, *Māntrika* (the South Indian title of the northern *Cūlikā Upaniṣad*), *Darśana* (or *Yogadarśana*), *Dhyānabindu*, *Haṃsa* (or *Haṃsanāda*), *Kṣurika*, *Mahāvākya*, *Maṇḍalabrāhmaṇa*, *Nādabindu*, *Pāśupatabrahmā*, *Śāṇḍilya*, *Tejobindu*, *Triśikhibrāhmaṇa*, *Varāha*, *Yogacūḍāmaṇi*, *Yogakuṇḍalī* (or *Yogakuṇḍalinī*), *Yogaśikhā*, and *Yogatattva*. The South Indian collections do not typically categorize the *Cūlikā/Māntrika Upaniṣad* as a *yoga* text.

The twenty-one *Yoga Upaniṣad*s provide a window into the complex history of the discipline of sacred sounds (*mantra yoga*) expounded in the North Indian versions of the texts, and the syncretistic forceful discipline (*haṭha yoga*) promoted in the South Indian collections. The impressionistic northern texts present overlapping perspectives on a tradition that practiced exercises of the vital breath (*prāṇa*, *vāyu*) and meditation (*dhyāna*). The threefold breath control of inhalation, retention, and exhalation (*pūraka*, *kumbhaka*, and *recaka*), which is not found in the classical *Upaniṣad*s, is present in the YU.

The unnamed passageways (*nāḍī*s) of the classical *Upaniṣad*s have been replaced with the systematic terminology of three primary passageways symbolized as the sun, moon, and fire. The term *kuṇḍalinī*, which is so important for many of the medieval yoga traditions, does not appear as a technical term in the early YU, but the texts employ mind, pointed flame, and vital breath (*manas*, *śikhā*, and *prāṇa*) in terms familiar to *kuṇḍalinī yoga*. There is no system of mystical circles (*cakra*s) in the northern texts. Esoteric body locations similar to those of the *cakra* systems are called *marman* ("vital point") and *dvāra* ("gate"). The texts do mention flowers (usually the lotus) employed as visualizations within the yogic body. The imagery of the "gates" of the body resonates with the imagery of the three *granthi*s ("knots") associated with gods Brahmā, Viṣṇu, and Śiva in later *haṭha yoga* and Tantric texts. There is no strong emphasis on gods in these early texts, although some mention various Hindu gods by name. They do not mention or discuss goddesses.

The yoga practices described in the northern texts focus primarily on recitation of the mantra *oṃ*. The purpose of silent meditation (with inner ear and eye) is to focus the *yogin*'s consciousness into a force that can escape the body at death through the cranial suture, or alternatively melt away in the region of the forehead. Vital breath, the *oṃ* sound, and subtle pathways are the clearly defined yogic concepts in these texts.

Apart from the terms referring to *oṃ*, the northern texts do not use a systematic vocabulary like those we find in some of the other yoga traditions. Systematizing yoga according to limbs appears in some of the early northern texts. In all cases, the system is six-limbed. The six-limbed system of yoga is first found in the *Maitrāyaṇīya* (or *Maitri*) *Upaniṣad*, and is later associated with the systems of Buddhist Tantric yoga, as well as with the yogic teachings of the twelfth-century *yogin* and Nāth Siddha, Gorakhnāth (the exact nature of each "limb" differs from one to another system, with some overlap). The basic imagery of these limbed systems is that of a wheel (mandala), wherein the "limbs" are spokes. Typically, these systems include breath exercises and body postures as their first two limbs, with the other limbs usually involving mental practices (reflection, meditation, etc.).

The expanded South Indian versions of the YU reflect the systematization and standardization of yogic language and practice between the thirteenth and seventeenth centuries. Various *yoga* texts incorporated this standardization. The eight-limbed path of Patañjali was transformed over time by elaboration into the eight-limbed path of Dattātreya or Yājñavalkya. The elaborate six-limbed *haṭha yoga* of the Nāth Siddhas, the eight-limbed paths, and other traditions developed during this period a consistent vocabulary of the subtle body and the practices and theories of yoga. The southern redactors of the YU appropriated and recast these systems and expanded the northern texts with additions from a variety of other texts and traditions.

The southern canon of YU quotes from more than two dozen known sources. The eleven expanded texts are often eight to ten times the length of the original northern versions. The additional ten texts, only attested in the southern collections, continue the pattern of the expanded texts, quoting many of the same sources and teaching the same combination of the discipline of reciting the *oṃ* sound (but with the addition of other special sounds, especially the *haṃsa* mantra) with the systems and practices of *haṭha yoga*. The established sources of the expanded texts fall into five categories: yoga texts, texts of medieval non-dual philosophy (Vedānta)—including devotional *Gītā*s, which are poems that usually depict a conversation between a god and a mortal—special ritual and mystical texts called *Tantra*s and *Āgama*s, and classical Vedic and Upanishadic sources.

Almost half of the additions, quotations, and paraphrased materials come from Nāth Siddha traditions—particularly from the writings attributed to Gorakhnāth, such as the *Gorakṣaśataka*—but also the later Nāth-derived *Haṭhayogapradīpikā*. A quarter of the remaining citations come from other kinds of yoga texts such as the Kashmiri *Laghuyogavāsiṣṭha*, the encyclopedic *Upāsanāsārasaṃgraha*, and the eight-limbed paths of the *Yogayājñavalkya* and *Yoga Śāstra* of Dattātreya. The remaining sources are a collection of other late medieval compilations that include diverse materials.

The translations that are included here represent the North Indian tradition of the YU. The northern texts appear to offer the reader authentic medieval brahminic understandings of yoga, whereas the southern texts are more like encyclopedias of pan-Indian yoga from the early modern period.

Although there are no formal divisions among the *Upaniṣads* that deal with yoga, the "*bindu*" titles of the northern canon appear to represent a coherent body of five texts dedicated to the discipline of reciting sacred sounds (*mantra yoga*). Their original titles were *Brahmabindu*, *Amṛtabindu*, *Dhyānabindu*, *Nādabindu*, and *Tejobindu*. The "*bindu*" of these titles has several connotations within the mystical traditions. *Bindu* means "drop, dot, or point." In these texts, this drop refers to the *anusvāra* mark, which is written above the syllable to denote the *m* in the mantra *oṃ*. The term *bindu* has many additional connotations. Accompanying meanings and metaphors include: life-giving drops of fluid (especially sexual fluids), a point at the center of a mystical diagram, any concentrated essence, the sexual organs of the god or goddess (especially in the Śākta-Śaiva traditions of the early Tantras), the one essential reality of reality, a point on which one should focus the eyes in meditation, and others. In all of these usages, the intention is to convey a sense of concentrated essence, the essential condition, the fundamental concept, point of focus, or the smallest coherent unit. All of the texts use the term *bindu* either explicitly or by implication to refer to the final silence that follows recitation of the mantra. It is the final act in mantra recitation, the final goal of the practice, and the final object of meditation. The *bindu* for these texts is the ultimate symbol of the highest intensity of human focus, which is conceived as leading a person to ultimate truth and immortality. Some of the texts also use the term *nāda*. "The buzzing reverberation" (*nāda*) of *m* (also denoted by the point—*bindu*—of the *anusvāra* placed above the syllable) adds another technical term to the mantra theory and practices of these texts. *Nāda* means the reverberation or humming sound that precedes the final melting into silence. The texts describe *nāda* as resembling the pealing of a struck bell; it is followed by the *bindu* of silence. The northern texts all show some similarities to the *bindu* texts. The remaining titles in the larger southern collection, however, include such diverse materials that they do not always show coherence as a body of texts.

The Texts Translated Here

BRAHMAVIDYĀ UPANIṢAD ("SECRET TEACHINGS OF THE ARCANE SCIENCE OF TRUE BEING")

The *Brahmavidyā Upaniṣad* exists in a short northern version of fourteen verses and a much longer southern version (B). The shorter northern text is exclusively devoted to analogies and allusions concerning the sacred sound, *oṃ*. The classical *Upaniṣads* had already broken the sacred syllable into its constituent sounds (*mātrās*) (*a* + *u* + *m*). After equating each of the sounds with three of the "four states"—waking, dreaming, and deep sleep—the ancient *Māṇḍūkya Upaniṣad* suggested that there was a fourth state that was without a sound. Following Olivelle's translation of *Māṇḍūkya Upaniṣad* 11, it is "the cessation of the visible world; auspicious; and unique." It is here that the *Brahmavidyā* takes up and extends the discussion. It adds a one-half sound: a point (*bindu*) was written above the syllable to denote the reverberation (*nāda*) of *ṃ*. The *a*, the *u*, and the *ṃ* are described in the text and they are associated in turn with texts, sacred fires, divisions of the cosmos, and gods. Most of these associations are modeled on discussions of the *oṃ* as found in the ancient texts called the *Brāhmaṇa*s and the classical *Upaniṣad*s. Here, the sound *a* is equated with the *Ṛgveda*, the householder fire, the earth, and the deity Brahmā (verse 5). The sound *u* is equated with the *Yajurveda*, southern fire, the mid-regions, and the deity Viṣṇu (verse 6). The sound *ṃ* is equated with the *Sāmaveda*, offertory fire, heaven, and the deity Īśvara (verse 7). The symbolism here shows the "connections" between the sounds comprising the *oṃ* and the whole of the cosmos. The texts are the holiest scriptures of Hindu lore. The sacred fires were the center of complex Vedic rituals: chants, songs, words were spoken over and into these fires as various liquids and other substances were poured. *Oṃ* was the most sacred of these sounds.

The inclusion of the half sound is original to the *Brahmavidyā*. The half sound has no correspondences. This is because it is considered transcendent and therefore possessed of no characteristic other than being identified with the unqualified ultimate form of existence, *brahman*. The *laya* (verses 13–14)—the "fading away" or "vanishing," of the sound *oṃ*—is compared to the slow fading of a bell. *Brahman* is the peace or stillness (*śānti*), wherein the sound fades away.

The southern version of the text has 111 stanzas that provide much greater elaboration for sound disciplines and reverberation disciplines (*mantra yoga*, *nāda yoga*). It includes speculations on *oṃ*, *kuṇḍalinī-śakti*, *haṭha yoga* practice, fivefold breath control, and renunciation. Two-thirds of the expanded verses (verses 14–80) reproduce the third chapter of the *Upāsanāsārasaṃgraha*, an anthology from around the sixteenth century. The expanded southern text was probably composed in the seventeenth or early eighteenth century.

The extended portions of the text explain the concepts of breath-power and harnessing the powers of mind and body through yoga. Much of this discussion proceeds by means of the metaphor of the migratory gander, or *haṃsa*. *Haṃsa* is the masculine form of the word for the migratory South Asian goose. The gander is a metaphor for the true self (*ātman*) and for the vital breath (*prāṇa*). Midway through the expanded text (verse 53), the teaching is re-framed in terms of a dialogue between a sage and his student, Gautama (in this, it is similar to the frame dialogue of the *Haṃsa Upaniṣad*). The *haṃsa* sound is important in many Indian esoteric traditions, from the Vedas to the Tantras. Many texts associate the in-breath and the out-breath with the mantras *haṃ* (I) and *saḥ* (that). Combined together, these mantras form *haṃsa*. Repeated in meditation (*haṃsa, haṃsa*: "gander, gander") the words take on the secret meaning of their reversal, *so 'ham*: "I am" or "I am That" ("I, *ātman*, am That, *brahman*").

The reader finds the *haṃsa* discourse in most of the expanded southern YU. In the expanded texts of the south, it takes on all the significations found in the Tantras and other medieval yoga canons. The expanded southern *Brahmavidyā* adopts another Tantric notion from its sources, stating that its "arcane science of the ultimate being" is good for people of "all walks of life." Although the text thus includes (via its sources) significant Tantric materials, it is conservative and Vedantic in its overall interpretation and tone.

AMṚTABINDU UPANIṢAD ("SECRET TEACHINGS OF THE IMMORTAL POINT")

The *Amṛtabindu* also appears in some collections under the older title "*Brahmabindu Upaniṣad*" ("Secret Teachings of the Point that is True Being"); this was probably its original title. The *Amṛtabindu* (*Brahmabindu*) is one of the earliest texts classified as a *Yoga Upaniṣad*. It is a text of twenty to twenty-four verses similar to the *Amṛtanāda Upaniṣad* (a different text, but also called *Amṛtabindu* in some manuscripts).

The *Amṛtabindu* begins its discussion by describing the mind (*manas*) as the source of both bondage and freedom. The *yoga* described in the *Amṛtabindu* focuses solely on recitation of, and meditation on, the sacred syllable *oṃ*. Pronouncing and repeating the mantra *oṃ* aloud is the preliminary practice. Once the mind rests in the heart through use of the *oṃ* mantra, the practitioner may progress to the soundless recitation. Tonal or sounded (*svara*) meditation is considered inferior to non-tonal or soundless (*asvara*) meditation. The text relies on the view that the *yogin* implodes the mind by first tuning it to the absolute sound, shape, and meaning of the *oṃ* sound. Once this inner tuning is complete, he "says" or "hears" the mantra without speaking until nothing is left in consciousness but the true, immortal, being.

Based on the principles expounded in the classical *Upaniṣad*s and the other *bindu* texts, the "*bindu*" in the title that leads to immortality (or to *brahman*, depending on the title of the manuscript) is the hum or nasalization that follows the *m*, which was written in Indic orthography by using a dot or point (*bindu*). When this humming sound fades away at the end of the recitation, then the silence that follows is the true object of mental focus and meditation. After the *yogin* masters the initial training of reciting the mantra that finishes in silence, then silence itself becomes the practice.

Here, it would appear that the true object of knowing is the sound that trails into silence (*bindu*). This silence is referred to as indivisible. It is precisely identical to the fundamental essence of reality (*parabrahman* and *ātman*). The metaphors working here involve reabsorption and concentration. The *yogin* concentrates all of himself: he becomes the smallest unit possible, the point (*bindu*). When he succeeds in shrinking and concentrating himself into this smallest point, he is nothing other than pure self, pure being (*brahman*).

The text's method is one of guiding the mind via the *oṃ* sound, first through recitation and then through silent mental exercise, to a singularly focused, absolute, eternal peace. Its brevity, simplicity, and contents represent exclusively Vedantic methods and goals of the classical type.

DHYĀNABINDU UPANIṢAD ("SECRET TEACHINGS OF THE MEDITATION POINT")

This text has northern and southern versions. The northern text contains twenty-one to twenty-three verses in two sections. The southern text contains approximately 106 to 107 verses (with mixed prose). The northern version begins with praise of the discipline of meditation (*dhyāna yoga*) for the removal of all evil or sins. Next, the text expounds (verses 4–6) on the order of *oṃ* recitation. First are the sounds (*akṣara*) *a* + *u* + *m*. Higher still are the nasalization (*anusvāra* or *bindu*) and its resonance (*nāda*). Higher than the reverberation or resonance (*nāda*), the syllable vanishes as the sound fades. Silence is the highest place. The text instructs the *yogin* to meditate on the silence after the sound has faded. Next (verses 7–10) follow a series of similes—fragrance of a flower, butter in milk, and so on—illustrating the subtlety and pervasiveness of *ātman*. Next, yogic inhalation, breath retention, and exhalation (*pūraka*, *kumbhaka*, and *recaka*) are associated with body location, flowers, and gods (these verses are similar to material in other texts of this genre).

It may be that this text's tradition of meditation imagines the three sounds of *oṃ* as originating in the three flowers, with the hum of the final resonance as the fourth flower. This would locate the *a* in the navel, the *u* in the heart, the *ṃ* between the brows, the reverberation either in the heart or at the top of the head, and the silence beyond body, form, flower, or sound. The text does not actually mention the sounds of *oṃ* as part of the initial meditation on the three flowers. The remainder of the text (verses 18–23) includes metaphors for *oṃ*, focusing on the silently reverberating point of *oṃ*. This point, the half-sound, draws the mind out of the heart up to the space between the eyebrows, where it melts away. One of the difficulties with this text is that it is unclear whether the various meditations (first, on the three gods; second, on the heart or head lotus; third, on the place between the eyebrows) should be practiced in sequence, or if they are three different disciplines. It could appear that they originated from separate practices, but that our author is bringing them together purposefully. However, this is unclear from the text itself.

This text's southern version, of approximately 106 to 107 verses (with mixed prose), examines meditation on the syllable *oṃ*. All of the supplementary verses and prose in this expanded text come from other known texts. With the exception of transitional phrases and other minor variations, the expanded southern *Dhyānabindu Upaniṣad* cites the *Gītāsāra* (ca. 1600–1650), chapter 6 of the *Vivekamārtaṇḍa*, the *Haṭhayogapradīpikā* (ca. 1450), and the *Rājayoga-prakaraṇa* (fourth) chapter of the *Upāsanāsārasaṃgraha*. Christian Bouy (see Further Reading) discusses these sources in depth. The southern version probably reached its present form by shortly after the mid-seventeenth century.

The southern version of the text begins with a forty-verse discourse on the *oṃ* mantra, combining the original text and the *Gītāsāra* with visualization meditations focused in the heart. This investigation of the mantra *oṃ* is similar to that of the other "*bindu Upaniṣad*s," but it is expanded by the contents from the *Gītāsāra*. The second half of the text is devoted to *haṭha yoga* and is largely quoted or paraphrased from chapter 6 of the *Vivekamārtaṇḍa* (the "original" *Gorakṣaśataka* of Gorakhnāth: see the chapter by James Mallinson in this volume) and the *Haṭhayogapradīpikā* (derived from Nāth Siddha texts). The *Dhyānabindu Upaniṣad* provides some details on a six-limbed *yoga* path (in the style of Gorakhnāth, as derived from the *Vivekamārtaṇḍa*) and discusses *kuṇḍalinī-śakti* and *khecarī mudrā*, with the standard descriptions of the pathways, vital breaths, and the six esoteric body centers (*nāḍī*s, *prāṇa*s, and six *cakra*s) known to the Nāths. There are also several verses devoted to *haṃsa* meditation. Unlike some of the other compilation texts, the editor does little with the expanded sources, copying them often verbatim from the Nāth sources.

The following translations are from *The Atharvana Upanishads*, edited by Ramamaya Tarkaratna, *Bibliotheca Indica: A Collection of Oriental Works*: volume 76 (Calcutta: Ganesa Press, 1872–74; reprint, New Delhi: Munshiram Manoharlal Publishers Pvt. Ltd., 1990); *Yoga Upanishads: With the Commentary of Sri Upanisad-Brahmayogin*, edited by A. Mahadeva Sastri (Madras: The Adyar Library and Research Centre, 1920, 1968); and K. Narayanasvami Aiyar, *Thirty Minor Upaniṣads: English Translation with Sanskrit Text* (Madras: K. Narayanasvami Aiyar, 1914; revised ed. Delhi: Parimal Publications, 1997).

Suggestions for Further Reading

For a somewhat free translation of the South Indian version of the texts, see T. R. Srinivasa Ayyangar, trans., *The Yoga Upaniṣads* (following the Commentary of Śrī Upaniṣadbrahmayogin), ed. G. Srinivasa Murti, revised 2d ed., Adyar Library Series, No. 20 (Madras: Adyar Library, 1952). For good quality translations of many of the North Indian versions, see volume 2 of Paul Deussen, *Sixty Upaniṣads of the Veda*, trans. V. M. Bedekar and G. B. Palsule (Delhi: Motilal Banarsidass Publishers, 1980, 1997). For good introductions to the *Upaniṣad*s in general, see Teun Goudriaan and Jan A. Schoterman, *The Kubjikā Upaniṣad: Edited with translation, introduction, notes and appendices* (Groningen: Egbert Forsten, 1994); Patrick Olivelle, trans., *Saṃnyāsa Upaniṣads: Hindu Scriptures on Asceticism and Renunciation* (New York: Oxford University Press, 1992); Patrick Olivelle, trans., *Upaniṣads* (New York: Oxford University Press, 1996); Christian Bouy, *Les Nātha-Yogin et Les Upaniṣads*, Publications De L'Institut De Civilisation Indienne, 62 (Paris: De Boccard, 1994); and Paul Deussen, *The Philosophy of the Upanishads.* 1906, trans. A. S. Geden (Reprint, Delhi: Motilal Banarsidass Publishers, 2000). For more on my work on these texts, see Jeffrey C. Ruff, "History, Text, and Context of the Yoga Upaniṣads," Ph.D. Dissertation, University of California, Santa Barbara [Proquest Dissertations and Theses Full Text 3073645]). For mantras, sacred sounds, and the types of *yoga*s represented in these texts, see André Padoux, *Vāc: The Concept of the Word in Selected Hindu Tantras*, trans. Jacques Gontier (Albany: State University of New York Press, 1989); and David Gordon White, *The Alchemical Body: Siddha Traditions in Medieval India* (Chicago: University of Chicago Press, 1996).

Translations

Brahmavidyā Upaniṣad, verses 1–13 (northern recension vv. 2–14)

I will proclaim here the mysterious teaching of the arcane science of true being; I will speak of the all-pervasive and amazing effects of that divine word called the eternal flame (*oṃ*).

Those who know the power of sounds say that the one imperishable syllable, *oṃ*, is true being. Here, I will tell you about that syllable: its letters, their positions, and the three measures of time.

It is proclaimed that there are three gods, three realms, three books of true knowledge (*Vedas*), and three sacred fires. Just as these, three are the sounds of that auspicious triple-sound (*oṃ*) and there is a half sound as well.

It is explained by those who know the power of sounds that the *Ṛg Veda*, householder's fire, the earth, and the god Brahmā are the same as the letter of the "a" sound.

Next, the "u" sound is taught to us as being the same as the *Yajur Veda*, the atmosphere, the southern fire, and the god, Lord Viṣṇu.

Last, the "m" sound is taught to us as being the same as the *Sāma Veda* and heaven, the offertory fire also, and Īśvara, the supreme god.

The "a" sound is imagined in the middle of the forehead, which we call the "conch-shell," there it appears in the middle of the circle of the sun. The "u" sound stands in the middle looking like the moon.

The "m" sound appears as a pulsating flame, resembling lightning. Now, these three sounds should be understood in this way as having the appearance of sun, moon and fire.

The half-sound sits above the humming syllable, *oṃ*, just as a flame burns in the space above a lamp.

Shining at the highest point, that pointed flame opens the solar pathway. That solar path, which is very fine like a lotus fiber, passes through the sun. This way leads to ultimate reality.

Having opened the most important of the 72,000 pathways, that passage which gives life to everyone, the pointed flame, in fact, stays there shining its light onto everything.

At precisely that time, he who seeks the universal lets the *oṃ* sound fade into peaceful silence, just as the sound of a bell fades to silence.

He is never-ending being, who, having sung this most amazing sound, then lets it fade to silence within. [This is] because the point where this meditation ends is never-ending being, and that is immortality.

AMṚTABINDU UPANIṢAD / BRAHMABINDU UPANIṢAD, VERSES 1–23

They teach that the mind is twofold: confused or clear. It is confused when obsessed with desires and wishes; it is clear when it is free from desires and wishes.

Because of this, it is easy to see that the mind is the origin of both bondage and freedom in everyone. The mind causes bondage when it is obsessed with stuff; the mind gains freedom when it is free from all that stuff.

Since freedom depends on a mind free of obsession with all that stuff that attracts and distracts our senses, one who aspires for freedom should free his mind from all that.

Banishing obsessions with worldly objects, withdrawing the mind into the heart, and having no random thoughts and feelings, he enters the supreme state.

Holding the mind still in the heart until all random thoughts and feeling have ceased: we can genuinely call that "deep knowledge" and "freedom." Anything else is clever talk and shallow speculation.

Neither thinking nor non-thinking, but paradoxically, thinking and non-thinking at the same time. Free from making choices one way or the other, one becomes the original being.

Gaining union with the soundless by means of the sound [*oṃ*], one enjoys the highest reality. By experimenting with stillness, non-being is understood as being.

That is what we mean by original self or genuine being: it is without divisions, without fluctuations, and without confusion. When one realizes, "I am ultimate being!" that very same person certainly enjoys a stable sense of his true self.

Changeless, infinite, without cause and incomparable, without limits, without beginning—awakened to this truth, one is set free.

There is no death, no becoming, no bondage, no seeker, no freedom nor wishing for it—that is genuine reality.

Recognize your true self as the same whether awake, dreaming, or even deeply asleep. There are no repeated births for one who rids himself of these three distinctions.

A singular being-self resides in each and every different being. Singular and multiple, like the moon reflected in a pond.

This is just like the space in a jar; when the jar is broken into pieces it is only the jar that breaks, not the space inside. Life is like the space.

All the forms of things are like the jar, mindlessly breaking into pieces over and over again; they are unaware, but life always knows living, just as space is always space.

Enveloped in creative expression, true self stays in the darkness of the small lotus blossom we call the heart, but when the confusion clears, then one sees only unity.

The imperishable sound [*oṃ*] is supreme reality. A wise person should meditate on that eternal unity which remains when the sound finally fades, if he truly seeks peace and quiet within his true self.

Two kinds of arcane sciences are necessary: that of the original sound and that of the supreme. One who properly tunes himself to the original sound also realizes the supreme.

After long practice and study of books, a truly wise person seeking deep knowledge and true judgment forgets most of the bookish stuff, just as when one keeps grain but throws away the husks.

The colors of cows are many, but the color of milk is one.

Signs and symbols are like the cows, deep knowledge is like the milk.

Just as butter is hidden in milk, true judgment flows inside everyone.

With the churning rope of deep knowledge and the paddle of mind one churns the *oṃ* in the heart. With this meditation, one can draw out the streaming one, the supreme self, undivided, still, and peaceful.

Thus, with this meditation, I am truly mindful that "I am genuine being."

The genuine being that dwells inside everyone is also everyone's true home. "I am that, the god of life! I am that, the god of living!"

DHYĀNABINDU UPANIṢAD, VERSES 1–8, 30–40 (VV. 3–18, 21–22 IN NORTHERN RECENSIONS)

Even if bad actions are like mountains extending for miles and miles, the discipline (*yoga*) of meditation opens a path through them. Nothing else ever opens this path.

The "point" is more important than the syllables, it is more important than the reverberation. When the syllables and sound ceases, then silence is the most amazing state.

A yogin loses all doubts if he concentrates on the highest, which is even higher than the unstruck sound of the heart.

Pure being is so subtle it is comparable to the tip of a hair being divided into a thousandth of a hundredth part, and then divided again by half.

A true self is in everyone, like the scent of a flower, like butter hidden in milk, like oil in sesame seeds, gold in ore, or a thread [strung] through beads. The one who knows this true self with his mind focused on genuine being is not confused.

Just as the oil depends on the seeds and the scent upon the flowers; so in the body of a person, the self is inside it and outside of it . . . in the whole and in the parts.

The true self exists everywhere . . .

While inhaling, one should visualize mighty Viṣṇu with four arms as resembling a flax flower at the level of the navel. While holding the breath, one should visualize grandfather Brahmā with four faces seated on a lotus in the heart, like red and white jewels. While exhaling, one should visualize the three-eyed one between the eyebrows sparkling like a flawless crystal, destroying all evil.

Below there is a lotus flower: the face of the blossom hangs downward with its stem going upward, just like a plantain flower. It is auspicious and contains all sacred sounds and divine powers.

It blooms for a century and is richly endowed with hundreds of petals, which cover its seedpod. There one should repeatedly visualize the sun, moon, and fire.

Then, by repeatedly saying the "heart-seed" (*oṃ*), one opens the lotus through the power of the sun, the moon and the fire. Through this practice, the eternal self is set free.

A person has true knowledge when he knows the mystical syllable (*oṃ*) with its three creators, its three places, and its three paths, to truly be the three and one half sounds.

A person knows the truth when he understands that the true point of the humming *oṃ* is silence. It is like the drop at the end of a long stream of oil or the gradual fading of the peal of a bell.

The *yogin* treading the path of yoga should draw up the vital breath just as a man would suck water through a lotus stalk.

Having concentrated the essence of the half-sound as the seed of the lotus, [one should] then draw it up through the lotus stalk by means of the sound and guide it in between the eyebrows where it dissolves into silence.

He should know that the middle of the eyebrows in the forehead, which is also the root of the nose, is the seat of immortality, the great dwelling place of true being.

—6—

The Sevenfold Yoga of the *Yogavāsiṣṭha*

Christopher Key Chapple

The *Yogavāsiṣṭha*, also known as the *Mokṣopāya*, was compiled in longer and shorter versions over the course of several centuries, most likely from the end of the Gupta period (ca. 500 CE) until it reached its expanded form by the eleventh century. Its philosophy combines aspects of Mahāyāna Buddhism with Advaita Vedānta and served as the foundation for the later school known as Emergence-through-Thought. It is also closely associated with the key ideas and vocabulary of Kashmir Śaivism. It was a favorite of important figures in the development of modern-day Hinduism, including Sri Ramakrishna and Swami Sivananda.

The *Yogavāsiṣṭha* contains more than sixty nested stories told by the sage Vasiṣṭha to his protégé, the young Lord Rāma. One day, a sage named Viśvāmitra asks Daśaratha, Rāma's father, to send Rāma into the forest to chase away troublesome characters who are disrupting the sages in their forest retreats. Rāma recoils at this idea and laments that all activities in life lead to suffering. Vasiṣṭha provides instruction that restores Rāma's confidence and resolve, empowering him to fulfill his dharma. As part of their dialogue (some 29,000 verses in the longer version), Vasiṣṭha talks about kings who change shape and lead alternative lives; a queen who becomes liberated and then helps her husband not only to become free but also to rule justly; and a young man, paralyzed by grief upon the death of his parents, who is coached back to emotional health by an older brother—who reminds him of all his various prior births, from an ant in a dunghill to a glorious swan—helping him regain his equilibrium. This and scores of other stories make the point that interactions with the world are shaped by the nature and quality of thought, and that through understanding one's motivations and intentions, one can gain perspective, turn to the sacred texts, and build and rebuild the world into a place of wholesomeness and freedom. The *Yogavāsiṣṭha* proclaims the possibility of becoming liberated in the embodied state and points to an ultimate *nirvāṇa* state after the body passes.

The practice of yoga at the time of *Yogavāsiṣṭha* was an engrained part of India's spiritual landscape. Numerous levels and stages of yoga were articulated by Hindu, Jaina, and Buddhist philosophers. The most widely known yoga was advanced by Patañjali (ca. 350–450 CE). His *Yoga Sūtra* sets forth both a threefold and an eightfold yoga system, which seem to serve as a template for other systems. These were developed by Patañjali in the context of earlier Upanishadic models. He most likely was aware of the Buddha's articulation of the eightfold path and the later ten Bodhisattva Bhūmis of Mahāyāna Buddhism, as well as the fivefold Jaina ethical code, rooted in nonviolence (*ahiṃsa*). In Jainism, Umāsvāti's fifth-century articulation of the fourteen stages of spiritual advancement (*guṇasthānas*) provides a parallel articulation of stages of spiritual advancement, as do the "yoga lists" of Haribhadra (ca. 750 CE) and Hemacandra (ca. 1150 CE).

One of the earliest systems of yoga can be found in *Maitri Upaniṣad* (6.18), which outlines a sixfold yoga beginning with control of breath and culminating in *samādhi*: (1) control of breath (*prāṇāyāma*), (2) inwardness (*pratyāhāra*), (3) meditation (*dhyāna*), (4) concentration (*dhāraṇā*), (5) contemplation (*tarka*), and (6) absorption (*samādhi*). This differs quite significantly from the yoga articulated a few hundred years later by Patañjali, which adds ethics (*yama*), observances (*niyama*), and physical postures (*āsana*), places meditation after concentration, and subsumes contemplation (*tarka*) within its descriptions of *samādhi*, albeit in variant linguistic forms (*vitarka, savitarka, nirvitarka*). Hence, Patañjali's eightfold yoga includes the following: (1) ethics (*yama*), (2) observances (*niyama*), (3) postures (*āsana*), (4) control of breath (*prāṇāyāma*), (5) inwardness (*pratyāhāra*), (6) concentration (*dhāraṇā*), (7) meditation (*dhyāna*), and (8) absorption (*samādhi*).

Patañjali's eightfold yoga becomes, in a sense, the gold standard for later systems, particularly as the Jaina philosophers advance their own interpretations of yoga. Haribhadra-sūri (ca. 700–770 CE) aligns the eight stages of yoga with his own imaginative rendering of Patañjali's eight stages in light of a parade of goddess-like stages that seem to capture the feeling-tone of each practice: (1) Friendly (*Mitrā*), (2) Protector (*Tārā*), (3) Powerful (*Balā*), (4) Shining (*Diprā*), (5) Firm (*Sthirā*), (6) Pleasing (*Kāntā*), (7) Radiant (*Prabhā*), (8) Highest (*Parā*). Haribhadra also provides lists for two additional eightfold yogas that seem to demonstrate the interest similarly shown by Vedāntins and Buddhists in utilizing the eightfold idea to advance their own systems.

Bandhu Bhagavaddatta uses terms that resonate with key ideas from Śaṅkara and others within the Vedānta school, with several terms employing the desiderative grammatical form: (1) No Aversion (*Adveṣa*), (2) Desire for Knowledge (*Jijñāsa*), (3) Desirous to Hear Truth (*Śuśrūṣā*), (4) Hearing Truth (*Śravaṇa*), (5) Subtle Awakening (*Sukṣmabodha*), (6) Reflection (*Mīmāṁsā*), (7) Perception of Truth (*Pratipatti*), and (8) Enactment of Absorption (*Sātmi Kṛta Pravṛtti*).

In accordance with his Buddhist approach, Bhadanta Bhāskara employs a sequence of negating terms before arriving at the state deemed "free of attachment." His list is as follows: (1) No Distress (*Akheda*), (2) No Anxiety (*Anudvega*), (3) No Distraction (*Akṣepa*), (4) No Interruption (*Anuttānavatī*), (5) Not Muddied (*Abhrānti*), (6) Not Finding Pleasure in Externals (*Ananyamud*), (7) No Pain (*Arug*), and (8) Free from Attachment (*Saṅga Vivarjitā*).

The later Jaina scholar Hemacandra-sūri (eleventh century CE) also employed the frame of eightfold yoga, which Olle Qvarnström has noted "serves the purpose of adapting Jainism to the prevailing religious environment as well as to the larger pan-Indian intellectual debate" (Qvarnström 2002: 9). Hemacandra's *Yogaśāstra*, one of the earliest handbooks to include information later popularized in the *haṭha yoga* texts, starts with an exposition of correct behavior correlating to Patañjali's *yama* and *niyama* (chapters one through three), moves into a description of yoga postures (end of chapter four), and describes various forms of breath control in great detail (chapters five and six) and inwardness and concentration (also in chapter six) before itemizing stages of meditation (chapters seven through eleven) and the final state of release (chapters eleven and twelve).

In addition to his well-known eightfold yoga, Patañjali also includes a threefold yoga at the beginning of the second section of the *Yoga Sūtra*. Known as Krīya Yoga, it specifies three core practices for the attainment of yoga: austerity, study, and devotion (*tapas, svādhyāya, īśvara-praṇidhāna*). Haribhadra also employs a threefold system, which he describes as Icchā, Śāstra, and Sāmarthya Yoga or alternately Icchā, Jñāna, and Krīya, as they are known in Tantra. These terms are similar to those found in Tantric traditions that were developing and gaining popularity throughout India during his lifetime. They refer to a desire to enter into the path of yoga, a willingness to follow the way of knowledge as articulated in the scriptures, and a resolve to take up the practices of yoga. This threefold system, as we will see, bears some similarities to the first three steps of the sevenfold yoga in the *Yogavāsiṣṭha*.

Another key to understanding yoga systems can be found in the section titles of the *Bhagavad Gītā* and the *Yogavāsiṣṭha*. Each text lies within the genre of epic literature and narrates a sequence of unfolding teachings conveyed by guru to disciple, specifically Kṛṣṇa to Arjuna and Vasiṣṭha to Rāma. In both instances, the texts begin with the collapse of the protagonist. In the words of

American psychologist William James, both heroes experience an episode of entering into the phase of the "sick soul." Arjuna balks at entering into what he perceives to be an unwinnable war. Rāma, a teenager, resists Viśvāmitra's request that he launch a campaign to purge the forest of unruly elements. Both these kṣatriyas push back against the performance of their dharma, becoming paradigmatic examples of human disaffection with worldly entanglements. Both are educated through the teachings of yoga to embrace their dharma, to engage the world, and to perform their duties from a place of freedom from attachment (*vairāgya*). The paradox of their eventual acceptance of responsibility for these grave tasks underscores the ongoing tension between worldly involvement (*pravṛtti*) and rejection of the world (*nivṛtti*). Non-attached action (*karma-yoga*) provides the bridge between involvement and rejection and helps make sense of these inherent contradictions. Each narrative talks about the ultimate goal of leaving the world in peace, yet both emphasize the necessity of living life fully.

Each chapter of the *Bhagavad Gītā* names a particular experience of yoga, beginning with the yoga of the despondency of Arjuna (chapter one) and then moving from the yogas of knowledge, action, the renunciation of action in knowledge, to the yogas of renunciation and meditation (chapters two through six). Devotional or bhakti yoga occupies the middle six chapters of the *Bhagavad Gītā*, focusing on knowledge, the imperishable *brahman*, the royal mystery, the yoga of manifestation, the yoga of the vision of the universal form, and the yoga of devotion (chapters seven through twelve). The final six chapters of the *Bhagavad Gītā* equip Arjuna for his return to the world of the battlefield. In these chapters, Kṛṣṇa teaches the yoga of the distinction between the field-knower and the field, the yoga of the distinction between the three *guṇa*s, the yoga of the supreme spirit, the yoga of the distinction between the divine and the demonic tendencies, the yoga of the distinction of the three kinds of faith, and the yoga of renunciation (chapters 13 through 18).

In the unfolding of the *Bhagavad Gītā*, Arjuna moves from his despondency and resistance through a progressive sequence of teachings. Kṛṣṇa reminds him of the core principles of knowledge (the soul cannot be killed), non-attached action, and meditation. These lead to a sequence of chapters on devotion, through which the visionary experience of Kṛṣṇa's divine identity re-orients Arjuna's grasp on reality. In the final chapters of the *Gītā*, Arjuna learns to see the world through the Sāṃkhya prism of the three *guṇa*s, and hence develops the sense of dispassion that equips him, as would be said in modern India, to "do the needful." In the process, Arjuna learns to operate from a much broader context (nothing is born, nothing dies) that allows him to advance the narrative of the story, and, by extension, serve as an example, albeit ultimately a tragic one, of how yoga requires engagement with the ways of the world, while retaining remembrance of one's ultimate position as a soul connected to the vast expanse of the cosmos. For Mahatma Gandhi, this metaphor served to inspire his nonviolent campaigns against injustice. Karma yoga allows reintegrating the vision of the totality (as seen in chapter eleven) into the realm of worldly engagement.

This lesson can also be seen in the *Yogavāsiṣṭha*. However, whereas the *Bhagavad Gītā*, a much shorter text nested in a huge narrative, ends with Arjuna finding the resolve to enter into battle, the *Yogavāsiṣṭha* retains its interest in and praise of *nirvāṇa* up to the end. Even though the reader knows that Rāma will eventually protect the sages in their hermitages and rescue his wife Sītā from Rāvaṇa's confinement in Sri Lanka, the writer of the *Yogavāsiṣṭha* constantly reminds the reader that all reality is fiction. In the spirit of Borges' magical realism, Vasiṣṭha tells dozens of stories that undermine the reader's (and Rāma's) sense of the fixity of things. One gets a sense that regardless of what happens, nothing is really happening; all things that occupy space simultaneously call out and point to the fluidity, evanescence, and ultimate freedom of every circumstance, every occurrence. Hence, the chapter flow of the *Yogavāsiṣṭha* follows a similar trajectory to that of the *Bhagavad Gītā*, but with a difference. Whereas Arjuna's ultimate embrace of the yoga of renunciation leads him back to the reality of the battlefield, Rāma's entry into *nirvāṇa* delivers him into a state of perpetual non-dual awareness. One could argue that both narratives see their protagonists engage in warfare and participate in princely and kingly duties. However, Arjuna proclaims later that he forgot Kṛṣṇa's lessons and he eventually suffers a stint in hell due to his misdeeds, whereas Rāma goes on to rule from a place of dispassion and freedom.

Rāma's spiritual or yoga journey can be summarized in the book (*prakaraṇa*) titles of the *Yogavāsiṣṭha*: (1) Rāma's Disaffection (*Vairāgya*); (2) The Behavior of the Seeker (*Mumukṣu Vyavahāra*); (3) Creation (*Utpatti*); (4) Existence (*Sthiti*); (5) Dissolution (*Upaśama*); and (6) Liberation (*Nirvāṇa*). These six sections of the *Yogavāsiṣṭha* provide a narrative arc for understanding the spiritual path. Rāma begins, as does Arjuna in the *Gītā*, in a state of deep questioning, rejecting the notion that any of his actions carry importance or significance. He then learns about the efficacy of human action and creativity (*pauruṣa*). He discovers that his thoughts and emotions construct the very world that he inhabits. Consequently, he learns about his intimate relationship with the creation and maintenance of the world. In story upon story, Vasiṣṭha demonstrates how the whims and desires of the past inform and create the present. Ultimately, Vasiṣṭha shows Rāma both how to create the narrative of human life and how to dissolve it. This skill, particularly as conveyed through womanist narratives that show the power of the goddess and self-liberation of Queen Cūḍālā, is then taken up by Rāma himself, who moves into a place of freedom, engages the all in the each, and sees the vast space of pure consciousness in all things.

In chapter 162 of the *Nirvāṇa Prakaraṇa*, Vasiṣṭha teaches a sevenfold yoga to Vasiṣṭha. It is particularly suited to help the reader understand the many dream narratives of the text and follows the overall philosophy of the *Yogavāsiṣṭha*: to the extent that a person can see beyond the world of appearances while embracing them, one can move with ease within and beyond all attachments, cultivating a life of perfect freedom, or at least a life that embraces moments of deep insight. The later school of Dṛṣṭi-Sṛṣṭi-Advaita-Vedānta relies upon the *Yogavāsiṣṭha* to explain and promote this method.

The sevenfold yoga of the *Yogavāsiṣṭha* begins with disenchantment. Big questions haunt one's awareness, dramatically posed in the critical question, "How can I go on living out these stale old karmas?" At this stage of renunciation, one decides to change and improve oneself. In the second stage, deep thinking, one cultivates concentration and meditation and fully takes on an ethical life. The third stage, non-attachment, signals a radical split from one's former identity. In this state, the ego dissolves, bringing great peace. All three of these stages of yoga are said to happen within the realm of waking consciousness. By living in this manner, one assumes great dignity, earning the respect of others. In the fourth stage, all things appear as if they were in a dream. In the fifth stage one gains deep peace, as if one were engaged in deep sleep. The sixth stage is described as being liberated while still in the body. In the seventh stage, one's body dissolves, and one merges with or returns to the universal consciousness.

The *Yogavāsiṣṭha* sets forth seven stages of yoga as follows: (1) Renunciation (*Nivṛtti*); (2) Deep Thinking (*Vicāraṇa*); (3) Non-attachment (*Asaṃsaṅga*); (4) The World as Dream (*Svapna Loka*); (5) Non-dual as if in Deep Sleep (*Advaita Suṣupta*); (6) Living Liberation (*Jīvan Mukti*); and (7) Freedom from the Body (*Videha Mukti*). In many ways, the first three stages are similar to the first three stages of Tantra and Haribhadra's threefold yoga. In Icchā Yoga, one desires to leave behind the sufferings and pains of the world. In Śāstra/Jñāna Yoga, one diligently dwells in the modality of correct insight and behavior. In Sāmarthya/Krīya Yoga, non-attachment arises spontaneously, allowing one to move through the world, unaffected by its negativities, like the Nonattachment Yoga of the *Yogavāsiṣṭha.*

The latter four phases demonstrate the special philosophy of the *Yogavāsiṣṭha.* Having disengaged from the fixity of things in the world, at the fourth stage one sees all things as if they are merely a dream. At the fifth stage, one is able to go beyond even the dream itself into a realm of utter peace. In a sense, these stages reflect verse 2.67 of the *Bhagavad Gītā*: "When others are awake, it is like night to the restrained one; when others are asleep, this person awakens." At the sixth stage, one resumes activity in the world, but only apparently so; in truth, one is liberated while yet living. At the seventh stage, one passes beyond, into the ultimate reality, safe from rebirth.

The beginning of the yoga of the *Yogavāsiṣṭha* mirrors Rāma's own experience. Rāma experiences a deep disaffection (*vairāgya*) for the things of the world. He does not wish to engage in the battle for which he has been recruited. Through his tutelage by Vasiṣṭha, he comes to learn of the power of human effort and the efficacy of human action, as well as the ability that one has to overcome the difficulties of the past. Repeatedly, Vasiṣṭha shows Rāma that the world is no more than a dream, a refrain repeated through the course of dozens of stories. Eventually, by seeing the relationship between his intentions and his mental conjurings and the creation of the world, Rāma transcends attachment and moves forward in the role of *jīvanmukta*—a status, incidentally, that remains with him through the remainder of the *Rāmayana.*

This translation is based on the Sanskrit for the text included in Wasudeva Laxamana Sastri Pansikar, ed., *The Yogavāsiṣṭha of Vālmīki with the Commentary Vasiṣṭhamahārāmāyaṇatātparyaprakāśa*, revised and re-edited by Narayan Ram Acharya Kavyatirtha (Bombay: Pandurang Jawaji, 1937; reprint New Delhi: Munshiram Manoharlal, 1981). The Sanskrit version reproduced in *The Yoga-Vasiṣṭha of Vālmīki: Sanskrit Text and English Translation,* edited and revised by Ravi Prakash Arya (Delhi: Parimal Publications, 1998) was also consulted. Several of my students contributed to the following translation, including Viresh Hughes, Jodi Shaw, Daniel Levine, Wynanda Jacobi, and Randall Krauss.

Suggestions for Further Reading

Partial translations of the text by Swami Venkatesananda can be found in *The Supreme Yoga: A New Translation of the Yoga Vāsiṣṭha*, 2 vols. (Shivanandanagar: The Divine Life Society, 2003); *The Concise Yoga Vāsiṣṭha* (Albany: State University of New York Press, 1984); and *Vasiṣṭha's Yoga* (Albany: State University of New York Press, 1993). An early English rendering of the text can also be found by Vihari-Lala Mitra, *The Yoga-Vāsiṣṭha-Mahārāmāyaṇa of Vālmīki* (Calcutta: 1891–1899, reprint Varanasi: Bharatiya Publishing House, 1976). A new critical edition of the entire text is under way in Germany under the direction of Walter Slaje.

For further reading, see the works of B. L. Atreya, particularly *The Philosophy of the Yogavāsiṣṭha* (Adyar: Theosophical Publishing House, 1936) and *Deification of Man: Its Methods and Stages According to the Yogavāsiṣṭha* (Moradabad: Darshana, 1963). Surendranath DasGupta devotes eighty pages to the *Yogavāsiṣṭha* in his *A History of Indian Philosophy in Five Volumes* (Cambridge: Cambridge University Press, 1932). More recent studies include T. G. Mainkar, *The Vasiṣṭha Rāmāyaṇa: A Study* (New Delhi: Meharchand Lachhmandas, 1977); Wendy Doniger O'Flaherty, *Dreams, Illusion and Other Realities* (Chicago: University of Chicago Press, 1984); Christopher Chapple, *Karma and Creativity* (Albany: State University of New York Press, 1986); Jürgen Hanneder, *Studies on the Mokṣopāya* (Wiesbaden: Harrassowitz, 2006); and Arindam Chakrabarti and Christopher Key Chapple, eds., *Engaged Emancipation: Mind, Morals, and Make Believe in the Mokṣopāya* (Delhi: Motilal Banarsidass, 2011). On the eightfold yoga of the *Yogaśāstra*, see Olle Qvarnström, *The Yogaśāstra of Hemacandra* (Cambridge, MA: Harvard University Press, 2002).

Yogavāsiṣṭha Book Six, Chapter 126

On the Seven Stages of Yoga

1. Śrī Rāma asked:

What constitute the seven stages of yoga practice?
How are the various stages of the yogin distinguished?

STAGE ONE: RENUNCIATION (NIVṚTTI)

2. Vasiṣṭha responded:

Listen to the characteristics of the two types of people.
The engaged ones (*pravṛtti*) draw near to heaven.
The renouncers (*nivṛtti*) are yearning for liberation.

3. What is this thing called *nirvāṇa*?
To me, it is stopping transmigration.
By contrast, the one who keeps doing what is to be done
stays engaged (in the world).

4. However, just as a tortoise withdraws it neck
and just as the ocean's tides fill any available opening,
so, after countless births, a person of great discernment is born.

5. (Such a person says): "Alas! I have had enough of the *saṃsāra*
caused by this weakness of mine.
How can I live another day, driven by these stale karmas?

6. What would be the highest [method] for release from pain?
What actions would lead to this superior liberation?"
The renouncer, it is recalled,
asks these ultimate questions and more.

7. "Having experienced this dispassion (*virāga*),
how will I cross over the ocean of *saṃsāra*?"
This, indeed, is the highest thought;
from it arises devotion to truth.

8. Having drawn into oneself due to dispassion (*virāga*),
one experiences fragrance-filled meditations,
an uplift of one's actions within the realm of forms,
moving forward with joy every day.

9. The one who continually questions the stupid actions of people
does not condemn their faults, but performs virtuous actions
(by way of counter example).

10. This person's mind is wary of busy tasks.
This person performs only mild actions,
is continually on guard against sin,
and looks away from shallow pleasures.

11. This person speaks delightful and affectionate words,
nurturing and leading to love appropriate to time and place.

12. Such a person has accomplished the first stage (*bhūmika*) of yoga
and serves wise people in thought, deed, and word.

STAGE TWO: DEEP THINKING (VICĀRAṆA)

13. Then one is led forward and seeks out the knowledge of the scriptures.
This person would become a deep thinker (*vicārin*)
and move in the direction of deliverance from *saṃsāra*.

14. It is said that this person already has attained the first stage.
Others are regarded to be self-obsessed.
This stage of deep thinking has two names:
"established in riches" and "arrived at the stage of yoga."

15. From the performance of concentration (*dhāraṇā*) and meditation (*dhyāna*),
and through keeping the company of revealed and remembered scriptures,
such a one is regarded silently and aloud as reaching toward the highest wisdom.
[Note that this person is performing the sixth and seventh limbs of Patañjali's yoga.]

16. This person knows the classifications of things
and the rules of proper conduct.
Having heard what is to be learned,
this person has command (over the mind)
like a householder manages the home.

17. Such a person leaves behind
conceit, pride, envy, delusion, and cupidity.
Like a snake shedding its skin,
this person escapes from attachment to externals.

18. From serving wise people, and following the guru,
scriptures, and clear thinking,
one discovers how to act
according to the unparalleled supreme secret.

STAGE THREE: NO ATTACHMENT (ASAMSAṄGA)

19. The third yoga stage is called "no attachment" (*asaṃsaṅga*).
In this, one arrives at an agreeable state, like [walking into] a bed of flowers.

20. The mind of this person focuses on the meanings of scriptural statements.
This person takes up company with those in ashrams [spiritual retreats]
who are calmed by their austerities and are making progress
in the narrative journey to the inner self.

21. Those who scorn *saṃsāra*
and are treading the path toward the release from desire
gather together in the refuge of virtue,
living in this way into the waning years of their lives.

22. Such people pass the time prudently
along with forest dwellers in their hermitages.

With the radiance of their pacified minds,
they are non-attached, happy, exuding auspiciousness.

23. From practicing the holy scriptures
and from doing meritorious actions,
this person consequently speaks well
and settles into seeing the truth of things.

24. Having obtained this third stage,
one experiences the awakening (*bodha*) of the Self
through two types of non-attachment.
Listen as I explain this distinction.

25. The two ways of non-attachment are equally splendid:
I am not the doer; I am not the enjoyer.
I am not oppressed nor do I oppress others.

26. With the intention of keeping a distance from the world,
one sees as equal all who have bodies and names.
Every one is formed by karma from past lives
and is indeed subject to God (Īśvara).

27. [Such a person continually asks:]
If I am happy, is it due to me? If I am sad, is it due to me?
If I experience pleasure, is it due to me?
If I experience displeasure, is it due me?
If things turn out well, is it due to me?
If things go wrong, is it due to me?

28. All that comes together eventually falls apart.
All thoughts that arise eventually dissipate.
Time swallows all existence, zealously and continually.

29. "It does not matter!" Through the practice [of this insight],
one enters the inner [realization] of non-existence.
Attaching the mind to the meaning of this phrase
is the same as [dwelling in] non-attachment.

30. Through the various steps of yoga
and through associating with great souls,
one separates oneself from unreliable people
and joins with those who have knowledge of the self.

31. Through creativity and effort
and from the frequent practice of yoga

one lives the life of a spotless doer,
having arrived at a place of firm meaning.

32. In the core [understanding] of the highest purpose,
one crosses the ocean of *saṃsāra*.
"I am not the doer—God is the doer,
but deeds belong to *prakṛti*."

33. Having indeed accomplished this highest transcendence,
one penetrates the meaning of all words.
One sits like a sage in peace.
This, it is said, is the best non-attachment.

34. This [state] is neither inside nor outside,
not below nor above, not in the quarters nor in the sky.
It is not with meaning nor is it without meaning.
It is not without awareness nor is it aware.

35. [Like the moon] it sits, radiating peace.
In darkness or in the clouds, it is the same,
without beginning or end, unborn, beautiful.
This, it is said, is the best non-attachment.

36. Delight, contentment, and joy
are caused by this spotless blossom [of non-attachment].
Conscious thought, though at first like a lotus, can start to cling
and contract into a necklace of obstacles.

37. As the lotus of discernment rises up inside,
it bursts like a flash of lightning in one's thoughts.
Non-attachment to the fruits
is the third stage of yoga.

REVIEW OF THE FIRST THREE STAGES

38. By performing yoga, through accumulated purity
and by the storehouse of one's good actions,
one arrives at the mysteriously fortuitous first stage.

39. The guardian Mothers say, "This stage is like a tender sprout.
The waters of discernment must be diligently
sprinkled on it to protect and nourish it."

40. By this gift, one becomes brilliant.
Through deep thinking (*vicāra*) one would be guided upward,
just as a gardener tends to his seedlings diligently, every day.

41. By holding onto this inner strength indeed,
one sets in motion an inexhaustible commitment.
From effort at the second stage (*vicāra*),
one reaches the third stage (*asaṃsaṅga*).

42. This third stage is non-attachment, which is higher.
The person at this stage shuns all remaining things
and dissolves all thought.

43. Śrī Rāma said:
What world would be the destiny of those
whose actions are vile?
Who are born in wicked families and are confused?
Who do not take up the company of yogins?

44. What path, O Bhagavān, will those follow
who have failed to attain the first, second, or third stage
at the time of death?

45. Vasiṣṭha said:
Saṃsāra is bestowed on the one who is deluded and taken by foolishness.
The consequence is hundreds of random births.

46. But possibly freedom from passion will arise
through association with the holy ones.
In this freedom from passion,
a person inevitably rises up to the level of one of these stages.

47. Thus, it is agreed upon in the scriptures
that *saṃsāra* can be ended.
The living being can be released from the body
by attaining a stage of yoga.

48. Through following the stages of yoga, one basks [in the benefits of]
past happy deeds, as if one were riding in the chariot of the gods
in the presence of those souls who protect the world.

49. It is as if one were dwelling in the fragrant groves on Mount Meru,
delighting in the company of a beautiful friend.

Thus, the accomplishment of good deeds
will prevail over the previous bad deeds.

50. The yogins, having vanquished the net of worldly enjoyment,
stand victorious in a blessed state.
Unsullied and of pleasant disposition,
these most excellent persons live on, protected [from negativity].

51. Having been born into yoga, they serve others
and encourage others to attain yoga.
These wise ones, due to their prior practice of meditation,
are on course within the stages of yoga.

DIGNITY IN YOGA

52. O Rāma, these three stages occur in the realm designated as the waking state.
This waking state is seen through the brilliance of the intellect,

53. Those who are disciplined through yoga
carry themselves in their solitude with dignity.
Having seen such people, the minds of the ignorant
are inspired to develop a desire for liberation.

54. This person desires to perform what needs to be done
and does not get involved with improper activity.
Standing up for refined conduct,
such a person is renowned as possessing dignity.

55. This person follows proper conduct,
studies the scriptures, and has a stable mind.
Due to this appropriate behavior,
such a person is renowned as possessing dignity.

56. In the first stage, the (seeds of yoga) sprout.
In the second stage, the (plant of yoga) grows.
In the third stage, it bears fruit.
This would be the unfolding dignity of yogins.

57. This dignified yogin, upon death,
carries pure intentions [to the next life].
After enjoying pleasure for a long time,
that person assumes [a life of] yoga again.

FOURTH STAGE: WORLD AS DREAM (SVAPNA LOKA)

58. From the practice of these three stages (of yoga),
one arrives at the destruction of ignorance.
Singular knowledge arises in the mind
like the splendor of the full moon rising.

59. Those yogins, their minds disciplined and
thoroughly free from dwelling on difference,
regard all things to be the same.
Through this, they enter the immeasurable fourth stage.

60. Standing in the non-dual vision,
with all thoughts of duality put to rest,
the yogins see this world as if it were a dream.
Through this, they enter the immeasurable fourth stage.

61. The first three stages (of renunciation, deep thinking, and
non-attachment)
take place in waking life. In the fourth stage, things are seen
as if they are dreams, like the falling away (of leaves) in autumn.
Thing gradually fade away as if into oblivion.

FIFTH STAGE: NONDUAL SLEEP (ADVAITA SUṢUPTA)

62. Having arrived at the fifth stage,
one is at the end of the remaining existence.
At this fifth stage, one reaches the level (*pada*)
that is called sleep (*suṣupta*).

63. That person stands in a state of utter non-dualism (*advaita-mātra*),
each part in perfect peace.
The appearance of dualism drops away,
and one awakens into inner joy.

64. In this fifth stage of deep sleep (*suṣupta-ghana*),
one's countenance takes on an inward stability,
transcending external concerns.

65. One achieves eternal, abundant peace through this.
One is perceived as if one were a sleeping owl.
In doing this practice one rushes to banish (worldliness) in this stage.

SIXTH STAGE: LIVING LIBERATION

66. The sixth stage is another name for the soul as it traverses these steps:
All form is seen as neither nonexistent nor existent.
One obtains action neither with an ego nor without an ego.

67. In solitude, with thoughts diminished,
one dwells in a state released from "oneness" or "two-ness."
With the knots of karma untied, one finds peace in the body,
living as a liberated soul.

68. Standing neither in *nirvāṇa* nor not in *nirvāṇa*,
one shines brightly,
outwardly free, inwardly free,
free like the piece of sky in a jar.

69. Full on the outside, full on the inside,
as full as a jar overflowing with water,
this person seems highly accomplished,
but also seems like nothing special.

SEVENTH STAGE: FREE FROM THE BODY

70. Having dwelt in the sixth stage,
one then attains the seventh stage:
this is called liberated, freed from the body.
This is the seventh stage of yoga.

71. Peaceful beyond words,
this state is beyond the horizon of the earth.
By some, it is called Śiva.
By others, it is referred to as Brahmā.

72. By some, it is determined to be female, others call it male.
Thought of in so many ways,
at the core of things, it is imagined as the Self.

73. How can this eternal, indescribable consciousness be described?
Its attainment has been spoken of in seven stages by me to you, O Rāma.

—7—

A Fourteenth-Century Persian Account of Breath Control and Meditation

Carl W. Ernst

While it is perhaps contrary to customary expectations, practices associated with *haṭha yoga* were in fact known outside of India in Muslim intellectual circles. The most important example of this phenomenon is the text known as the *Amritakunda* or *Pool of Nectar*, which circulated in Arabic, Persian, Ottoman Turkish, and Urdu versions from the seventeenth century onward, in Persia, Turkey, and North Africa as well as in India. The Muslim readers of these texts understood them differently according to their presuppositions. Some were attracted by the occult and magical powers promised by the yogis, who in these texts are invariably called jogīs, in North Indian pronunciation. Others saw in these writings significant parallels to the philosophical and mystical traditions current in Persia, which were particularly associated with Sufism and Neoplatonism. Over time, accounts of yogic meditation practices were increasingly Islamized, so that eventually it became difficult to recognize anything particularly Indian or foreign about them. Although descriptions of jogīs are relatively common in Islamicate literature, the word "yoga" (*jog*) hardly ever occurs, but it appears to be regularly represented by the Arabic-Persian term for ascetic practice, *riyāzat*.

The text translated here is the earliest known description of yogic practices found in the writings of Muslim authors. It is a short passage found in a voluminous encyclopedia compiled in Persia by a noted Shi`i scholar and physician, Shams al-Dīn Muhammad ibn Mahmūd Āmulī, who died in Shiraz in 1353. For decades he had taught in the academies established by the Il-Khan Mongol rulers of Iran. While half of this encyclopedia focuses on the Islamic religious sciences, half of it is concerned with the sciences of the ancients, which for all practical purposes included philosophy, science, and the arts. The passage translated below occurs in the section on natural sciences, which includes medicine, alchemy, interpretation of dreams, astronomy, occult sciences, veterinary science, and agriculture.

Amuli focuses on two elements associated with the yogic tradition: the control of breaths, and meditative practices associated with the cakras. The material that he briefly summarizes here is known to exist in longer versions, most notably the Persian text acquired by the Italian traveler Pietro della Valle in southern Persia in 1622, which bears the Hindi title *Kāmrū bījākṣa*, or *The Kāmarūpa Seed Syllables.* That work seems to have been composed by a Persian intellectual in India who became interested in yogic practices of breath control and the summoning of the female spirits known as *yoginī*s. Amuli directly refers to that text, and he also repeats its emphasis on associating these teachings with the goddess Kamak (also known as Kāmākhyā). Breath control is said to be employed by *jogī*s for prolonging life and for divination, and the breaths are divided into five types corresponding to the physical elements; numerous examples are provided to show how breath coming from the left or right nostril can predict the future or provide answers to questions. The notion of five breaths appears to be connected to the classic Indian division of breaths into *prāṇa*, *apāna*, *vyāna*, *samāna*, and *udāna*, as outlined by Kenneth G. Zysk. The use of breath for divination, particularly for predicting death, seems to reflect widespread Hindu and Buddhist Tantric practices found in India and Tibet, as Michael Walter has shown.

The section on breaths is followed by a brief discussion of the "science of imagination" (Arabic *wahm*), which deals with the ascetic lifestyle and the cultivation of the "water of life" (Persian *āb-i hayāt*) to overcome death; the latter is a deliberate parallel for the nectar (*amṛta*) sought in yogic practices. This passage also includes a description of a method for predicting the time of death by concentrating on the afterimage of one's shadow, and it contains an account of nine psychic centers corresponding to the *cakra*s of *haṭha yoga*, each of which is associated here with a vivid image. Other texts such as the *Amritakunda* give more extensive and varied accounts of *cakra* meditations, and they also associate them with *yoginī* goddesses, but they continue to employ the term "imagination" for the power that animates all of these extraordinary manifestations. The text concludes on a derisory note, dismissing the entire subject as a waste of time. Although at least one nineteenth-century Orientalist scholar (Alfred von Kramer) saw this passage as proof of the Indian origins of all the mystical practices of Muslim Sufis, in retrospect it appears instead to indicate a relative lack of comprehension of the technical and theoretical aspects of yoga.

The Persian-language source from which this translation is taken is Shams al-Dīn Muhammad ibn Mahmūd Āmulī, *Nafā'is al-funūn fī `arā'is al-`uyūn*, ed. Mīrzā Abū al-Hasan Sha`rānā (Tehran: Kitābfurūshī Islīmiyya, 1379/1960), 3:360–65, collated with a seventeenth-century manuscript in the collection of Dr. Taufiq Sobhani (Tehran).

Suggestions for Further Reading

The basic problems in understanding Muslim interpretations of yoga are sketched out in Carl W. Ernst, "Situating Sufism and Yoga," *Journal of the Royal Asiatic Society*, Series 3, 15:1 (2005), pp. 15–43. The history of the most important transmission of a yogic text in Muslim contexts is presented in Carl W. Ernst, "The Islamization of Yoga in the Amrtakunda Translations," *Journal of the Royal Asiatic Society*, Series 3, 13:2 (2003), pp. 199–226. A more extensive version of the text translated below, discovered by Pietro della Valle in the seventeenth century, is discussed in Carl W. Ernst, "Being Careful with the Goddess: Yoginis in Persian and Arabic Texts," in *Performing Ecstasy: The Poetics and Politics of Religion in India*, ed. Pallabi Chakrabarty and Scott Kugle (Delhi: Manohar, 2009), pp. 189–203. The use of breath in Tantric divination is discussed by Michael Walter, "Cheating Death," in *Tantra in Practice*, ed. David Gordon White, Princeton Readings in Religions (Princeton, NJ: Princeton University Press, 2000), pp. 605–23. Kenneth G. Zysk provides an overview of the five breaths in "The Science of Respiration and the Doctrine of the Bodily Winds in Ancient India," *Journal of the American Oriental Society* 113/2 (1993), pp. 198–213. Nile Green describes nineteenth-century Muslims interested in yogic techniques in "Breathing in India, c. 1890," *Modern Asian Studies* 42:2-3 (2008), pp. 283–315.

The Science of Breath and the Science of Imagination

The former is an expression for the knowledge of the breaths and the proofs thereof. The latter is [an expression for] the knowledge of the summoning of imaginations and managing ascetic practice in that. These two sciences are famous among the Indians, and any one who attains perfection in these two they call a jogī; they consider him among the company of spiritual beings. They say that Kamak Dev has established both sciences.

They call spiritual beings (*rūhāniyān*) "*dev*," and they say that Kamak is still living, abiding in the town of Kamru in a cave. To satisfy their needs, they go to the door of that cave, and some claim that they see her. Every day the emperor of that realm sends pure foods and fresh drinks there, which they place at the door of the cave, where they immediately disappear. Many people have witnessed this affair. The explanation of both sciences is exhaustively discussed in the book *Kāmrū bījākṣa*, which is the most famous of their books. Here, allusion will be made to each of these in a separate section, God willing.

PART ONE, ON THE SCIENCE OF BREATH

Know that the breath sometimes comes from the right side, and sometimes from the left side, and sometimes it is from both nostrils. They relate the right nostril to the sun, and the left to the moon, and they say that in one day 21,600 breaths come forth, or 900 every hour, more or less.

As they say, sometimes in one hour 1,600 breaths come forth, and during two hours, the breath comes from a single nostril. Sometimes it happens that over three days the breath goes from one nostril. There are some jogīs who take no more than a single breath in a day and night, one in the morning and one in the evening. Thus they say that when one reaches this stage, in six months it becomes easy. They consider obtaining this stage to be the cause of long life, the cure for all illnesses, and the attainment of complete happiness.

According to them breath is of five kinds:

1. The earthy breath, and they say that that breath goes towards the ground, and they say it is yellow in color.
2. The watery breath, and that is the breath which goes straight. They say that it is white in color.
3. The fiery breath, and that is the breath that goes upward. They say the color of this breath is red.
4. The airy breath, and that is the breath that goes crooked. They say this breath is green.
5. The heavenly breath, and this breath goes inward. They say its color tends towards whiteness.

They say that whenever the breath goes to the right side, it is a good sign for all of the following: the beginning of affairs, seeing kings and sultans and nobles, asking them for one's needs, going to battle, buying horses and beasts of burden, going to warm climates, cutting nails, branding animals, curing the sick, getting bled, farming, companionship and friendship, looking for lost items, and going north and east.

If it comes from the left side, it is a good sign for planning a trip especially to the west, buying and wearing new clothes, making jewelry, taking children to school, making agreements, marriages, construction, and trade.

They say that the earthy and watery breaths are a sign for abundant fortune and happiness. The fiery and airy breaths are a sign for depression, trouble, and illness, and the heavenly breath is a sign for confusion and impediment in one's affairs.

They say that when a questioner asks about the nature of a subject, if the earthy breath appears, the subject concerns plants; if it is airy or watery, the subject concerns animals; if it is fiery, the subject concerns minerals; if it is heavenly, it concerns no subject. When someone asks about affairs or a need, if the name of the questioner has an odd number of letters and the breath comes from the right side, that affair will come out right; but if a need arises, and if the name has an even number of letters and the breath comes from the left side, that affair will not come out right and the need will not be fulfilled.

If one asks about a sick person, and the name of the sick person has an odd number of letters, and the breath of the questioner and the person questioned comes from the right side, the sick person will become well; if the name of the sick person has an even number of letters, and the breath of both is from the left side, that sick person is in danger.

If they ask which of two opponents will triumph, [and] if the questioner has come from the side where the breath is increasing, the person whose name he says first will triumph. If the questioner comes from the side where the breath is decreasing, the person whose name he says last will triumph.

If they ask about a pregnant woman, [and] if the questioner has come from the left side, and the breath is increasing from that side, that child will be a girl; if he is coming from the right side, and the breath from that side is increasing, it will be a boy.

If they ask about a foreign army, and the questioner is from the left side, and the breath goes from that side, that army will come; if the breath does not come from that side, or itself decreases, that army will not come.

If they ask about a missing person, whether he is living or dead, [and] if the questioner comes from the side where the breath is decreasing and sits on that side where the breath is increasing, the person is living; if he has come from the side where the breath is increasing and sits where the breath is decreasing, that missing person will not come back. If he comes from the side where the breath is decreasing and also sits on that side, the missing person is dead.

If they ask about someone kidnapped or escaped, and the questioner comes from the side where the breath is increasing, he will come back. If he is from the side where the breath is decreasing, he will come back later.

They say if one's breath is disturbed, so that for an entire day and night one cannot tell [from] which [side] the breath comes, it is proof that one will have a strong child. If both breaths for a day and night are equal, it is a sign of madness. If for four hours continuously breath comes from the left side, it is auspicious for him. If it is for eight hours, one of his friends will be injured. If it comes for nine hours, one of his relatives will suffer affliction. If it comes for ten hours, he will be afflicted. If it comes for twelve hours, a powerful enemy will appear. If it comes for a day and a night, death is to be feared.

They say when one person fears another, if, at a time when the breath comes from the left side he goes to a garden and picks 120 colored blossoms and sits by running water, casting them into the water one by one in the name of that person, he will become kind and no dread or fear will remain.

They say that if at a time when the breath comes from the right one has intercourse with a woman, a male child will come. If the breath comes from the left side, the child that will be born is female. May the breath be blest, the step fortunate, and the outcome praised.

PART TWO, THE SCIENCE OF IMAGINATION

The basis of this division in their view is ascetic practice. The lowest stage in ascetic practice is that one choose seclusion and abstain from eating meat, drinking intoxicants, and sexual intercourse. One sleeps little, enjoys sweet fragrances, avoids frivolity, eats little, does not dress in clean or perfumed clothes, and does not mix with anyone. If someone gives him the worst possible injury, he does not seek retribution or become concerned about it. The highest stage is that one is satisfied with fish for daily food, sleeps only one hour a week, and only breathes twice a day, so that his state is perfected, he controls the universe, and after that he does as he pleases.

One of the marvelous things told there is that they say if, at the time of weakness and the sign of death, one imagines that the water of life is flowing within oneself, and one becomes firm in this imagination and makes it continuous so that there is no interruption in his concentration, he will be released from that weakness and death will be repelled. He carefully follows this very method so that he lives, but when he grows tired of himself and no longer is busy repelling [death], he will be destroyed.

Some say such-and-such a person will never die; rather, when he becomes pure of all obscurities, he will no longer need food and drink, but will become purely spiritual and hidden from the eyes of men.

They say if one does not know how much of his life remains, when the sun has risen and is high, one goes to the desert and faces west, opposite one's shadow on the ground, standing straight and motionless. One places both hands on the knees, as when one bows [for Islamic ritual prayer], summoning this imagination without permitting any other thought. Then one raises the head and gazes at the shadow. If he sees the shadow whole in body, it is a sign that he has [much] life remaining. If he sees that he lacks a hand, two years remain to him. If he sees that he lacks a foot, one year remains.

They say that the places of the imagination are nine:

1. The first is the skull.
2. The second is between the two eyebrows.
3. The third is the throat.
4. The fourth is the slender hole near the nostrils, which is in the gullet, and which leads to the brain.
5. The fifth is the heart.
6. The sixth is the belly.
7. The seventh is the navel.
8. The eighth is the genitals.
9. The ninth is the seat.

The imagination of the skull is like the moon become full. The imagination of the eyebrow is like the sun. The imagination of the throat is like light. The imagination of the nostrils is like darkness. The imagination of the heart is like a burning lamp. The imagination of the belly is like a burning candle. The imagination of the navel is like the rays of the sun. The imagination of the genitals is like fire. The imagination of the seat is like moonlight.

They have demonstrated every one of these subjects, but since discussion of that cannot conceivably be very useful, this will be sufficient.

Yoga in Jain, Buddhist, and Hindu Tantric Traditions

8

A Digambara Jain Description of the Yogic Path to Deliverance

Paul Dundas

Jainism, a religious tradition whose historical origins reach back to the sixth or fifth centuries BCE and which takes its name from the Jinas, the omniscient teachers who are regarded as transmitting its truths throughout eternity, is typically Indian in its mapping out of a gradualistic path that can lead each human being to a state of moral and cognitive perfection and thence to deliverance from rebirth. Intrinsic to this path, one would suppose, must be some basic set of psychophysical transformative techniques that enable the practitioner to break free from spiritual shackles (particularly relevant in Jainism where the karma that diminishes the self's pristine functions is conceived of as a substance) and advance beyond the constraints of an undeveloped mode of being. Unfortunately, identification of a quintessential type of regularly enacted yogic technique within Jain tradition is not a straightforward matter, and it must be admitted that Jainism's general tendency to privilege the practice of modes of asceticism such as fasting over extended meditative activity has contributed to an unwillingness on the part of scholarship to countenance any clear alignment of Jain spiritual exercises with the much better known and widely studied Hindu yoga and Buddhist meditation. Nonetheless, the existence of an extensive pre-modern literature in Sanskrit, Prakrit, and other languages makes it clear that Jain practitioners have for centuries been preoccupied, at least at an idealized level, with the appropriate methods for bringing about inner cultivation and the restoration of the self's innate qualities.

The first evidence for some sort of meditative culture within Jainism occurs in the early scriptures written in Ardhamāgadhī (a vernacular-derived literary dialect), where the term *jhāṇa* and forms grammatically connected with it occasionally appear. This expression ultimately derives from the Vedic Sanskrit *dhī*, "inspiration brought about by superhuman forces," and is ubiquitous in Theravāda Buddhist literature, where (with the slightly different Pāli spelling of *jhāna*) it signifies a heightened but transient form of awareness akin to trance. The early Jain scriptures (whose origin in some form can be located approximately in the third or fourth century BCE) regularly refer to the "bright" (*sukka*) *jhāṇa*, which denotes a situation just short of death in which physical and mental activities have all but run their course and the meditator is grounded in complete existential stillness. Rather than being an advanced mode of experience which could be further cultivated, bright *jhāṇa* appears to have been envisaged as the state reached through the final relinquishing of karmic accretions whereby the senses have become inoperative, an inner attainment not unlike the advanced (and controversial) Buddhist meditative state called "attainment of cessation" (*nirodhasamāpatti*). Somewhat later and more schematic Ardhamāgadhī texts view bright *jhāṇa* as the culmination of a fourfold structure in which three antecedent mental meditations are styled respectively as "anguished" (*aṭṭa*), "fierce" (*rodda*), and "virtuous" (*dhamma*), with each of these four states of *jhāṇa* being further subdivided into four specifically focused varieties.

There can be no doubt that *jhāṇa* as described in early Jain texts does not readily conform to the conventional understanding of meditation as a type of inner reconfiguration. The first two varieties, in particular, reveal by their designations "anguished" and "fierce" that they were conceived of as relating to psychologically unproductive and self-preoccupied states of mind, harmful to oneself and others and engendering deleterious karma, which characterize much of the unawakened human condition. Both are to be abandoned as symptomatic of an individual's location on the spiritually inadequate early stages of the path to liberation (envisioned in standard Jain soteriology as involving ascent through fourteen successive stages called *guṇasthānas*). Virtuous *jhāṇa* involves pious activity and reflection relating to the excellence of the Jain religion and also consideration of the individual's moral actions and isolated location in a vast cosmos where rebirth as a human being is very rare. While this type of *jhāṇa* may have obviously positive transformative qualities when compared with the anguished and fierce types, it is in essence little more than a series of contemplative exercises, albeit of a relatively advanced sort. By around the middle of the first millennium CE, Jain teachers were stipulating that only those in possession of a particularly developed (and idealized) "diamond-hard" physical structure were authorized to cultivate the last two subvarieties of bright *jhāṇa*, and eventually the attainment of this culminating type of *jhāṇa* as a whole, along with deliverance itself, came to be regarded as an unrealistic aspiration in this particular debased era in which the *arhat*s, or omniscient ones, could no longer exist.

The term "yoga" is commonly employed in Jainism to refer to the physical, mental, and vocal modalities of the body brought about by any karmically induced movement of the incorporeal self (*jīva*); it can also denote the combination (*yoga*) of right faith, right knowledge, and right conduct, the so-called Three Jewels. The highly influential Haribhadra (ca. eighth century CE) seems to have been the first member of the Śvetāmbara sect to identify yoga in its more familiar sense of a structured sensory and physical discipline oriented toward gnosis as the necessary condition for deliverance from rebirth. Haribhadra's creative perspective on yoga is most clearly exemplified in his "Collection of Views on Yoga" (*Yogadṛṣṭisamuccaya*) in which he juxtaposes his own interpretation of Jain practice with aspects of yogic methods found in a variety of Hindu and Buddhist systems to produce an integrated soteriological path of eight stages, most likely consciously reflecting Patañjali's model in the *Yoga Sūtra*, which privileged truth and moral and practical efficacy over sectarian allegiance. A later Śvetāmbara monk, Yaśovijaya (1624–1688), who seems to have viewed himself as extending Haribhadra's intellectual enterprise, produced two little-studied commentaries on the *Yoga Sūtra*, and elsewhere in his writings he speaks approvingly of Patañjali as an authoritative teacher who was genuinely oriented toward deliverance. However, Śvetāmbara philosophers have generally been uneasy about excessively facile equivalences between Jain and non-Jain soteriological path structures, and the Samkhyan ontological categories to which Patañjali's yoga system is to a large extent linked have been consistently deemed unacceptable.

The religious experience of Jains is a much more complex historical and social phenomenon than the simple essentializing designation "Jainism" would permit, and in light of the extensive contribution of monks of the Digambara sect to Jain yogic culture, it would be particularly misguided to view this subject through an exclusively Śvetāmbara prism. The bifurcation of the early Jain community was undoubtedly a long, drawn-out process, with its most obvious feature—namely, the emergence by around the fifth century CE of separate renunciant orders in which monks either were "white robed" (*śvetāmbara*) or "naked" (*digambara*)—obscuring major sectarian differences relating to control over an emerging canon of scriptural texts. The Digambaras rejected the Ardhamāgadhī scriptures of the Śvetāmbaras and instead based their claims to represent authentic Jainism on extensive texts written in a dialect called Śaurasenī. According to their monastic redactors, these were drawn from the residue of a group of fourteen scriptures known as the Pūrvas, which supposedly had been preached by the Jinas, but which were subsequently lost due to temporal decline. These Digambara texts, which relate to ontological, cosmological, and disciplinary matters, are invariably highly technical and, viewed historically, no doubt reflect the various totalizing intellectual projects that were a feature of Indian religio-philosophical systems in the early centuries of the first millennium CE. In particular, the "Scripture in Six Parts" (*Ṣaṭkhaṇḍāgama*), the most significant early Digambara work, evinces a strong analytical preoccupation with the self and the complex modifications it undergoes through beginningless interaction with the multifarious varieties of karma.

This intense focus on the nature and centrality of the self is a defining characteristic of Digambara Jainism as a soteriological path and finds its most compelling articulation in the Śaurasenī writings of Kundakunda. The dating of this celebrated but mysterious poet remains a subject of scholarly disagreement; the standard Digambara location of him in the second or third century CE is almost certainly too early, and there can be no doubt that some of the works attributed to him are apocryphal, while others have been subject to interpolation. Nonetheless, these considerations in no way diminish the power of Kundakunda's yogic vision and the influence his major works were to have on later Digambara tradition. Kundakunda proposes a radical soteriology, which relates not to an external goal but to innermost experience wherein the self as both agent and object of knowledge is the only significant reality and represents by its own nature the very state of deliverance itself. Jain teaching proposes that the self in its purest form is non-material, omniscient, and in possession of the qualities of perfect insight, bliss, and energy, and that these attributes have been either drastically diminished or totally eliminated because of karmic accretions peculiar to each individual. Kundakunda employs a perspectivist framework to establish that from the higher or absolute standpoint, (called *niścayanaya*) everything external or "other" (*para*) to the self has merely a provisional transactional validity, which should be understood on the basis of the worldly standpoint (called *vyavahāranaya*). In this light, only the self in its purest form can claim soteriological salience. Such an interiorization of truth as a form of yogic reality entails that ostensibly central Jain disciplinary practices such as fasting are only valid in the transient world of rebirth, whereas the self in its authentic form is unconditioned by any external factors, whether morally positive or negative, and so can never be truly modified by ascetic activity or karmic influx. Deliverance is accordingly envisaged by Kundakunda as the direct experience by the self of its own pure and unconditioned nature as a totally independent entity.

Kundakunda's strongest premodern influence was to come at a time when Digambara Jainism had very much declined in significance, at least in terms of numbers of adherents. In the seventeeth century, the Adhyātma ("Spiritual") movement, a group of lay intellectuals based in Jaipur and Agra, extensively reframed (often on the basis of earlier Sanskrit interpretations) and disseminated in vernacular poetic form a number of his works, including his "Essence of the Doctrine" (*Samayasāra*). The Adhyātma movement's deritualized and introspective brand of Digambara Jainism remains significant to this day. Learned Sanskrit commentaries on Kundakunda's works are nowhere to be found until the tenth and eleventh centuries, another argument for pushing his dates forward. At about the same time a number of Sanskrit poetic treatises appeared, which integrated Kundakunda's insights concerning the true nature of the self into a more developed yogic path, while also displaying a revived interest in *dhyāna* (the Sanskrit equivalent of *jhāṇa*), a topic which by this time had largely become redundant in mainstream Śvetāmbara discourse. The *Tattvānuśāśana*, or "Instruction in Reality," is an impressive example of such a treatise.

Rāmasena was a Digambara monk who can probably be dated to some time in the first half of the tenth century and is otherwise largely obscure. Quotations from the "Instruction in Reality" found in the works of the thirteenth-century lay scholar Āśādhara establish an upper limit of 1228 for Rāmasena's poem, beyond which it seems to have been little known until modern times. The rather mundane title of the "Instruction in Reality" obscures the fact that this work is not a simple discussion of the various categories of reality (*tattva*s), which are the routine subject of Jain philosophizing, but rather deals with the deepest dimensions of experience when stripped of all material and pyschological cloaking. It should, however, be emphasized that the "Instruction in Reality" is not some sort of personalised description of Rāmasena's own yogic realization. Autobiographical accounts of religious experience were unknown in Jainism prior to the seventeenth century, and Rāmasena should best be regarded as providing a kind of blueprint describing the various transformative stages that cumulative Digambara tradition suggested were likely to be passed through by the practitioner, who is variously designated in the "Instruction in Reality" as "monk" (*muni*), "yogin," "ascetic," and occasionally "good man" and "adept" (*sādhaka*). Rāmasena's regular use throughout the poem of the optative mood, which can have both an injunctive and a potential sense in Sanskrit, is indicative of his generalized presentation of yogic practice.

Although Rāmasena does sporadically engage in the philosophical schematizing characteristic of Jain ontological analysis and occasionally acknowledges the traditional gradualist structure of the fourteen stages to deliverance (e.g., at verse 221), his overall strategy in the "Instruction in Reality" is to describe the self and the pyscho-physical world within which it is located in terms of the two levels of truth as established in Kundakunda's interpretation of the soteriological path. The poem thus falls into approximately two halves, the second of which is translated below, together with a short section from the first half. In conforming to what might be dubbed a "mystical pattern" that intensely refocuses Jainism's basically dualist worldview, Rāmasena makes clear that when it is considered from the higher perspective to be an immanent experience (rather than something spatially or psychologically external), full engagement with the self in its true form through *dhyāna* affords immediate deliverance (verses 143–58 and 218–23). Nonetheless, Rāmasena also deploys to striking effect Jainism's standard soteriological vision of the siddha, the liberated self, as disembodied and completely free from the occluding effects of karma, rising to the crown of the universe to remain for eternity with the other liberated selves (verses 231–46). Most significantly, Rāmasena draws on the resources of a mantric culture that had developed within Digambara Jainism in the latter part of the first millennium CE. Here, the power of extended liturgical utterances—such as the most important Jain mantra, the "Homage to the Five Supreme Beings" (that is, liberated selves, arhats, teachers, preceptors, and monks), or the single word "arhat" (sometimes used in the spelling "arha" or "arhaṃ")—could be ritually harnessed and absorbed, thus enabling access to various forms of advanced attainment (verses 183–86). Simply labeling passages describing these procedures as "Tantric" may not be rigorous enough, since even in scholarly discourse this designation has frequently become little more than a generic term for a whole range of yogic activities, from the mildly esoteric or interiorized to the wildly antinomian. However, there can be no doubt that, in common with other contemporary Digambara writers on yoga such as the circa tenth-century Śubhacandra, whose seminal "Ocean of Knowledge" (*Jñānārṇava*) remains untranslated into any western language, Rāmasena deploys a strongly ritualized idiom. Much of this may derive from Saivism, such as the monastic yogin's manipulation of mantras within mandalas, his use of ritually demarcated space, the practice of magic rites, and temporary transformation into various superhuman figures such as the twenty-third Jina Pārśva, the divine bird Garuḍa who is the enemy of poisonous snakes (thus enabling the curing of diseases), the god of love, and Indra, the king of the gods (verses 200–216). However, subtle body systems, which were a feature of Hindu *haṭha yoga* and also permeated Buddhism from around the eighth century, find no place in Rāmasena's description (see the elliptical verse 181). There can, nonetheless, be occasionally identified a slight Buddhist tinge to the "Instruction in Reality," as for example when Rāmasena refers in a positive sense to *nairātmya*, the "absence of self" (verses 174 and

176), an expression regularly used in Buddhist discourse but at variance with the Digambara perspective, as well as to *mahāmudrā* (verse 202), a term frequently occurring in Vajrayāna Buddhism in the sense of direct experience of non-duality, but here most likely denoting a ritually instrumental hand gesture (*mudrā*).

At the outset of the "Instruction in Reality" (verses 1–80; not translated below), Rāmasena establishes that the Jinas, the omniscient teachers, have described the path to deliverance in basic terms of abandoning what is karmically negative and espousing what is karmically positive. Then, after briefly referring to the role of the two levels of truths in providing a more profound soteriological framework for what is to follow, he proceeds to describe the virtuous type of *dhyāna* as the most appropriate form of meditative activity for those on the intermediate stages of the path in current times. No doubt in acknowledgment of Patañjali's system (if not that of the Śvetāmbara teacher Haribhadra), Rāmasena refers to the "eight limbed" means of practicing yoga, which is linked with *dhyāna* as involving a totally stable control of the mind and orientation toward the self. This necessary conquest of the senses can be facilitated by *svādhyāya* ("study of texts"), which entails either a simple recitation of the "Homage to the Five Supreme Beings" mantra or the study of scriptures. Rāmasena continues by establishing (verses 82–96; cf. verses 218–23 and 229) that, contrary to the traditional view, there is nothing that precludes the practice of dhyāna in this particular temporal phase, and he accordingly describes the appropriate physical and mental environment for this. After providing this general account of the necessary preliminaries to *dhyāna*, Rāmasena then identifies (verses 100–37; not translated below) as particularly efficacious foci for meditative energy syllables of power, such as those constituting the name "arhat," which can be ritually superimposed on various parts of the body, and the fully visualized figure of the Jina with his many distinguishing marks and superhuman attributes. However, these objects of *dhyāna*, powerful and lofty though they might be, relate to what is different from the self when envisaged from the worldly perspective. The remainder of the "Instruction in Reality," Rāmasena asserts, will pertain to the innermost self as viewed from the absolute perspective.

The "Instruction in Reality" has not hitherto been translated into a western language. Rāmasena's language, while grammatically relatively simple, is nonetheless tightly packed and, a few similes apart, shows little sign of any developed aesthetic concerns. Repetition is an important part of its idiom, and it is accordingly not easy for a translator to differentiate between frequently recurring and seemingly interchangeable words used by Rāmasena to refer to "the self," such as "*sva*" (literally "one's own"); "*ātman*" (which can have a reflexive sense of "oneself" as well as signifying "the self"); and "*jīva*," a term of Jain ontology literally denoting "life" or, more technically, "life-monad" (see verse 152), one of the six fundamental entities in the Digambara Jain description of reality (the others being motion, stasis, atoms, space, and time). I have, however, avoided translating any of these Sanskrit expressions as "soul," since for many modern readers this has become either an excessively overcoded or near meaningless term. For convenience, I have translated *dhyāna* throughout as "meditation."

Rāmasena's *Tattvānuśāsana* was first edited in 1918 on the basis of a single manuscript by the celebrated Digambara paṇḍit Nathuram Premi (Bombay: Manikcand-Digambara-Jain Granthamala, vol. 13, pp. 1–23), who attributed the work to a teacher called Nāgasena. A much fuller edition based on several manuscripts was published in 1963 (Delhi: Visevamandir Trust) by another prominent Digambara scholar, Jugalkishor Mukhtar, who as early as 1920 had made a convincing case for identifying the work's author as Rāmasena. Impressive though Mukhtar's extensive Hindi commentary undoubtedly is, there remain difficulties with some of his readings of the Sanskrit text, and in preparing the translation below I have accordingly availed myself where it seemed appropriate of the 1993 edition of the *Tattvānuśāsana* by Bharatsagarji (Datiya: Bharatvarsiya Anekant Vidvat Parisad), who, however, follows Premi in attributing the work's authorship to Nāgasena.

Suggestions for Further Reading

Appreciation of Rāmasena's "Instruction in Reality" and its milieu is enhanced by familiarity with other Digambara poems of similar theme and style. The eleventh-century *Dhyānastava* of Bhāskaranadi has been edited and translated into English by Suzuko Ohira (Varanasi: Bharatiya Jnanapitha, 1973) who also provides a valuable introduction. One of the most interesting texts of the Digambara yogic tradition is Yogīndu's *Paramātmaprakāśa*, which has been elegantly translated into French by Nalini Balbir and Colette Caillat as *Lumière de l'Absolu* (Paris: Éditions Payot & Rivages, 1999). This anthology of one hundred verses, composed in the medieval literary language called Apabhraṃśa, is often dated to the sixth century CE, but it is more likely approximately contemporary with the "Instruction in Reality." While Yogīndu unquestionably stands in the same Digambara yogic tradition as Kundakunda and Rāmasena, his verses also contain notable similarities with the *dohā* songs of the late Buddhist siddha poets. See Friedhelm Hardy, "Creative Corruption: Some Comments on Apabhraṃśa Literature, Particularly Yogīndu," in *Studies in South Asian Devotional Literature: Research Papers 1988–1991*, ed. Alan W. Entwistle and Françoise Mallison (New Delhi and Paris: Manohar and École Française d'Extrême Orient 1994), pp. 3–23. Rāmasena's approximate contemporary, the Śvetāmbara teacher Hemacandra, had a particularly encompassing sense of what was entailed by yoga, as is evinced by his *Yogaśāstra*, effectively a summa of Jain practice. Possible overlaps between this work and Rāmasena's "Instruction in Reality" in respect to advanced yogic cultivation can be gauged from Olle Qvarnström, "Jain Tantra: Divinatory and Meditative Practices in the Twelfth Century *Yogaśāstra* of Hemacandra," in *Tantra in Practice*, ed. David Gordon White (Princeton, NJ: Princeton University Press, 2000), pp. 595–604.

There exists no systematic discussion of the historical development of meditation and yoga in Jainism in any western language, although a useful if insufficiently analytical beginning has been made by Sadhvi Uditaprabha "Usha" in her Hindi study, *Jain Dharm meṃ Dhyān kā Aitihāsik Vikās Kram* (Byavar: Muni Sri Hajarimal Smrti Prakashan, 2007). It should be noted that, its title notwithstanding, R. Williams' *Jaina Yoga: A Survey of the Medieval Śrāvakācāras* (London: Oxford University Press, 1963) in fact relates to the monastic literature legislating for lay behavior which barely mentions the topic of meditation. This work can, however, be consulted for a description of *sāmāyika*, the brief period of mental and physical withdrawal from worldly concerns which is the form of contemplative activity most frequently engaged in by devout Jains, even if it plays no part in Rāmasena's description of the yogic path. See Williams, *Jaina Yoga* (pp. 131–39). The role of meditation in early Jainism and its commonality with styles of brahminic yoga are considered by Johannes Bronkhorst, *The Two Traditions of Meditation in Ancient India* (Stuttgart: Franz Steiner 1986, pp. 29–41). Haribhadra's approach to yoga is discussed by Christopher Key Chapple in *Reconciling Yogas: Haribhadra's Collection of Views on Yoga* (Albany: State University of New York Press, 2003). For the historical position of the Digambaras within Jainism, see Paul Dundas, *The Jains*, 2d ed. (London and New York: Routledge, 2002), pp. 46–49 and 120–25; and for a clear overview of Digambara yogic practices, see P. S. Jaini, *The Jaina Path of Purification*, 2d ed. (Delhi: Motilal Banarsidass, 2001), pp. 251–58. The best account of Kundakunda's works is provided by W. J. Johnson, *Harmless Souls: Karmic Bondage and Religious Change in Early Jainism with Special Reference to Umāsvāti and Kundakunda* (Delhi: Motilal Banarsidass, 1995). The seventeenth-century Adhyātma movement of Digambara laymen and its aftermath are described in the fascinating study by John E. Cort, "A Tale of Two Cities: On the Origins of Digambar Sectarianism in North India," in *Multiple Histo-*

ries: *Culture and Society in the Study of Rajasthan*, ed. Lawrence A. Babb, Varsha Joshi, and Michael W. Meister (Jaipur and New Delhi: Rawat Publications 2002), pp. 39–83.

Rāmasena: Instruction in Reality, Verses 82–96 and 143–247

THE LEGITIMACY OF MEDITATIVE PRACTICE

82. Those who assert that this is not the appropriate temporal period to engage in meditation themselves proclaim their ignorance of the Jain doctrine.

83. In this respect the supreme Jinas no doubt do forbid the practice of bright meditation today, but they have authorized the performance of virtuous meditation for those proceeding along the two advanced paths intended for laymen and monks, which respectively involve the suppression and total elimination of karma.

84. The traditional statement that meditation is for the person of a diamond-hard body was made with reference only to bright meditation as practiced while on these two advanced paths, and does not prohibit those on the lower stages from engaging in less advanced types of meditative practice.

85. Even if there are at this moment no meditators fully immersed in the ocean of the scriptures, why should others of more limited scriptural knowledge not meditate in accord with their ability?

86. If today there are none who follow advanced methods, why can other ascetics not practice according to their ability?

THE APPROPRIATE CIRCUMSTANCES FOR MEDITATION

87. He who practices continually, following the instruction of a qualified teacher, will see the conditions for meditation arise through his skill in mental focus.

88. As branches of learning, no matter how extensive, become fixed in the mind through repetitive study, so meditation becomes fixed for practitioners.

89. When a meditator with the appropriate characteristics endeavors to meditate, let him be of firm resolve and, after making due preparations, engage in practice in the following manner:

90. In an empty house, or in a cave, by day or alternatively by night, beyond range of women, animals, those of ambiguous gender, insects and plants, and low caste people also,

91. Or in some other place, reputable, pure, level, free from all animate and inanimate hindrances to meditation,

92. Seated at ease on the ground or on a rock, or standing, with body straight, upright and extended, limbs motionless,

93. With eyes firmly fixed on the tip of the nose, breath measured, engaging in mental abandonment of the body in a manner free from the thirty-two faults,

94. Carefully withdrawing the thieving senses from external objects, removing thought from all things and focusing it solely on the object of meditation,

95. Giving up sleep, fearless, continually energetic, one should meditate upon one's self or what is different from it in order to bring about inner purity.

96. According to scripture, meditation is twofold when viewed from the absolute perspective and the worldly perspective respectively. The former depends upon one's self, the latter upon what is different from that.

143. He who desires to meditate, confidently knowing his self and what is different from it as they both are, should understand, should witness only his self, abandoning anything else as worthless.

144. Before this, he should prepare and train himself by considering scripture. Then, attaining one-pointedness in respect to that, he should not think about anything further.

145. He who does not initially engage in reflection upon scripture out of fear of indulging in inadequate conceptualization is continually deluded about his self and thinks about the external only.

THE SELF AS OBJECT OF MEDITATION

146. Therefore, in order to destroy delusion, to bring consideration of what is external to an end, and to bring about one-pointedness, he should concentrate upon his own self first of all in the following manner:

147. "I am sentient, of innumerable space points, free from corporeality, a pure self whose nature is that of the liberated self, characterized by knowledge and insight.

148. I am not what is other, the other is not me, I am not part of the other, the other is not within me. The other is other and I am I. The other belongs to the other and I am mine.

149. The body is one thing and I am another; I am consciousness while the body is unconscious. It is manifold and I am single; it is transient and I am eternal.

150. I will not be an unconscious thing, nor am I an unconscious thing. I consist of knowledge; no one belongs to me and I belong to no one.

151. The connection of owner and owned that I had with my body and the confusion about the apparent unity of the two derive from another cause, not from one's own true nature.

152. In this world, seeing by the self within the self that same self which consists of knowledge of the actuality of fundamental entities such as the life-monad, I am then indifferent to material objects.

153. I am the true entity, I am consciousness, I am the knower and seer. I am eternally neutral. I am measured by the body I have taken to myself, and beyond that I am incorporeal, like the sky.

154. Being existent, I accordingly exist continually from the fourfold perspective of form, place, time and nature. From the standpoint of the form, place, time and nature of what is other, however, I am very much non-existent.

155. I am not my body and sense organs, since they do not know anything, have not known anything and will never know anything.

156. I am truly that entity which is consciousness, which knew thus previously, which will know in another manner and actually knows in this manner at this very moment.

157. This world is neither to be innately wished for nor hated, but to be viewed with equanimity. I am not one who desires or hates, but rather one who is naturally indifferent.

158. The body and senses are separate from me and I am truly different from them. I am nothing of these and they are also nothing of me."

THE NATURE OF EXPERIENCE OF SELF

159. So, having correctly considered that one's self is different from anything else and making one's inner disposition identical with it, one should not think about anything else.

160. Absence of thought is not a simple absence for Jains, as it is for those of false religious views. Rather it is an experiencing of oneself in the form of insight, knowledge and equanimity.

161. The yogin's experience of himself by the self and his being the agent of experience is called "self apperception" (*svasaṃvedana*), an understanding of oneself akin to seeing.

162. This has no other cause because it takes the form of knowledge of one's own self and what is other. Therefore one should abandon thought and experience it through consciousness of the self.

163. Because the self takes the form of insight, knowledge and equanimity, in knowing and seeing one becomes neutral. Let that self—which is consciousness in both general and specific terms—be experienced by one's own same self.

164. With the self one should perceive the self which is always different from all those inner states that arise from karma, its nature knowing, neutral.

165. So then one can experience freely one's neutral nature in the self, which is lacking any obsession with the false and what is wrong knowledge.

166. It certainly cannot be witnessed with knowledge gained from the senses because it lacks form and other tangible aspects. Sensory judgments cannot themselves actually see because they are imprecise conjectures.

167. However, when both senses and mind have been restrained, that which is beyond the senses is particularly clear. Witness that form which is to be experienced internally with consciousness of one's self.

168. Although the body is not luminous, consciousness in the form of knowledge can be seen spontaneously, shining in its independence.

169. If the self that consists of knowledge is not experienced by the yogin when in deep concentration, then he is not meditating but merely indulging in delusion-like swooning.

170. In experiencing that self, he reaches a state of supreme one-pointedness and thus attains bliss based on the self, which is beyond the range of speech.

171. As a lamp in a windless place does not flicker, so this yogin who is grounded in his own self does not abandon one-pointedness.

172. And then for that one who sees his own self in himself nothing appears other than supreme one-pointedness, even though external objects continue to exist.

173. Hereby the self, while empty of other things, is not innately empty. This self, whose nature is both empty and non-empty, is apprehended by the self alone.

174. And from it comes that beholding of the self, properly excluded from other things, called the vision of the non-dual, complete selflessness that effects deliverance.

175. All internal states are in some way separate from each other. In the same manner as the external world is not truly connected with self, so the self is not connected with the world.

176. Selflessness means non-existence of other selves and that relates to the actual existence of one's own self. So insight into one's own self is true insight into selflessness.

177. In viewing the self when it is combined with what is different from it, one beholds what is dual. In seeing what is separate from other things, one sees the self as non-dual.

178. In seeing the self exclusively, one destroys karmic stains that have been

accrued. Having dispelled the state of "I" and "mine," one also wards off future karmic stains.

179. The more the meditator gains fixity in his own self, the more the conditions of his concentration will appear clearly.

180. This is the object of the two types of meditation, the virtuous and the bright. Understand the difference between the two in terms of differences in purity and practitioner.

TECHNIQUES OF MEDITATION

181. This meditation upon the self will be difficult to achieve through exclusive reliance on an understanding of a subtle body. Even what is known by the wise is not perceived quickly.

182. Therefore the intelligent should practice meditation based on an apprehension of the gross elements. For they can be perceived, manipulated and give visible and invisible results.

183. At the beginning of that practice one should successively focus upon the elements of wind, fire and water in order to create an appropriate body and effect purification.

184. Having filled and sustained the syllable "a" with wind, having burnt karma with his own body by means of the fire of the syllable "r," and having expelled the ash,

185. The mantric syllable "ha," pouring ambrosia on the self, must be meditated upon in the sky after one has constructed a new body, itself nectar and refulgent.

186. Then with utterances of the mantra of Homage to the Five Supreme Beings sequentially combined with the syllables of the five objects of meditation placed on the five main places on the body, after performing the ritual of integration,

187. One should then meditate upon the self as the *arhat* with his designated marks, or as the liberated self that has destroyed all karma, incorporeal, blazing with knowledge.

188. It might be argued that in meditating upon the self as *arhat* when it is not actually that eminent figure, yogins, while no doubt otherwise receptive, might be confused about whether they in fact are coming into contact with him.

189. That objection is incorrect. For I am referring at this juncture to the inner *arhat*, that is to say the self which is intent on meditation on the *arhat*. In this way one comes into contact with the *arhat* within that very self.

190. The yogin becomes identical with that inner state by which the self

develops. And thus, pervaded by meditation on the *arhat*, the self is by its nature the inner *arhat*.

191. The one who knows the self becomes identified with that inner state; through it he meditates upon that form which is the self, which is like crystal with all its attendant qualities.

192. Alternatively, it can be said that the self's modifications, future and past, which constitute the *arhat*'s nature, always exist substantially in all entities.

193. So this future modification that is the arhat is always present substantially among those qualified to gain deliverance. What confusion could there be for the yogin in meditating upon this?

194. Furthermore, if this were actually to be confused, then no result would come about from it. Thirst is never dispelled by a mirage.

THE IMMEDIATE RESULTS OF MEDITATION

195. Results appear in many guises, calm and fierce, for meditators according to their particular contemplative focus.

196. Being meditated upon by those who enter a state of concentration after gaining the instruction of a teacher, this self of limitless power bestows liberation and material enjoyment.

197. That self when meditated upon in the form of the *arhat* and the liberated self brings about liberation for the one experiencing his final body. For the person who has gained merit through meditation upon it, there arises worldly experience of what is different from the self.

198. Knowledge, good fortune, health, gratification, prosperity, good looks, fortitude and whatever else is esteemed in this world come about for the one who meditates on the self.

199. Having seen one who is suffused with meditation on the self, the great planets tremble. Ghosts and witches are put to flight, while fierce creatures instantly become tame.

200. The meditator, with mind pervaded by contemplation of that god who is able to perform any action, becomes identified with him and so achieves his desire.

201. Deploying the mighty hand gesture, the mighty mantra and the mighty mandala, the yogin, in becoming Lord Pārśva, is in possession of a body made fully integrated.

202. And in directing his mind as appropriate on meditative foci such as fire, he quickly governs and controls the powerful planets.

203. Himself now becoming Indra in the middle of the great mandala, with

crown, earrings, and holding a vajra-weapon while wearing yellow clothes and other ornaments,

204. Garnering his breath, with fingers in the "stopping" gesture, uttering the mantra that effects immobility, with mind concentrated he performs all the magic rituals of immobilization.

205. Spontaneously becoming Garuḍa, the divine bird and enemy of serpents, he destroys poison in an instant, and then having become the god of love he leads the world into his power.

206. Turning into the god of fire, he accordingly becomes surrounded with hundreds of blazing flames, and on enveloping a sick man with them he can quickly remove a feverish chill.

207. Becoming composed of nectar and raining ambrosia down on that same sick man, the yogin then takes his burning fever into himself and dispels it.

208. Having then become composed of the Ocean of Milk, laving the entire world, the yogin performs calming and restoratative rituals for embodied creatures.

209. Why say more? The yogin can take the form of a god and bring about whatever he desires to perform.

210. Calm when engaged in calm action and fierce when engaged in fierce action, this adept yogin accordingly masters calm and fierce actions.

211. Attracting, bringing into one's power, immobilizing, causing stupefaction, moving at speed, removing the effects of poison, calming, bring about aversion, disturbance and restraint:

212. Meditators can perform magic actions of these sorts. They give rise to no ambivalence because a state of complete integration has come to fruition for such yogins.

213. Filling the body with breath, expelling and retaining it, burning, inundating, unifying, magical gestures, mantras, mandalas and foci of contemplation,

214. The appearances of gods who oversee action, their external characteristics, throne, authority, vehicle, energy, birth, name, refulgence, location in the cardinal directions,

215. The number of their arms, faces and eyes, their nature, fierce or otherwise, color, touch, voice, state, clothing, ornament and weapon—

216. Knowledge of things of this sort and whatever else is described in texts relating to mantras that bring about calm and fierce action: such are the attendant features of meditation,

217. For meditation is the principal cause of whatever result comes about in this world and whatever result comes about in the next world.

THE NATURE OF BRIGHT MEDITATION

218. The main motivating factors for meditation are the following: the instruction of a teacher, faith, continual practice and a firm mind.

219. Yogins should not grasp after the worldly result that arises from meditative practice. It has been described simply to demonstrate the mighty power of meditation.

220. The fierce or anguished type of meditation is for those who desire mundane results only: therefore abandon these and practice the virtuous and bright forms.

221. The neutral knowledge of reality, which comes about in the eighth stage of the path and beyond and is pure because the stains of both good and evil have disappeared, is called bright.

222. It is bright because of its conjunction with pure qualities, completely spotless and still, like a ray of light from a precious stone, owing to the destruction or quiescence of the dustlike passions.

223. Adopting the Three Jewels of right faith, knowledge and practice, and abandoning the cause of bondage, practice meditation continually, O yogin, if you seek deliverance.

DELIVERANCE

224. For the yogin occupying his final body, his delusion disappearing because of the excellence of his meditative practice, deliverance comes about at that very moment, while for the one who is not occupying his final body it will come gradually.

225. To be precise, for the one who is not occupying his last body but who practices meditation continually, there will be a wearing away and warding off of all types of bad karma.

226. Merits in abundance flow in at every instant through which the yogin can first be reborn as a deity of great power among the gods in heaven.

227. There he dwells for a long time, drinking the ambrosia of pleasure enjoyed by the gods, delighting all the senses and extremely pleasing to the mind.

228. Then having descended to a happy rebirth in human form as an emperor or some such person and enjoying that existence for a long time, he abandons it of his own volition and takes initiation as a naked monk.

229. With body now hard as diamond, after engaging in the fourfold bright meditation and destroying all eight types of karma, he then attains imperishable deliverance.

230. Deliverance is complete separation from the cause of connection between self and karma. It results in qualities such as complete knowledge born of the total destruction of karma.

231. Through destruction of the binding of karma and through natural upward motion, the self, now liberated, in one instant rises to the crown of the world.

232. For so long as a mortal is in the world of rebirth there is physical contraction and expansion brought about by karma. In the state of liberation, however, these factors do not exist because of the destruction of those karmas that are their cause.

233. Thereupon, with a shape slightly smaller than the dimensions of his body that has been just abandoned, he remains there as a liberated being, constituted by his own qualities.

234. The mortal for whom karma has disappeared exists then in his own shape. There is no absence, nor lack of consciousness, nor consciousness without object.

235. The nature of every self reveals both itself and what is other. However, like the disc of the sun, its act of revealing does not derive from anything else.

236. When karma has disappeared, the self exists in its own form, just as a jewel exists through its innate causes when the dust clinging to it has disappeared.

237. It is not deluded, does not doubt, does not consider its own aims, is neither attached nor feels hatred, but exists in itself continually.

238. It then remains in a state of neutrality, a lord among the liberated, completely knowing and seeing the self, an object of knowledge in terms of past, present and future, just as it is.

239. And there, not regressing to rebirth, it experiences unchanging happiness consisting of limitless knowledge, insight, energy and desirelessness beyond the ordinary senses.

240. It might be asked what sort of happiness there can be in the state of deliverance for liberated selves who transcend the senses, since pleasure can only come about for one experiencing objects by sensory means.

241. If you think this to be so, then your view is no better than delusion, since even now, dear friend, you do not understand the nature of happiness and suffering.

242. The bliss of deliverance is known to be dependent on the self; it is without affliction, beyond the senses, unperishing and arising from the destruction of the noxious karmas.

243. A worldly pleasure that is passionate, transient, arising from both one-

self and what is different from that when conceived superficially, the cause of desire and vexation,

244. The basis of delusion, treachery, intoxication, anger, illusion and greed: this is in fact what suffering is, since it is the cause of the binding of further causes of suffering.

245. The pleasure that comes from the objects of the senses embodies the power of delusion. A sweet savor arising from something bitter is the result of the illusory influence of saliva.

246. The pleasure of emperors and of the gods in heaven is not equal to a fraction of the bliss of the liberated selves.

247. Therefore deliverance is described as the highest among the aims of men. And it is to be gained by the followers of Jain teachings only, not by others who hate the self.

—9—

Saraha's *Queen Dohās*

Roger R. Jackson

The *Queen Dohās* is part of a profound and paradoxical poetic trilogy celebrating the experience of the naturally awakened mind, purportedly sung for the people, queens, and king of an Indian city by a great adept (*mahāsiddha*) of Buddhist Tantric yoga named Saraha, the "Arrow Shooter."

The siddhas—traditionally said to number eighty-four—are venerated throughout the Tibetan cultural sphere as the supreme practitioners of the esoteric and often controversial systems for spiritual unification—yoga—that arose among Buddhists in north India in the final centuries of the first millennium CE. Their lives, as recounted in countless Tibetan hagiographies, exemplify the Tantric ideals of uncompromising wisdom, fearless compassion, and a willingness to employ any means, no matter how unconventional, to attain divine gnosis (*jñāna*) and hasten the liberation of deluded beings who wander from life to life. Their translated songs, ritual manuals, treatises, and commentaries are at the heart of the Tantra section of the Tengyur (*bstan 'gyur*), the portion of the Tibetan Buddhist canon devoted to explanation of the sūtras and Tantras taught by the Buddha and collected in the Kangyur (*bka' 'gyur*) portion of the canon. And, the various guru lineages they comprise serve as an important basis of inspiration and legitimization for Tibetan Buddhist religious orders, the most important of which are the Old Translation school—the Nyingma, and the New Translation schools—the Kagyü, Sakya, and Geluk.

Saraha is among the siddhas most celebrated by Tibetans, in part because he is regarded as one of the first—perhaps as early as the second century CE. He is renowned for his expertise in the highly elaborate and esoteric Yoginī Tantras, but primarily he is seen as the founder of a tradition of theory and practice focused on the "Great Seal," Mahāmudrā. First mentioned in early Tantras and gaining special prominence in the Yoginī Tantras, Mahāmudrā can denote many things—including a yogic hand gesture or a consort in sexual yoga practice—but it most often refers to the innately void, luminous, and blissful nature of the mind, a set of contemplative practices through which mind's nature is directly comprehended, and the liberated state of buddhahood achieved through that practice. In short, Mahāmudrā is the experience of the "natural mind." It became an important topic of discussion in Tibet, especially among the New Translation schools, and is central to the Kagyü order, which views the ground, path, and goal of Buddhist practice—whether based on the Tantras or the sūtras—in terms of Mahāmudrā. All Tibetan traditions regard Saraha as the source of a lineage that in India includes the great philosopher Nāgārjuna, the mountain hermit Śavari, the oil merchant and Yogī Tilopa (10th–11th century), and the scholar-turned-siddha Nāropa (956–1041); and in Tibet the great translator Marpa (1012–1097), the cave-dwelling poet-saint Milarepa (1052–1135), and the founder of institutional Kagyü, Gampopa (1079–1153).

Finalized in the early fourteenth century, the Tengyur contains some twenty-five works attributed to Saraha, most of which were introduced to Tibet in the eleventh and twelfth centuries. Around half are ritual or exegetical writings dedicated to such Tantric buddha-deities as the compassionate bodhisattva Avalokiteśvara, the protector Mahākāla, or the wrathful Yoginī Tantra deity Buddhakapāla ("Buddha Skull"). The other half are poetical texts, sometimes denoted as "adamantine songs" (*vajragīti*) or "performance songs" (*caryāgīti*) but most often identified by the common medieval Indian verse-form in which nearly all Saraha's songs were composed, the *dohā*. *Dohā*s are rhyming couplets—sometimes discrete, sometimes in connected series—that employ both common imagery and esoteric references to instruct their listeners or readers. The most important of Saraha's *dohā*-collections are those comprising the Core Trilogy (*snying po skor gsum*): the *People Dohās* (*dmangs do ha*), *Queen Dohās* (*btsun mo do ha*), and *King Dohās* (*rgyal po do ha*). The *People Dohās* is by far the best known of the three, but the other two have been influential as well.

Accounts of Saraha's life are many and various. In the best-known version, traceable to the eleventh-century Nepalese master Balpo Asu, he is a south Indian brahmin for whose sake a bodhisattva manifests as a female arrow-maker to teach him how to construct an arrow, and then to explain to him the symbolic Buddhist meaning of the arrow-making process and the arrow's various parts. Saraha is instantly liberated, and goes to live with the fletcheress in a cremation-ground, where he enjoys Tantric gatherings and sings adamantine songs. Beseeched by his subjects, the king tries to bring Saraha back to the brahmin fold. In response, Saraha teaches 160 *dohās* on Buddhist practice to the common people, eighty to the queens, and forty to the king himself.

Saraha remains in the kingdom, singing songs and performing good works, before dissolving into the enlightened realm in a "rainbow body."

Another well-known version of Saraha's life, found in Abhayadatta's twelfth-century hagiography of the eighty-four siddhas, depicts him as a brahmin living in the east Indian city of Roli. He practices Hinduism by day and Buddhist Tantra by night. Accused by other brahmins of indulging in drink, he is exonerated after effortlessly passing physical trials. He converts the people, queens, and king through his *dohās*, and then goes away with a fifteen-year-old girl, who serves as his cook, consort, and teacher. One day, as his companion is cooking radishes, Saraha enters a twelve-year contemplation. When he emerges from it, he asks her if the radishes are ready. She notes drily that they wouldn't keep and are now out of season, and upbraids him for his attachment, at which he attains Tantric awakening, the "accomplishment of Mahāmudrā" (*mahāmudrā-siddhi*), and together they ascend to the paradise of the awakened "sky-travellers" (*ḍāka*s or *ḍākinī*s).

Unfortunately, much of what Tibetan tradition claims about the life and works of Saraha is unreliable. As recent research has shown, Saraha is almost impossible to locate in time and place, and his works are in some cases of dubious authenticity. Kurtis Schaeffer has argued that "Saraha" is in fact largely a product of early first-millennium Tibet. Legends of his deeds cannot be traced earlier than the eleventh century, and the South Asian authors of these early hagiographies, such as Balpo Asu and Abhayadatta, were probably writing within a Tibetan cultural milieu, perhaps even in the Tibetan language. The same ambiguities attend much of Saraha's literary corpus. We have found very few Indic-language versions of works attributed to him, and possess most of his output only in Tibetan. As Ronald Davidson has noted, one hallmark of Tibetan interactions with Indians was the production of "grey texts," which purported to be Indian compositions translated into Tibetan but were actually Tibetan writings created by Indian scholars working in Tibet or by Tibetans collaborating with Indians. Tibetan scholars seeking to establish the Indian pedigree of canonical texts were well aware of this, and there was serious debate in Tibet over whether the *Queen* and *King Dohās* were composed by Saraha or by Balpo Asu, who introduced them to Tibet in the eleventh century; similar questions could be raised about other "Saraha" works.

Saraha is not, however, simply a Tibetan invention. His name turns up in at least one Indian guru lineage list, and a number of performance songs under his name in Old Bengali and several quite divergent versions of the *People Dohās* in the closely related Eastern Apabhraṃśa language have emerged from manuscript finds over the past century—evidence that "Saraha" was indeed known in India. Although many uncertainties remain about the provenance and authenticity of the writings attributed to him, in the absence of conclusive proof that he is *not* the author of the works under his name, we may provisionally draw some conclusions about him. If some form of Eastern Apabhraṃśa or Old Bengali was in fact a language he used, Saraha may have been a native of the eastern Gangetic region, where these languages were prevalent for several centuries before and after 1000 CE. Since he is named in texts datable to the mid-eleventh century and is the author of a commentary on the *Buddhakapāla*, a Yoginī Tantra of the late ninth or early tenth century, we may tentatively conclude that he lived sometime between 900 and 1050 CE. Finally, the meaning of Saraha's name suggests that at some point in his life he may have been either an archer or a fletcher. And he was, of course, a singer of songs and a writer of Tantric texts.

If Saraha was a denizen of the eastern Ganges region—present-day West Bengal and Bihar—during the tenth or early eleventh century, he probably lived under the aegis of the Pāla Empire, which dominated the area to one degree or another from the eighth through twelfth centuries, and was the last significant Indian dynasty to promote Buddhism. The Pāla realm covered the traditional heartland of Buddhism, including the site of the Buddha's awakening in Bodh Gayā, the former royal capital of Rājagṛha, and the great monastic university at Nālandā. Though their military and political fortunes waxed and waned, a succession of Pāla kings maintained and enhanced the ancient Buddhist sites; founded new monasteries and universities, such as Odanatapuri and Vikramaśīlā; supported the development of a distinctive, ornate school of sculpture and architecture; and assisted in the transmission of Buddhism to Tibet, first in the eighth century and then again during the eleventh and twelfth centuries.

The Buddhist culture of the Pāla dynasty was complex and somewhat polarized. On the one hand, great temples such as the Mahābodhi at Bodh Gayā thrived, and the monastic universities of Nālandā, Odantapuri, and Vikramaśīlā attracted students from throughout Asia to study the classics of Buddhist philosophy and master important Buddhist rituals. The curriculum at the great universities covered the monastic vows and basic categories of Foundational ("Hīnayāna") Buddhism, the philosophical speculation and ethical reflection of the Great Vehicle, Mahāyāna, and the panoply of esoteric approaches to metaphysics, contemplation, and ritual subsumed under the name Adamantine Vehicle (*vajrayāna*), Mantra Way (*mantranaya*), or Vehicle of the Tantras (*tantrayāna*). While the universities must at times have been hotbeds of argumentation and experimentation, they were above all institutions devoted to the preservation and transmission of mainstream academic and ritual traditions, and it should not surprise us that some Buddhists chafed at their restrictions and felt that genuine spiritual liberation only could be found outside their walls. This was particularly true of those attracted to the esoteric and sometimes transgressive ideas and practices found in the emerging Mahāyoga and Yoginī Tantras. Like the sūtras of Foundational and Mahāyāna Buddhism, these texts were treated as academic subjects in the universities, but their countercultural discourse made them far less amenable to full domestication.

The bearers of the Pāla Buddhist counterculture were the siddhas, who in many respects presented a radical alternative to the elite Buddhism of the Pāla court, the great temples, and the monastic universities. If their hagiographies are to be believed, some were brahmins, rulers, merchants, or monks, but most siddhas—whether by birth or choice—worked humbly as hunters, fishermen, weavers, wine-sellers, launderers, potters—or fletchers. They lived alone or in small communities of male and female practitioners, convening regularly for initiation ceremonies and Tantric ritual feasts. They were devoted to their gurus, practiced assiduously, and challenged the social and religious conventions of the day by drinking liquor, mocking brahmins and scholars, consorting with low-caste lovers, frequenting forests or cremation grounds, and singing songs that celebrated spontaneity and spiritual freedom. Primarily, they were adherents of the advanced Buddhist Tantric systems associated with the buddha-deities Guhyasamāja, Hevajra, and Cakrasaṃvara (also known as Heruka). The last two were especially favored, and their prominence shows that the religious milieu of the siddhas—hence of Saraha—was above all that of the Yoginī Tantras.

The Yoginī Tantras, which also include the systems of Caṇḍamahāroṣaṇa, Buddhakapāla, Vajrayoginī, and Kālacakra, were the final, and most controversial, flower of Tantric Buddhism in India. Most of them were composed between the eighth and eleventh centuries, and show signs of influence by Hindu Śaiva Tantras of the same era. Along with selected Mahāyoga Tantras (especially the *Guhyasamāja*), they were categorized by the Tibetan New Translation schools of the eleventh and following centuries as Unsurpassed Yoga Tantras (*niruttarayogatantra*). These were considered the Buddha's supreme teachings, for their rejection of arid scholasticism, their embrace of the sensory world, their employment of techniques for sublimating such basic drives as aggression and sex, their gnostic exploration of the nature and potential of the mind, their techniques for manipulation of the subtle or psychic body, and their insistence upon the Tantric yogi's freedom from normal social and religious constraints. Taken together, these were said to provide the surest means to buddhahood—Mahāmudrā—in a single life.

Their rhetoric notwithstanding, the authors of the Yoginī Tantras and related literature implicitly drew on the Foundational Buddhist articulation of the primacy and spiritual potential of mind; the distinction between a miserable cycle of rebirths (*saṃsāra*) and a calm and blissful liberated state (*nirvāṇa*); and the delineation of the path to freedom in terms of morality, concentration, and insight into the absence of an enduring self (*anātman*). They explicitly identified with Mahāyāna assertions that all beings possess buddha nature (*tathāgatagarbha*) and that the ideal practitioner is the selfless bodhisattva, who, motivated by the altruistic awakening mind (*bodhicitta*), engages the conventional world and works through skillful means (*upāya-kauśalya*) for the sake of wandering beings, while seeing that the nature of all phenomena—dharmas—is voidness (*śūnyatā*) and/or conception-only (*vijñaptimātra*). Like other Mahāyānists, they saw buddhahood as consisting of two bodies: a void, non-conceptual, omniscient, all-pervasive Dharma Body (*dharmakāya*), and a Form Body (*rūpakāya*) divisible into an Enjoyment Body (*sambhogakāya*) that teaches advanced bodhisattvas and an Emanation Body (*nirmāṇakāya*) that manifests in multiple ways for myriad beings. To these, an "Essential Body" (*svabhāvikakāya*) sometimes was added, either as the void aspect of the Dharma Body or as the unity of Dharma, Enjoyment, and Emanation bodies.

As in other, earlier Tantric systems, the central practice in the Yoginī Tantras is "deity yoga" (*devayoga*), whereby the practitioner assumes the mental, verbal, and physical attributes, and creates the environment, of the buddha-deity he or she will soon become. In this sense, where practitioners of sūtra-based traditions traverse a path that leads to a goal, Tantric practitioners take the goal and make it their path. Tantric practice invariably involves finding a qualified guru; receiving from him or her a ritual initiation (*abhiṣeka*) that introduces the deity and the deity's sacred environment, or mandala; and then, with the guru's guidance, undertaking the contemplative ritual, or *sādhana*, of the deity. In a typical *sādhana*, one reduces ordinary appearances to voidness; then from voidness recreates one's environment as a mandala and oneself as the deity; populates the mandala with its other inhabitants; utters evocative and powerful mantras; adopts bodily postures (*āsana*) and ritual hand-gestures (*mudrā*), utilizes symbolic implements such as a *vajra*, bell, or hand-drum; and finally dissolves the whole visualization back into voidness. In general, the Tantric practitioner maintains the "divine pride" that his or her body, speech, mind, environment, and companions all are sanctified and pure, and employs all possible means—including magic—for both worldly aims and the liberation of beings. This "dress-rehearsal" for awakening eventually will lead to the performance of actual buddhahood.

The Yoginī Tantras (like the Mahāyoga Tantras) add depth and complexity to these basics. Their deities are wrathful, sexually charged, and in many cases female: *yoginīs* or *ḍākinīs*. The guru is regarded as the deity incarnate, to whom one vows absolute obedience and loyalty. The higher initiations require the disciple to ingest fluids produced by the guru's ritual intercourse with a consort (*mudrā*) and to practice sexual yoga him- or herself, so as to sample the blissful gnosis whose perfection will be the aim of yogic practice. As in other Tantras, the basic Yoginī Tantra *sādhana* (the "generation phase" of practice) involves visualizing oneself as a deity at the center of an elaborate mandala, transforming one's way of seeing oneself and the cosmos in anticipation of changing one's actual mode of being in the final phase of the path. Advanced yogis are enjoined to adopt a lifestyle that deliberately cultivates eccentric and sometimes transgressive behavior, living in charnel grounds and practicing such "pure lamps" on the path as the ingestion of urine, feces, semen, blood, and marrow, or the flesh of human, cow, elephant, dog, and horse. They also are urged to undertake a series of transformative psychophysical yogas (the "completion phase") within the subtle body, with its network of channels (*nāḍī*s), focal points (*cakra*s), breath-related energies (*prāṇa*s), and hormonal "drops" (*bindu*s). Through forceful breathing or mantra-recitation, one brings the body's disparate energies from the side channels (the "sun" and "moon") into the central channel (*avadhūtī*), and moves drops up or down between the cakras to produce a series of four ecstasies (*ānanda*) and reveal the natural mind: a nonconceptual, non-dichotomous, and blissful gnosis that comprehends the voidness and luminosity of mind and all phenomena (*dharma*s)—also called the innate (*sahaja*), the primordial (*nija*), the real (*tattva*), suchness (*tathatā*), the ultimate sphere (*dharmadhātu*), mind itself (*cittatva*), truth (*arthatva*), actuality (*dharmatā*), the natural state (*svabhāva-sthiti*), the core (*garbha*), awareness (*vidyā*), luminosity (*prabhāsvara*), and Mahāmudrā. This gnosis usually is facilitated by sexual yoga with a consort, and may be deepened through contemplations that simulate the death-process—for the mind's true nature is said to be most manifest during sex and dying. Finally, gnosis is used as a basis for the attainment of Mahāmudrā: the transformation of the mind into a buddha's Dharma Body and the physical body into the Form Body, an achievement sometimes referred to as the "fourteenth stage" of bodhisattva practice.

It is immensely difficult to achieve buddhahood through Yoginī Tantra processes, for it requires a combination of devotion, wisdom, compassion, discipline, and skill that few possess. Yet paradoxically, the gnosis one seeks to uncover through Tantric practice is simply the natural mind, just as it has always been: primordially undivided, concept-free, luminous, void, and blissful. And while the siddhas advocated and practiced the Yoginī and other Tantras in their full complexity, they insisted at the same time that we must not complicate practice too much, and that if we dispense with conceptuality, abandon elaborate techniques, ignore traditional categories, and simply allow the mind to abide in its naturally awakened state, we will be buddhas right here and now. Like that of Zen, this Tantric "rhetoric of immediacy" is liable to misunderstanding, and begs a number of important questions: Is it really that easy? Are conventional concepts truly useless? Who is qualified for a practice so direct? Still, it formed an important part of late Indian Buddhist philosophical and contemplative discourse, and was carried over into Tibet, where, under one name or another—most often Dzokchen (*rdzogs chen*) or Mahāmudrā—it became more or less prominent in every Buddhist order. As noted earlier, Mahāmudrā was particularly central to the Kagyü, for whom it involved an unmediated experience of the natural mind taught as surely in the sūtras as in the Tantras. As we also know, the founder of the Mahāmudrā lineage in India was Saraha, and the texts comprising his Core Trilogy—the *People*, *Queen*, and *King Dohās*—were the Indian Mahāmudrā sources par excellence.

The *Queen Dohās*—more properly titled *A Dohā Treasury of Song-Instruction* or *An Inexhaustible Treasury of Song-Instruction*—are the least known or discussed of the Core Trilogy poems, and may not even have been composed by Saraha; yet they provide a sublime articulation of many of the Yoginī Tantra and Mahāmudrā themes outlined above, utilizing metaphor and simile, paradox and indirection, and a wide array of Buddhist terms to instruct the yogi in the proper way to buddhahood. The poem's eighty verses are divided into eight groups of ten, with each decade prefaced by the exclamation, "Amazing, the secret language of ḍākinīs!" The Tibetan commentator Karma Trinlepa (Karma 'phrin las pa, 1456–1539) gives a title to each of the eight sections, and we will follow these in outlining the poem's argument.

Section 1, "The Natural State," begins with homage to the "lord of bliss" who embodies the triple refuge of buddha, dharma, and saṅgha, and Saraha's promise to explain "the abiding state of naturally non-dichotomous Mahāmudrā." He goes on to outline many of the major themes to come: the natural purity of the mind, the essential voidness of dharmas, the futility of examining the mind's innate nature intellectually, the destructiveness of dichotomous thinking, and the bliss and freedom enjoyed by the yogi who has understood all this.

In section 2, "Pitfalls," each verse begins with the exclamation "Alas!" With a variety of evocative similes, Saraha warns the yogi against the spiritual mistakes that can divert one from the path, including mental distraction, excessive desire, obsession with hopes and fears, overconfidence in contemplation, failing to properly serve the guru, neglecting to receive initiation, discarding advice that has been imparted, breaking one's vows, engaging in base behavior, and losing oneself in complication.

Section 3, "Contemplation," is rife with paradox. It encourages the yogi to contemplate "non-dichotomous gnostic comprehension," even though that state utterly evades contemplative effort. It suggests the mind can be understood through sūtras on Perfect Wisdom, but insists its true nature is unattainable through any Tantra or treatise. Mind itself is said to be all there is but in fact "there is no mind." However, the yogi who transcends passion and hate, who relies on the guru and a consort, and whose mind is untroubled, reaches the "adamantine peak of the natural state," and is free to act like a drunk and live like an aimless river, full of gnostic bliss.

Section 4, "Encounter," begins with the claim that adamantine gnosis requires no Tantric rigamarole, that it is "lovely in its natural state." It should be the yogi's sole concern, and the guru's instruction is the only way to approach it. The guru gives instruction on seeing the sensory world as nothing but gnosis, and ultimately the guru *is* that gnosis, so all reality is "guru pointed out by guru." In the final verses of the section, Saraha begins to describe the eccentric yogi who, "aware that all things are suchness," roams the town, enters the royal palace, flirts with the women, and attains great bliss through the practice of sexual yoga at a Tantric feast.

In section 5, "Connection," Saraha continues his account of the eccentric yogi. He details the ideal qualities of a Tantric consort (here called *mahāmudrā*)—low-caste status, youth, physical beauty, passion, a mind "little given to concepts"—and then describes how the yogi initiates her, grants her gnosis, collects her "queenly fluids," and "fades into conceptless space." Saraha also describes the yogi's behavior more generally: with his hair in a topknot, adorned with copper and bone, and wrapped in animal skins, he frequents the bazaar, practices in the charnel-ground, and dances and sings at musical gatherings: "behaving without regard for dos and don'ts . . . his mind perpetually crazed, he performs the basest of deeds yet is free."

Section 6, "Commitment," focuses on the guru, who through initiation and instruction "shows all the manifold dharmas to be of a single taste," and "turns ignorance into awareness." The guru is said to be a king among physicians, and likened to a boat that "delivers us from *saṃsāra*'s deep vast sea." His gnosis shines like the sun, and he knows how to change all things into bliss as an alchemist turns metals to gold. The nectar of the guru's speech is the source of all realizations and attainments, so one should worship him at the crown of one's head and serve him devoutly and without ceasing.

In section 7, "Results," Saraha details the outcome of the practices taught by the guru. Often described as Mahāmudrā, here it is identified both with the mind's innate luminosity and the traditional buddha bodies of the Mahāyāna: "non-dichotomy devoid of is and isn't" is the Dharma Body, the mind's inherent bliss is the Enjoyment Body, "manifold guises for wandering beings" are the Emanation Body, and the gnosis of the indivisibility of these three is the Essential Body. The Dharma Body perfects one's own aims, while the Form

Bodies perfect the aims of others—and the unified gnosis that is the Essential Body renders worldly dangers harmless and destroys our greatest enemies: conceptuality and belief in self.

Section 8, "Instruction," concludes the poem by first reiterating a number of basic points: the yogi should not think in terms of virtue or vice, waste his time on labeling or logic, seek release from hopes or fears, or go on a spiritual quest, but rather let the mind settle into its space-like nature. Saraha adds that "mind at its core is free from virtues and faults," so even serving the guru, practicing contemplation, or behaving eccentrically are "based on falsehood and contrivance," and must be transcended, so that the yogi may reach the fourteenth and highest stage of the Tantric path, be "set in the inmost citadel of gnosis sublime," and "win Mahāmudrā for wandering beings."

What, then, is the yoga propounded by Saraha in the *Queen Dohās*? We may reasonably infer that it is above all that of the completion phase of the Buddhist Yoginī Tantras, during which—with initiation, instruction, and blessing from the guru—one attains buddhahood by revealing within the subtle body the innate bliss-void gnosis that is the true nature of ourselves and all things. This gnosis emerges through a variety of advanced techniques, including practicing sexual yoga, emptying the mind of concepts, and allowing awareness to settle into its primordial luminous nature—all within the context of the carefree, wandering life of an eccentric yogi. At the same time, because the key to achieving liberation is the realization of a voidness in which all conventions are obliterated, Saraha provides a counter-discourse wherein all ideas and practices, including those of the Yoginī Tantras, are negated as a "falsehood and contrivance" based on dichotomous thinking, which must be dropped in favor of the immediate and liberating experience of the natural mind: Mahāmudrā.

These two views of the path—as complex and subtle or simple and direct—appear to be in tension, but in the end they are complementary, for complex Tantric yogic practices never will succeed unless they, like everything, are dissolved at the appropriate time into the single taste of voidness; while a direct approach to innate gnosis, simple as it sounds, is virtually impossible without the profound preparation of body and mind that only the Tantras provide. Balancing the two, Saraha suggests, is the yogi's—and our—central task. If we wandering beings understand his song aright—and can maintain a stance that includes at once both affirmation and negation, devotion and critique, imagination and non-conceptuality, engagement and detachment, activity and inner stillness—then we will rest at ease in the natural mind from which we never strayed, and the Great Seal we never lost, Mahāmudrā, will be ours at last.

The translation that follows, from the Tibetan, is based primarily on the edition contained in the Derge Bstan 'gyur: Tōhoku catalogue no. 2264, rgyud 'grel, zhi 28b6–33b4; in A. W. Barber, ed., *The Tibetan Tripiṭaka: Taipei Edition* (Taipei: SMC, 1991, vol. 28, pp. 173/56/6–175/66/4). I have compared it with the version in the Peking Bstan 'gyur: Peking catalogue no. 3111, rgyud 'grel, tsi 34a2–39b5; in D. T. Suzuki, ed., *Tibetan Tripiṭaka: Peking Edition* (Tokyo: Tibetan Tripiṭaka Research Foundation, 1957, vol. 69, pp. 85/5/2–88/1/5). In the dozen-plus instances where a Peking reading seemed preferable to the Derge's, I have adopted it. I also have consulted the Tibetan commentary by Karma 'phrin las pa: *Btsun mo do ha'i ṭī ka 'bring po sems kyi rnam thar ston pa'i me long*, in *Do ha skor gsum gyi ṭi ka 'bring po sems kyi rnam thar ston pa'i me long: A commentary on the three cycles of dohā composed by the great Saraha* (Thimphu: Druk Sherig Press, 1984, pp. 217–315).

The Indic-language original of the *Queen Dohās*, assuming there was one, would have consisted of a series of rhymed couplets, but when *dohā*s and most other Indic verse forms were translated into Tibetan, they were split into four lines; my translation reflects the Tibetan approach. I have tried to render Saraha's verses in a style that is true to the original but also reflects his informality and directness: the poem, after all, was meant to be instructive without being pedantic. For a philosophically complex translation of the text, keyed to Karma 'phrin las pa's commentary, see Herbert Guenther, *Ecstatic Spontaneity: Saraha's Three Cycles of Dohā* (Berkeley: Asian Humanities Press, 1993, pp. 123–49). Finally, a note on gender: Although men and women could and did practice Tantra, most of the literature assumes a male subject. This is clearly the case in the *Queen Dohās*, so I have for the most part rendered pronouns accordingly.

Suggestions for Further Reading

For a critical perspective on Saraha, see Kurtis Schaeffer, *Dreaming the Great Brahmin: Tibetan Traditions of the Buddhist Poet-Saint Saraha* (New York: Oxford University Press, 2005). On the era in which Saraha was introduced to Tibet, see Ronald Davidson, *Tibetan Renaissance: Tantric Buddhism in the Rebirth of Tibetan Culture* (New York: Columbia University Press, 2005). For a complete translation of the Core Trilogy, see Herbert Guenther, *Ecstatic Spontaneity: Saraha's Three Cycles of Dohā* (Berkeley: Asian Humanities Press, 1993); for the *People Dohās* only, see David Snellgrove, "Saraha's Treasury of Songs," in Edward Conze, ed., *Buddhist Texts Through the Ages* (New York: Harper & Row, 1954), Roger Jackson, *Tantric Treasures: Three Collections of Mystical Verse from Buddhist India* (New York: Oxford University Press, 2004), and Schaeffer,

Dreaming the Great Brahmin; for performance songs, see Per Kværne, *An Anthology of Buddhist Tantric Songs: A Study of the Caryāgīti* (Oslo/Bergen/Tromsø: Universitetsforlaget, 1977).

For background on Saraha's Indian context, see S. B. Dasgupta, *Obscure Religious Cults* (Calcutta: Firma KLM Private Limited, 1969 [1946]); James Robinson, *Buddha's Lions: The Lives of the Eighty-Four Siddhas* (Berkeley: Dharma Publishing, 1979); David White, *The Alchemical Body: Siddha Traditions in Medieval India* (Chicago/London: University of Chicago Press, 1996) and *Kiss of the Yoginī: "Tantric Sex" in Its South Asian Contexts* (Chicago /London: University of Chicago Press, 2003); David Snellgrove, *Indo-Tibetan Buddhism* (Boston: Shambhala, 2002 [1987]); Ronald Davidson, *Indian Esoteric Buddhism: A Social History of the Tantric Movement* (New York: Columbia University Press, 2002); and Rob Linrothe, *Holy Madness: Portraits of Tantric Siddhas* (New York/Chicago: Rubin Museum of Art/Serindia Publications, 2006).

Translations of Yoginī Tantras include David Snellgrove, *The Hevajra Tantra: A Critical Study*, 2 vols. (London/New York: Oxford University Press, 1959); Christopher George, *The Caṇḍamahāroṣaṇa Tantra, Chapters I–VIII. A Critical Edition and English Translation* (New Haven: American Oriental Society, 1974); Shiníchi Tsuda, *The Saṃvarodaya Tantra, Selected Chapters* (Tokyo: The Hokuseido Press, 1974); and David Gray, *The Cakrasaṃvara Tantra: A Study and Annotated Translation* (New York: American Institute of Buddhist Studies, 2007). On Mahāmudrā, see G. N. Roerich, *The Blue Annals* (Delhi: Motilal Banarsidass, 1976 [1949]); Dakpo Tashi Namgyal, *Mahāmudrā: The Moonlight; Quintessence of Mind and Meditation*, trans. Lobsang Lhalungpa (Boston: Wisdom Publications, 2006 [1986]); and Roger Jackson, "Mahāmudrā," in Lindsay Jones, ed., *Encyclopedia of Religion*, 2d ed., vol. 8, pp. 5596–6001 (Detroit: Wadsworth Gale, 2005).

Saraha's Queen Dohās

[TITLE INFORMATION]

In the Indian language: *Dohakoṣopadeśagītināma* [*A Dohā Treasury of Song-Instruction*]. In the Tibetan language: *Mi zad pa'i gter mdzod man ngag gi glu zhes bya ba* [*An Inexhaustible Treasury of Song-Instruction*].

[TRANSLATOR'S HOMAGE]

I prostrate to the ever-youthful Mañjuśrī.

[SARAHA'S SONG]

[1. THE NATURAL STATE]

Amazing, the secret language of ḍākinīs!

1. Bowing deeply before the bodhisattva,
The lord of bliss whose nature is buddha,
Dharma, and saṅgha, I will explain
The abiding state of naturally non-dichotomous Mahāmudrā.

2. Beings are entwined like trees by vines,
And parched in the miserable desert of grasping at self;
Like a prince without a country and apart from his father
They have no occasion for bliss, their minds in torment.

3. "Gnosis of suchness won't come by examination;
It's free from deeds and gathers no karma."
When Saraha, who knows for himself, declares this,
All the scholars' hearts are full of poison.

4. Mind itself, truly authentic, is hard for everyone to comprehend;
It's the unstained core, unblemished by extremes.
From the start its nature can't be examined in any way;
If examined, it's the bite of a poisoned snake, that's all.

5. All dharmas assumed by cognition are void on their own;
They're free from conditions, so none exists as we think.
When you know their suchness, their natural state of release,
There is no seeing or hearing, so there's no disharmony.

6. All who conceive of "things," low like cattle;
Those who conceive of "no-things" are more foolish still—
While those who exemplify these as a lamp lit and doused
Abide in naturally non-dichotomous Mahāmudrā.

7. What arises as a thing is quelled in no-thing,
And that very sagacity free from either stance—
[Even] when it examines the minds of fools—
Is the instant of release described as Dharma Body.

8. The childish say, "There's a level of bliss apart
From that release"—but that's the same as water in a mirage;
Inquire of thought, which is just this primordial gnosis,
Where all stages, paths, and buddhas have a single taste.

9. A man who comprehends this is unbound;
Not clearing dust away, he's not begrimed by dust at all.
Where's the demarcation between affliction and the cure?
A person who tries to find it is bound within saṃsāra.

10. Earth, water, fire, wind, and space
Don't exist apart from the innate's single taste.
Not conceiving becoming and nirvāṇa as two —
This, it's explained, is the abiding state of the ultimate sphere.

[2. PITFALLS]

Amazing, the secret language of ḍākinīs!

11. Alas! Look at how the real points to itself by itself:
You have to look with an undistracted mind. When you don't,
Your distracted mind won't comprehend the real,
And you'll lose the jewel of the real in the thicket of things.

12. Alas! Don't be impassioned about what it is you desire:
When thought is impassioned with an object of passion,
It's an illness besetting sublime blissful mind,
A blow to stainless mind by the sword of desire.

13. Alas! Don't look at cause and result as two:
There is no cause for a thing to arise, nor any result;
If the yogi's mind is drunk on the poison of hope and fear,
Then the state of innate gnosis will be bound.

14. Alas! Don't say "the natureless real exists in contemplation":
If contemplator and contemplated are conceived as two,
Then dichotomous thought discards the awakening mind—
Such a person sins against himself.

15. Alas! Those preparing for knowledge should partake as they can
Of nectar drops from the guru's mouth;
If your service is untimely when you know the time and means,
You're like a blind man trying to rob the royal coffers.

16. Alas! A person bereft of the precious initiations
Is like a lowly servant aspiring to be king;
Confused about the Tantras of awareness-bearers,
He's condemned by ḍākas and plunges into adamantine hell.

17. Alas! If you've learned sublime meaning from virtuous friends
But don't hold it sacred, discarding it with a mind that's debased,
You're like a person half-blind being led into danger:
A great eon through, you bring yourself nothing but pain.

18. Alas! If you come to the place you've been shown but don't keep your vows,
You're like a man condemned by the king and seized:
Your life-breath seized by the iron hooks of ripening [acts],
Molten metal poured into your mouth—this is hard to bear!

19. Alas! If you comprehend the abiding state but your conduct's debased,
You're like a king who's deposed and made a sweeper;
Discarding that bliss that can't be exhausted,
You're bound by involvement with samsaric pleasures.

20. Alas! A yogi who's seen his own mind without complication
But strives nonetheless to complicate things,
Is like someone who's found a jewel and goes looking for trinkets:
Try though he might, he never [reaches] the place at the core.

[3. CONTEMPLATION]

Amazing, the secret language of ḍākinīs!

21. The gnosis that tries to hold the awakening mind
And comprehends awakening mind without even trying
Arises from nectar in the mouths of the holy
And shines in between the sun and moon.

22. It emerges from the focal points of a trustworthy person;
From a qualified *mudrā* [emerges] a unified mind:
Through her, form and other phenomenal things change their color;
Know this through instruction that pacifies.

23. Seeing for certain the actuality of luminous [mind],
You'll thoroughly comprehend the time and means of serving the guru;
The mind that applies to all is obtained
From *Perfect Wisdom* and other sūtras—contemplate it clearly.

24. The mind that can't be viewed as outside or in
Can't be considered anything by anyone—there is no mind.
I lift this song to the adamantine peak of the natural state:

Contemplate bliss as being like an aimless river.

25. The mind swayed by complication where crowds collect:
It's stable by nature, it doesn't project or engage;
Release the core of mind to do what it will:
Mind like a drunk who is free from deeds.

26. Contemplate gnosis unblemished by extremes,
Mind without contemplation or contemplated has no nature;
The ultimate beyond hope and fear is the adamantine mind:
Even if it goes to hell, there is no pain,

27. And if it dwells in sublime results, there's nothing more to gain.
So, beyond the help and harm brought on by pleasure and pain,
Through good behavior or bad it doesn't wax or wane:
This non-dichotomous gnostic comprehension is all there is.

28. If you claim that buddha is greater, know you're deluded;
When deedless thought seeks nothing at all,
There is no need to seek virtue, for there's no disharmony there.
You won't attain the real through any Tantra or treatise;

29. Mind without hate or desire is free from the stain of cause;
Experiencing great gnosis that looks at nothing,
The yogi who quells *saṃsāra*'s poisons—
Whether [straight] like a monk or [bent] like a bow—reigns in every realm.

30. The yogi who does not close his eyes or contemplate
Should [go] to distant spots and open places,
And, his unstained thought beyond passion and hate,
Contemplate the essence of utmost mind.

[4. ENCOUNTER]

Amazing, the secret language of ḍākinīs!

31. Devoid of mandalas or fire offerings,
Quite without mantras, *mudrās*, and consecrations,
It can't come about through any Tantra or treatise:
This adamantine gnosis is lovely in its natural state.

32. The sublime precious symbol that yields understanding at once
Is like a snake in a basket, lovely to none but [its owner].

Essence points to essence through the pure sublime guru;
Comprehending, he points it out to others, and thereby points to himself.

33. It's fine to engage with sounds and such that link
The three drops—potent like space, jewel,
And sun—with thought, remembering, and unremembering;
All dharmas assume the same taste, as [metals] turned gold by elixir [are the same].

34. When you train on the path, primordial gnosis is your sole concern;
He who shows the path by symbols is the pure sublime guru.
Rely on form, sound, smell, taste, touch, and dharmas:
All dharmas are unconditioned; they do not arise.

35. The fortunate are wise to unarising
And so perforce are wise to everything arisen.
Gnosis without distinctions is oneness alone;
The naturally settled mind pervades itself.

36. Knowing the single nature of apparent "self" and "other,"
Take unwavering hold of the real alone;
[Grasping] itself is a sickness of mind—release it,
And when you crave nothing, you'll lay hold of bliss.

37. Mind is devoid of all harmful actions;
It's not begrimed by deeds like getting or taking.
Free from effort, not occasional, not accidental, not conditional,
This seal of manifold appearance is a grand show indeed.

38. Seeing everything close-up at the holy one's timely [prompt],
You'll know there is no phenomenon that's not the guru;
The finger pointing to sky does not see sky;
So it is with guru pointed out by guru.

39. The eccentric yogi whose mind [roams] the town
Enters the royal palace and flirts with the women;
As someone who's eaten sour food sees food as sour,
He's aware that all things are suchness.

40. In the place adorned for a ritual feast,
He sees great bliss during sex;
Yogis possessed of symbols and vows
Welcome becoming and peace as the same: Mahāmudrā.

[5. CONNECTION]

Amazing, the secret language of ḍākinīs!

41. A yogi in whom gnosis has risen fears nothing,
So with godlike means, he should seek out [a woman] born at the margins;
Going to a low-caste town, he should little by little
Beguile her with agreeable [words], then grant her the supreme.

42. As much as he can, he should give to her gifts that betoken
Reverence, with a mind lacking "mine."
Wandering all about, he should examine [women's] marks:
By caste, by color—their collection of marks—he gradually comes to know them.

43. His very own daughter, mother, sister, or niece;
Low-caste women, laundresses, whores, or pickers of rags;
Women black, white, red, yellow, or dark maroon;
And women with moles: these are *mudrā*s for easy connection.

44. Sixteen years old, most beautiful, with golden-brown hair.
Fragrant as a blue lotus, breasts firm and strong, waist slim,
Hips broad, vagina concealed, lustrous with passion,
She's clearly devoutly consigned to [the yogi's] lustrous, potent secret.

45. Trusting, steadfast, little given to concepts:
The *mudrā* with these three signs should be ripened by initiation;
When [the yogi] takes hold of her qualities, he should grant her gnostic awareness,
And on that occasion take hold of the *mudrā* of primordial gnosis where all tastes the same.

46. The Mahāmudrā who concentrates queenly fluids:
Once [the yogi's] collected them [from her], he fades into conceptless space.
Sometimes he frequents the bazaar, and truly looks
At how things truly are, letting truth be freely displayed.

47. Sometimes he goes to the charnel-ground, and practices the pure lamps,
And sleeps with a carefree mind in ghost-haunted places;
He makes friends with outcastes, and draws the corpse-cart along;
"This is behavior unbecoming"—he's not to be held to that standard.

48. He joins in musical gatherings, amusing himself with song, dance, and flute;
Through the dance of Heruka, songs raised to the six [*yoginīs*], and such,
He should never tire in the least of uplifting his mind.
He should blanket his shoulders and bedeck his limbs with copper,

49. Tie his locks atop his head with a ring,
And adorn all his limbs with pieces of bone,
Then wrap his torso with elephant hide above and tiger skin below,
And wield in his hands a trident and bell.

50. Behaving like a crazed elephant and acting dumb,
Behaving without regard for dos and don'ts, like an elephant
Plunging on impulse into a pond: his mind perpetually crazed,
He performs the basest of deeds yet is free, says Saraha.

[6. COMMITMENT]

Amazing, the secret language of ḍākinīs!

51. He who shows all the manifold dharmas
To be of a single taste is the holy guru himself;
That sublime noble lord who's akin to the bill of a swan [in extracting essence]
Should with reverent mind be raised to the pure place at your crown.

52. Unified mind: it's the guru who points it out,
The place where it's shown is the pupil's heart.
Comprehending that, the kindly hero
Destroys all pain in an instant;

53. Observe this, and repay the kindness he's shown
By constantly serving that king of physicians.
He's the sublime boat that delivers us
From *saṃsāra*'s deep, vast sea—there is no other;

54. So trust that holy vessel, and honor unflinchingly in every way
The mighty boatman who's gained great bliss.
By the pure radiance of his sun-like gnosis
That person sublime turns ignorance into awareness;

55. Always serve the wheel-turning king who's wise in the ways
Of changing all dharmas to bliss as elixir turns [metals] to gold.

Mind like a river submerges dichotomous views,
Possessed of gnosis, rejecting nothing, and blemish-free;

56. Cognition that's uncontrived and cognition whose state's transformed
Emerge from nectar in the holy guru's mouth.
"Mind" and "mental events": these
Labeled conventions [become] the yogi's friends.

57. The lotus mouth of the guru is the agent of change,
And through it, all are transformed into spiritual friends.
Hidden in every Tantra, apart from convention,
The secrets of the buddhas are known to none.

58. Seeing with the eye of instruction and filled with initiation's taste,
When you touch the dust of the [guru's] feet, gnosis becomes awareness.
Shoot the arrow of voidness at the manifold things,
And induce the void experience by means of appearance,

59. And with wisdom that knows, see appearances for what they are.
The source of that wisdom is the master pure and unsurpassed;
Through his methods all afflictions are made sublime,
And no conceptual torment can change them back.

60. [Wisdom] surely emerges from the [guru's] core instruction;
And surely is gained through that noble lord's might,
So all who are blessed to belong to his line,
And are learned in time, means, and service, should always serve.

[7. RESULTS]

Amazing, the secret language of ḍākinīs!

61. Comprehending the natural sameness of wisdom and means,
You'll attain the innate through luminous mind;
It emerges by developing like the waxing moon,
And its brightness grows like rice in sunlight and moon.

62. The root of every attainment is the adamantine master,
The perfectly pure cause at the base of all results;
To act in accord with the Well-Gone One's words
The bodhisattva, the lord of bliss, has spoken well.

63. The Dharma Body, Complete Enjoyment and Emanation Bodies,
And the Essential Body are clearly known through cause and result;

Non-dichotomy devoid of "is" and "isn't" is the Dharma [Body],
Its essential bliss is the Great Enjoyment [Body],

64. Its manifold guises for wandering beings are the Emanation [Body],
And the very gnosis [that knows] they're indivisible is the [Essential] self of them all.
The nature of creature and creator cannot be conceived,
But the might of developing [mind] submerges all fear,

65. And results are two: perfecting the aims of oneself and of others.
Though imagined in terms of cause and result, [the bodies] are undivided in essence.
The twofold Form Body emerges by force of prayer and compassion:
Like a perfect vase, a wishing tree, a precious jewel,

66. The [Enjoyment] Body no one can apprehend is most lovely;
[The Emanation Body] appears for disciples in manifold forms,
All of them emanations beyond conceiving.
Cultivate the gnosis that's unthought and self-emergent,

67. And you cultivate results without exception.
The path that's the core of the unsurpassed Mahāyāna:
Take it as the path to these results, and abide in result without beginning.
The perfection of others' aims is the sublime result:

68. It mainly emerges through purification and other [ways].
The great release, where action is pure, surely is gained
Through the might of unceasing mind that's bereft of hope.
When in some great person this divine substance rises,

69. All poisons without exception are instantly quelled and dissolved;
Lions, crazed elephants, tigers, and bears,
Wild beasts, venomous snakes, fire, and ravines,
The king's condemnation, poison, and thunder and lightning—

70. All are the Essential [Body], hence do no harm.
Destroying the great enemy—concepts—it destroys all enemies;
Suppressing the poison of self-view it suppresses all poisons,
So sanctify this jewel that is your mind.

[8. INSTRUCTION]

Amazing, the secret language of ḍākinīs!

71. Whoever's aware of the secret of body, speech, and mind,
Is a person in whom there's no poison-fed stupor;
While someone who thinks of actions in terms of virtue
And vice—whatever he tries to do, he's a poison-addict, I say.

72. A person behaving that way only binds himself,
And sick with incessant longing, plunges into *saṃsāra*.
Through logic [you get] what's unneeded, and destroy what sufficed before;
Imagine something, and images impede your freedom.

73. Even the label "good" is a sickness plunging you into *saṃsāra*,
And when you label an act as "evil," its fruition still can't be stopped.
The mind that doesn't label abides like space;
Space is unabiding, the real is bereft of conventions.

74. The free mind settles into its nature
Just as it's always been: without need to label or examine.
The result is unimpeded and abides on its own from the start,
So you need not be bound to cures for your hopes and fears.

75. And so with every symbol and term you impose:
They are not correct, while what is, is the object of every sage.
Cause and result undivided—this is mind at its core;
To experience it, you don't need to look everywhere.

76. Serving the holy, listening [to instruction], and adopting what you've heard;
Obtaining blessings because "virtues arise from initiation";
Resting in cognition in concentration, then [engaging in] application and contemplation;
Behaving eccentrically, [thinking] it will lead to security—

77. All those are practices based on falsehood and contrivance;
Mind at its core is free from virtues and faults.
Truth itself requires no deeds at all,
While the mind that's done with deeds is great bliss sublime.

78. Those obsessed with the five sciences and such are in a demon's grasp;
Their minds are filled with the poison of grasping at things.

It's right for those whose minds reject externals and stay within,
Who practice at the core, to think on precisely this.

79. Clearing away the husk of logical complication,
Comprehending this unsurpassable core
Of truth that rises from your pure primordial senses,
You'll abide on the fourteenth stage.

80. A yogi desiring great gnosis
May proceed by stages or at once;
Set in the inmost citadel of gnosis sublime,
He must win Mahāmudrā for wandering beings.

[Derge:] Received/requested by the Indian master Vajrapāṇi and Lama Asu.

[Peking:] This completes the *Treasury of Song-Instruction* of the great lord of yoga Saraha the Great, a writing of the ultimate level that authentically points to the real.

—10—

The Questions and Answers of Vajrasattva

Jacob P. Dalton

Yoga, as union of practitioner and deity, can raise some perplexing theoretical questions. From the perspective of yogic union, if one's body, speech, and mind are already identical to those of the Buddha, why bother with ritual performance? If there is no distinguishing sacred from mundane, why create a distinct ritual space? Why look to a teacher for advice? Why seek the blessings and accomplishments of one's deity? These are precisely the kinds of questions posed in the ninth-century Tibetan text, *The Questions and Answers of Vajrasattva*. Ultimately such questions may be irresolvable, as they are in many ways inherent to Buddhist practice, to the paradox of discovering the deity within, of striving for a goal that is already present. Certainly similar issues continue to haunt yoga practitioners of today. But such questions may be particularly vexing for beginners, for those who are new to the conceptual systems of yoga and are therefore not yet familiar with the tradition's standard responses. Precisely such a situation may have been behind our *Questions and Answers*.

In the late eighth and early ninth centuries, Tibetans were encountering the Buddhist Yoga and Mahāyoga ("Great Yoga") Tantras for the first time. They were at once attracted to the mystery and power of these esoteric texts, and confused by their paradoxical and sometimes even antinomian implications. Perhaps because of the latter, early Tibetan enthusiasms for the Tantras seem to have worried the imperial court. Royal pronouncements were issued, restricting the translation and circulation of these dangerous texts. Official catalogues of Tibetan Buddhist translations explicitly excluded the more extreme Mahāyoga Tantras from their lists, and when the Tantras were translated, their most offensive passages were carefully censored. The transgressive and antinomian teachings of the Tantras appear to have threatened the court's wider project to promote Buddhist monasticism, ethics, and pious worship among the populace.

Nevertheless, within the court and among the aristocratic families of central Tibet, the Tantras remained popular and continued to be studied throughout Tibet's early imperial period (a period that ended around the mid-ninth century). *The Questions and Answers of Vajrasattva* is a testament to their popularity. The very fact of its existence already suggests a continuing interest among Tibetans of the first half of the ninth century; moreover, a colophon appended to one version of the text explains the author's aim in composing it:

> As may be deduced from the title, the compilations and Tantras in the Mahāyoga class can disagree from one text to another, so this [work] has been taught in order to clarify any obscure points among the Tantras or doubts that may arise. [Also] regarding its purpose, it was taught for the Nanam (Sna nam) and Dong (Ldong) clans and for the minds of future generations of yogis, with the aim of clarifying any unclear, doubtful, or difficult points. This aim, which is present from beginning to end, has been formulated into fifty-three questions in verse, each in two parts—a question and an answer.

The text was written for two clans in particular, both well-known aristocratic families that enjoyed close ties to the imperial court. It was perhaps with this audience in mind that Pelyang, in verse forty-two, suggests that the proper performance of yoga brings power, "in mind and in clan." In any case, Pelyang's text seems to indicate that the court's proscriptive edicts were not meant to ban the Tantras completely, but merely to restrict their circulation to its own inner circles.

As the colophon suggests, *The Questions and Answers of Vajrasattva* is arranged into a series of fifty-one questions and their answers (despite the above-translated colophon's count of fifty-three). Buddhist catechisms of this sort were popular in early Tibet. Within the Dunhuang archive alone we find the *Passages from Eighty Sūtras* (*Mdo sde brgyad bcu khungs*), another early Tibetan work that focuses on the practice of yoga from a non-Tantric perspective, as well as a second catechism (in India Office Library [IOL] Tib J 419/6) on the practices of the Mahāyoga Tantras. It seems that catechetical writings helped early Tibetans to make sense of Buddhism, and in this sense it is perhaps worth noting the prevalence of similar question-and-answer texts in modern books seeking to bring Buddhism to the west; see for example the books of Lama Yeshe, Chögyam Trungpa, and Joseph Goldstein.

The colophon to the *Questions and Answers of Vajrasattva* attributes the work to one Pelyang (Dpal dbyangs), also referred to as the Learned Nyen Pelyang (Mkhan po Gnyan dpal dbyangs) in Nubchen Sangye Yeshe's early tenth-century *Lamp for the Eye in Contemplation*. Nyen Pelyang appears to have been active in central Tibet during the first half of the ninth century. His teachings must have wielded considerable authority in his day, and several additional works on Tantric Buddhism are attributed to him in the Tibetan canon. Pelyang's other writings refer regularly to the *Guhyagarbha Tantra*, a Mahāyoga Tantra that exerted considerable influence in early Tibet and was closely associated with the emergence of the Atiyoga, or Dzogchen ("Great Perfection"), meditation traditions.

Within the *Guhyagarbha* and other early Mahāyoga Tantras dating from around the late eighth century, two complementary strands of rhetoric may be discerned: one that emphasizes the importance of adhering to the proper (and often complex) ritual procedures, and another that suggests such conventional concerns are unnecessary. The two strands may be mapped onto the two truths of earlier exoteric Buddhism, that is, the conventional and ultimate truths, but the distinction was also fed by the inherent tensions with which we began. Yoga at once involves conventional practices that facilitate realization of one's innate union with the deity and implies that the innate nature of that union renders such practices ultimately irrelevant. While both of these rhetorical strands are common in the Mahāyoga Tantras, the somewhat later treatises of the so-called Atiyoga class focus more exclusively on the ultimate perspective of the second strand. The *Questions and Answers of Vajrasattva* may reflect a moment in Tantric Buddhism's development when this kind of Atiyoga rhetoric had yet to separate fully from its Mahāyoga origins.

The *Questions and Answers* itself states in its opening lines that it was written for "those wishing to understand with awareness the way of the supreme Mahāyoga," and throughout it employs the ritual terminology of the Mahāyoga Tantras. Despite the work's technical language, however, its view of ritual is very much rooted in an ultimate perspective, so much so that its early readers understood the text, in certain parts at least, to be teaching Atiyoga. A tenth-century Dunhuang manuscript containing the *Questions and Answers*, for example, includes the copious interlinear notes of an unidentified author. According to this interlinear commentator, the view of Atiyoga is explained by the following lines in verse thirteen:

> Simply appearing as oneself: this is the true body (*dharmakāya*),
> Realized to be changeless like the sky.
> In propitiation (*sevā*), when no action or actor is perceived,
> There are neither words nor effort: this is the supreme propitiation.

Later, the same interlinear commentator reads the final line of verse thirty-one as another reference to Atiyoga. In answer to a question about the place of effort in yoga, we read:

With regard to whatever is to be accomplished,
Rest with effort in meditative equipoise again and again.
By cultivating [in this way], one becomes [worn like] a riverbed, little by little,
Until, without effort, one becomes spontaneously accomplished.

In this verse we see Pelyang taking what may have been a diplomatic position on the sudden-gradual debate that so concerned early Tibetans, as he allows for gradual progress along a path that culminates in a moment of sudden enlightenment. The resulting breakthrough, says our commentator, is equivalent to "the meaning of Atiyoga."

Despite Pelyang's acknowledgment in this verse that some effort and gradual training may be required, at least initially, he devotes most of his *Questions and Answers* to a more ultimate and immediate perspective. In this spirit, verse twenty-four explains that the yogi must discard as mere delusion all philosophical distinctions, even those of the two highest philosophical schools in early Tibet, the Yogācāra-Madhyamaka and the Sautrāntika-Madhyamaka. Similarly in verse nineteen, all meditation is impossible, while in verses seven and eight nothing is ever achieved.

Pelyang brings this same paradoxical logic of ultimate yoga to bear in his evaluation of pre-Buddhist Tibetan religious practices. In verse thirty-six, he introduces the issue of whether a proper yogi should worship the native gods and demons of Tibet. In the system of Yoga, he explains, "For one who has pledged to Samantabhadra-Vajrasattva, the worship of mundane gods and *nāgas* ("dragons") as higher beings is like a king performing the acts of a commoner. Do not beseech [such beings even] for your provisions; it conflicts with the purpose of Yoga." Here Pelyang takes an unusually hard line against the religious practices of pre-Buddhist Tibet. Many early Tibetans perceived Buddhism as a threat to the welfare of their native gods. As Buddhism continued to spread within Tibet over the following centuries, this tension was largely resolved by Buddhists' general acceptance of worshipping local spirits for mundane and material purposes, with the caveat that such practices would not bring the practitioner any closer to enlightenment. But Pelyang stakes out a more extreme position, refusing to grant even mundane value to spirit worship, and to justify his view Pelyang applies the rhetoric of the ultimate yogic perspective: given the innate union of oneself and one's deity, such lowly practices are irrelevant at best, and a transgression of one's yogic commitments at worst.

From such a standpoint, all religious practices apart from complete and perfect yoga are misled and can bring only worldly (*laukika*) benefits. One may gain wealth, cure an illness, or ensure a good harvest; one may be reborn as a god in heaven, or even attain the sublime meditative states of Brahmā (as in verse twenty-nine); but one will never achieve transcendent (*lokottara*) buddhahood. Only by overcoming all conceptual distinctions by means of Buddhist yoga can one comprehend the ultimate.

Even as the *Questions and Answers* insists on the irrelevance of lesser practices, it clearly speaks within a Yoga, or Mahāyoga, Tantric ritual context. It employs numerous technical terms and makes regular reference to Mahāyoga's complex ritual apparatus. One such term—or pair of terms—that may need explaining is "propitiation and accomplishment" (Tib. *bsnyen sgrub*; Skt. *sevā-sādhana*). In earlier *dhāraṇi*-based and Tantric ritual texts, this pair marked the two fundamental stages of ritual practice. During propitiation, the practitioner would make offerings and, in particular, recite the mantras of the deity in order to purify and empower herself for the next stage. Then during the stage of accomplishment, she would direct the power gained through propitiation toward a specific purpose, be it gaining wealth, harming enemies, achieving enlightenment, or whatever. Around the second half of the eighth century, this crucial terminological pair was expanded to four stages, those of propitiation, near propitiation, accomplishment, and great accomplishment. The resulting tetrad was then applied in different ways in a variety of ritual settings, and Pelyang makes reference to them.

Similarly in verse thirty-nine, Pelyang recommends the use of the profane "inner sacramental substances," typically consisting of semen, menstrual blood, feces, urine, and human flesh. Similarly too, verses forty-three to forty-seven comprise a sustained discussion of the "*vidyādhara* levels," the stages of realization to be scaled by the successful Mahāyoga practitioner. And verse eighteen refers to the "thusness concentration" (*tathatā samādhi*), a formless meditation on emptiness that opens many Mahāyoga ritual procedures, and that is typically followed by two further concentrations, an "all-illuminating concentration" and a "causal *samādhi*," which effect the generation of a visualized mandala.

Despite its ultimate perspective, then, the *Questions and Answers of Vajrasattva* functions within a more-or-less familiar ritual framework; it remains very much part of the Buddhist *dharma* ("teachings," or "truth"). Indeed, the word "dharma" itself appears throughout the text, both as a stand-alone term and within two crucial nominal compounds. The first of these, *dharmadhātu*, refers to the "space of truth," the enlightened realm of emptiness, while the second, *dharmakāya*, refers to the "truth-body," the most unelaborated form of the Buddha. The *dharmakāya* generally occurs as part of a triune set and is thus often associated with two further buddha-bodies: the *sambhogakāya* ("complete enjoyment body") that describes the blissful deities that appear as forms of clear light in the pure visions of practitioners, and that are so often depicted in Buddhist paintings; and the *nirmāṇakāya* ("emanation body"), that indicates the Buddha's coarser emanations, its bodies of flesh and blood. Clearly the Buddha in this system of yoga, as in Mahāyāna Buddhism more generally, extends far beyond the historical personage of Śākyamuni who lived some 2,500 years ago. Here the Buddha is more of an abstract force that may be represented by anyone who has successfully followed the Buddha's example, who is a *tathāgata*, "one who has gone thusly," or a *sugata*, "one who has gone well."

In the *Questions and Answers*, this ultimate Buddha is condensed in the person of Vajrasattva, the deity whose name appears in the title of our text and who is identified with Samantabhadra in verses three and thirty-six (cited above). The "*vajra*" in "Vajrasattva" is a central concept in Tantric Buddhism, and it covers a broad semantic field. As a thunderbolt, it is the weapon traditionally brandished by the bodhisattva Vajrapāṇi. Diamond-hard, it is also wielded as a ritual implement by Tantric practitioners. It represents the male aspect of enlightenment, to be paired with the female aspect that is represented in ritual by a bell held in the practitioner's other hand. Thus Vajrasattva, literally the "Vajra-Being," is the personification of this *vajra*, of the adamantine essence of enlightenment. He represents the highest buddha of the Buddhist Yoga-Tantra pantheon. As such, he incorporates all other buddhas and embodies the ultimate perspective from which distinctions between Vajrasattva and all other buddhas, between oneself and one's deity, and indeed between anything and anything else, is utterly unnecessary. It is from his perspective that the *Questions and Answers of Vajrasattva* communicates.

The translation below is based on my own unpublished critical edition of the *Rdo rje sems dpa'i zhus lan*. In creating the edition, I drew primarily upon the Dunhuang manuscripts, Pelliot tibétain 837 and IOL Tib J 470 (the latter being a direct copy of the former), as well as the canonical version found in the Peking *Bstan 'gyur* (Q. 5082).

Suggestions for Further Reading

For a more in-depth study of the *Questions and Answers of Vajrasattva*, see Kammie Takahashi, "Rituals and Philosophical Speculation in the *Rdo rje sems dpa'i zhus lan*," in *Esoteric Buddhism at Dunhuang: Rites and Teachings for this Life and Beyond*, edited by Matthew T. Kapstein and Sam van Schaik (Leiden: E.J. Brill, 2010). On the relationship between Mahāyoga and Atiyoga texts in early Tibet, see Sam van Schaik, "The Early Days of the Great Perfection," *Journal of the International Association of Buddhist Studies* 27.1 (2004): 165–206.

For further remarks on Mahāyoga and the *Thugs kyi sgron ma* by Gnyan dpal dbyangs, see Jacob Dalton, "A Crisis of Doxography: How Tibetans Organized Tantra during the 8th–12th Centuries," *Journal of the International Association of Buddhist Studies* 28.1 (2005): 115–82. For a preliminary study of the above-mentioned *Passages from Eighty Sūtras* by Spug ye shes dbyangs, see Helmut Tauscher, "The *Rnal 'byor chen po bsgom pa'i don* Manuscript of the 'Gondhla Kanjur'," in *Text, Image and Song in Transdisciplinary Dialogue*, edited by Deborah Klimburg-Salter, Kurt Tropper, and Christian Jahoda (Leiden: E.J. Brill, 2006), pp. 79–103.

The Questions and Answers of Vajrasattva

For the sake of those wishing to understand with awareness
The way of the supreme Mahāyoga,
Some doubts that might occur in one's mind
Are posed as questions by a student to a virtuous teacher.

Not contradicting the definitive scriptures, and
Following the awareness of reality,
These verses on instrinsic awareness and related [topics]
Are taught in accordance with the way things are.

1. Who is Vajrasattva?

The intrinsic space of unborn wisdom
Is the meaning of the unchanging and indestructible "vajra."
"Being" (*sattva*) is the vajra wisdom.
Because he benefits beings, he is known as "Vajrasattva."

2. Why is it said that Vajrasattva is the vajra mind of all the *tathāgatas* of the three times, and [also] that he is the lord of body, speech and mind?

In the realization of the unborn by the conquerors of the three times, these are equivalent.
The nature of all, he is the mind of the ocean of *tathāgatas*;
Because he becomes the very basis for all the signs
Of the body, speech, and mind, he is called their lord.

3. What is meant by the statement, "Vajrasattva is the nature of all beings and all phenomena"?

All phenomena and limitless beings
Are of one taste in the unborn space of the ultimate.
Therefore that same reality of the conquerors of the three times
Is the state of Samantabhadra-Vajrasattva.

4. What does it mean that the five wisdoms are taught to be the five buddha families?

Unborn wisdom is equal to the *dharmadhātu*.
Its good qualities manifest in five aspects;
Precisely those are the characteristics of the five wisdoms,
Taught as the five families of conquerors, by those of skillful means.

5. What is the difference between the *dharmadhātu* wisdom and the mirror-like wisdom? Why is the *dharmadhātu* called "wisdom"?

Because there is no difference between wisdom and the *dharmadhātu*,
Unborn wisdom is known to be like a mirror.
Because wisdom is inseparable from the state of awareness,
The *dharmadhātu* is called the wisdom of reality.

6. It is said that by cultivating one's single tutelary deity, one cultivates all the *tathāgatas*. What is meant by this?

The five families of the conquerors and so on,
And all the *mudrā*s [i.e. female consorts] of means without exception,
Are of one *vajra* taste in the *dharmakāya*;
The way they appear is not the way they are.

Thus the cultivation of a single conqueror
Is not just [the cultivation of] that one; it is the state of them all.
In the yoga endowed with this awareness,
Not a single *sugata* remains uncultivated.

7. What does it mean when it is taught that there is no attainment of enlightenment?

That which abides naturally as the sky,
Cannot be a cause for becoming the sky.
The sky of mind itself, the space of enlightenment,
Cannot be a cause for accomplishing enlightenment.

This mind itself which without basis or root,
Is, like the sky, not purified by cleansing.

Within enlightenment, which is free from production,
There is no enlightenment that comes from causes and effects.

8. Well then [if there is no cause and effect], how are the accomplishments attained through the practice of mantra?

Because one just abides naturally,
There is not the slightest particle of attainment.
Even so, one's efforts and devotions just as they are,
Are the blessings, in the manner of a wish-fulfilling jewel.

9. [So] what is different about how the accomplishments are attained by the yogi?

To use a metaphor, just as a king appoints a minister,
The attainments are granted from above—this is the outer way.
When the kingdom is ruled through having been offered by the people—
This is the unsurpassable way of the self-arisen Great Perfection.

10. Even if a yogi is clear about the view, if the signs and indications do not arise, isn't this a method incapable of attainment?

Because the nature of the conquerors is nothing but knowledge and concentration (*samādhi*),
If those are present, then any outer signs or indications are irrelevant.
To use a metaphor: Once someone desiring fire has found fire,
Then the presence or absence of smoke as a sign of fire would be irrelevant.

Consequently, without a mind that projects and yearns for signs and indications,
And without hoping that one [day] these will appear from elsewhere,
The buddhas of the three times have made the two [yogas] their main practice.
Being aware that [the signs] arise from themselves, they view them and persevere with equanimity.

11. Is accomplishment gained only through the cultivation of knowledge and concentration, or does it also come through the blessings [of the deity]?

Just as everything appears through the spread of deluded conceptualizations,

Accomplishment is gained through knowledge and [one-pointed] concentration alone.
Even so, just as the sun and moon are reflected in clear water,
The compassionate blessings [of the wisdom deity] arise in one who is without sin.

12. When the blessings are to arise, do they arise because one has developed aspirations for them, or no matter what one does?

When dirty water becomes clear,
No effort is required for the reflections of the sun and moon to arise.
Similarly, when one's own mind has been purified through yoga,
No effort is required for the conquerors' blessings to arise.

13. Will one draw near to the Sugatas no matter how the propitiation is performed?

Simply appearing as oneself: this is the true body (*dharmakāya*),
Realized to be changeless like the sky.
In propitiation, when no action or actor is perceived,
There are neither words nor effort: this is the supreme propitiation.

An intelligent one who is endowed with this kind of realization
Clearly cultivates the three types of conceptual *mudrā*.
Striving and unrelenting without distraction,
One is endowed with all the rituals and is near to the wisdom deity.

14. At the time of propitiating the wisdom deity, if one begins with some minor [preparatory] rites, would this be an obscuration?

Apart from cultivating body, speech, and mind,
One should not search elsewhere for accomplishments to achieve.
If one does not begin with an opposition between what is the [ritual] space and what is not,
Then one is inseparable from the practice of cultivation, whereby there are no obscurations.

15. When there are explanations saying that the tutelary deity is to be cultivated as a *saṃbhogakāya* with peaceful attributes, that the action deity is to be cultivated as wrathful, and so on, are these kinds of [explanations] definitive or not?

The primary [deities] and their emanated entourages, all the peaceful and wrathful ones,
Are of one taste in the *dharmakāya*. They are equal in their skillful means, in teaching for the benefit of beings.
Because of that, the *sugatas* are indeterminate at their fundamental root;
They are nothing but [one's own] dispositions and inclinations—whatever is wished for.

16. Having settled on a tutelary deity, is it an offence if one cultivates another [deity]?

Due to their [skillful] means, [deities] are demonstrated variously, yet they are one within the space [of reality].
Within that [too], the conceptualization, avoiding, and taking of entities, and the limitless obscurations
Are inseparable. For one who realizes that, to cultivate all the buddhas
In accordance with one's karmic continuum is not a fault but the supreme root of virtue.

17. It is said that if one has a high enough view, it is acceptable not even to have a tutelary deity. How can this be?

When one realizes that there is no self to rely on a tutelary deity,
And that one is primordially of the nature of Vajrasattva,
That very realization is the state of all the conquerors.
Thus, other than that, there is neither practice nor practitioner in propitiating the deity.

Just as Vajrasattva, for example, does not have a tutelary deity,
One who is endowed with realization does not focus on a deity separate from one's own sphere.
Depending on how the taming activities for the sake of beings are to be performed,
The conquerors enter the various concentrations of the oceans of buddhas.

18. How is the thusness concentration cultivated?

Uncontrived by the conquerors of the three times,
One's own mind is unborn from the beginning.

Since one's own unborn mind is reality (*dharmatā*),
There is no need to cultivate reality.

19. Well then, is it suitable for one just to sit there without meditating?

If a basis for expression existed,
Then the meditator would also exist.
Since in truth the mind is unborn,
Then what would it mean to remain without meditating?

20. So then is it important for one's mind to have been altered by a master?

The mind that maintains a self posits consciousness as the basis for valid cognition.
The root is non-realization and consciousness is like the leaves.
If, through a lack of confidence, one yearns for the teachings and is not a master oneself,
It is very important to have one's mind altered by an intelligent being so that it accords with the unmistaken truth.

21. It is said that if a yogi is capable in knowledge and concentration, he is equivalent to a buddha. What does this mean?

The nature of the body is illuminated as [having] the marks and signs.
The nature of the speech is endowed with the seed syllables of [the deity's] emanation.
The nature of the mind is realized as unborn space.
Because the unequal are equal, one is said to be equal to a buddha.

22. What is the purpose of performing projection and reabsorption? Within that which is already pervaded by the *dharmakāya*, does not projecting-and-reabsorbing contradict the logic of reality?

Whatever is projected and reabsorbed, from wherever and to wherever,
Is of one taste within the state of Samantabhadra.
Therefore within space, the projection and reabsorption of that same space is not observed.
Nonetheless, that does not stop [its efficacy] as a method—the reasoning is just that.

23. So then what are the good qualities in performing projection and reabsorption?

In order for something to appear where there is nothing at all,
Whichever [buddhas] are assembling emanate and project for the welfare of beings.
Then the many *sugatas* are reabsorbed once more,
Making one splendorous like the conquerors, that is, for one's own welfare.

24. For those who practice mantra, which is better, to view in accordance with the Yogācāra-Madhyamaka or the Sautrāntika-Madhyamaka?

The way of those who perform Secret Mantra
Overpowers the methods of conceptual concentrations.
Therefore [such people] do not view with even the slightest ideation.
All such concentrations
Are unrelated to the mind, so not one is established.

25. Even if conventionally one views [everything] as Mind-Only, if phenomena are utterly nonexistent, how can there be any concentration? It makes no sense.

[Even when] other concentrations unrelated [to the mind] are cultivated,
Nothing occurs in that other sphere.
Not even the non-existence of things
Can appear to the mind itself.

26. For those who perform Secret Mantra, how important are the logical discussions of the sūtras?

Merely by pronouncing words that are harmonious and pure,
The afflictions will not be overwhelmed and liberation will not occur.
[But] for an intelligent person who renounces the coarser dharmas and pride,
The logical discussions on the nature of awareness can be extremely important.

27. What is the root of the faults that make one unequal to the Noble Ones?

The solitary root that is the evil cause of cyclic existence
Is a lack of awareness of one's own mind, clinging to a self.
Because this great poison exists in the hearts of beings,
They do not attain the final path and are forever being born and dying.

28. If non-conceptual calm abiding on external objects is okay, then couldn't one be liberated even with a view of self-clinging?

If self-clinging has been thoroughly abandoned,
There will be no clinging to phenomena whatsoever.
As long as self-clinging continues to act as a cause for mind,
Even the attainment of a [state of] mountain-like calm abiding will not be liberating.

29. It is said that through the meditative states (*dhyāna*), the super-knowledges and magical powers are attained. So is non-seeking through calm abiding sufficient?

The meditative states of Brahmā's realm and so forth may be spontaneously accomplished,
There may be lights and colours and one may be endowed with the super-knowledges,
But if a self is conceptualized and the latent predispositions are not abandoned,
Sentient beings will continue to fall into the hells and not hear the teachings.

30. So one should not seek one-pointed calm abiding or concentration?

Calm abiding endowed with unmistaken realization,
A concentration that illuminates the conceptual *mudrā*—
To possess an aim like that is the supreme path of enlightenment;
Again and again it should be enhanced.

31. Is the spontaneously accomplished concentration accomplished with effort or without effort?

With regard to whatever is to be accomplished,
Rest with effort in meditative equipoise again and again.
By cultivating [in this way], one becomes [worn like] a riverbed, little by little,
Until, without effort, one becomes spontaneously accomplished.

32. Is it not contradictory to explain the cause of effortlessness to be accomplished through effort?

In his direct perception of sentient beings accomplishing through effort,
Is it false that the conqueror is spontaneously accomplished?
By striving at the letters and so forth,
Through repeated cultivation, there seems to be effortless arising.

33. Is the statement that one need not protect one's *samaya* ("vows") contradictory or not?

In accordance with the intentions and the actions of one who has mastered no self,
[When] one does not cling to self, one's three doors [of body, speech, and mind] are free of offense;
Not even the slightest particle arises, and there is no need to observe and protect.
Thus ask yourself whether it is contradictory to cling to an "I."

34. How should the appearance of one's body in the *mahāmudrā* [i.e., the form of the deity], and the [mental] mandala of one's concentration be viewed?

The physical body and the *mahāmudrā* both
Are equivalent as aspects of the mind, so the body itself does not exist.
So too the bending and laughing emanations of the mandala
Are aspects of the concentration and thus one's own mind.

Mind and the characteristics of its aspects are indivisible.
The appearances of self and other are of equal status,
So neither one's body nor the principal [deity] can be identified as "this."
So too, everything is the body [and] everything should be viewed as [mental] emanations.

35. Is [it] however [the case that] one acts in accordance with the system of Yoga?

[One's] insight and concentration are the mind and the body of the conqueror.
Ever undeterred, there is no aspiration.

Like a great conqueror, one subdues the earth,
Commanding and ruling over all without exception.

36. There are yogis worshipping the gods [and demons] of Tibet. Is this in agreement with the system of Yoga, or not?

For one who has pledged to Samantabhadra-Vajrasattva,
The worship of mundane gods and *nāgas* as higher beings,
Is like a king performing the acts of a commoner.
Do not beseech [such beings even] for your provisions; it conflicts with the purpose of Yoga.

37. The bodies of noble beings often appear crushed beneath the feet of the wrathful deities. In cultivating [the deity] like this, is there not conflict?

In the ultimate, which is of one taste, without high or low,
If an intellect that has abandoned fixated concepts of self and other
Understands all to be means, then there is no conflict.
By gaining power over conceptual differences, nothing is discerned.

38. By performing propitiation for one *tathāgata*, are the Tantras for the activities of all [the buddhas] accomplished?

In performing the propitiation of some *tathāgatas*,
If one has distinguished the profound and vast view,
Then just by beginning all the Tantras for the activities of the many conquerors,
The learned explain that everything is accomplished.

39. Following a great observance (*mahāvrata*) of the inner sacramental substances, is it the case that one does not gain accomplishment without further cultivation?

In the teachings on the substances of accomplishment,
There is practicing accomplishment and cultivating knowledge and concentration.
Without those, there will be no accomplishment; one will be like an animal.
Therefore perform the yoga in conjunction with the ritual necessities.

40. Following [the attainment of] the great powers, does it matter if one does not understand the dharma?

Unrivalled in the triple world, the powers of the conquerors
Arise from their understanding and realizing the nature of phenomena.
Since they lack these and do not have *bodhicitta*,
What is the point of the powers of the *yakṣa* and the *rakṣasa* [demons]?

41. What can be taken as a valid sign of yoga endowed with awareness? Is it sharper vision and so forth?

Realization of the unborn meaning is the eye of knowledge and wisdom.
Through the power of yoga, the divine eye is completely purified,
But otherwise those things that are common in the ordinary world—
Sharper vision and so forth—are not valid signs of yoga.

42. How should one act to become powerful?

An intellect that has realized an unerring view, the meaning of the two truths, and
The inseparable equality of oneself and the buddha,
One who possesses the secret mantras, *mudrā*s, concentrations, and ritual procedures,
And who never stops cultivating and accomplishing, will become powerful in mind and in clan.

43. How does it mean that buddhahood may be accomplished in a single lifetime?

In this very residual body,
The *vidyādhara* [level] of mastery over life may be attained.
In the lifetime of such a *vidyādhara*,
One can attain unsurpassable enlightenment.

44. What is the meaning of "*vidyādhara*"? What are the levels?

One who has realized the characteristic of knowing awareness
"Holds awareness" (*vidyādhara*) of the mantras and practices.
One who has ripened the vajra-bearers, i.e. the deities and so forth,
In accordance with her [buddha-]family, is on the levels of a *vidyādhara*.

45. How does one traverse and dwell upon the *vidyādhara* levels?

Because anything suitable to appear as a mental level,

Is an aspect of one's own mind, it is not a mental level.
Wherever that mind, that does not abide anywhere, may travel,
It ripens according to its karmic lot and is nothing but an appearance.

46. According to the way of Mahāyoga, what is the end of cultivating? How is one said to arise as a *vidyādhara*?

By cultivating one's own body in the *mahāmudrā* of the conqueror,
One becomes a manifest deity,
Endowed with the marks and signs and the higher perceptions.
Such a person is called a *vidyādhara* of the *mahāmudrā*.

47. If the ripening of other roots of virtue occurs in future lifetimes, why is the *vidyādhara*-hood that results from practicing mantra achieved in this lifetime?

For certain special virtues and sins,
The results can ripen in this lifetime.
So for the special practice of Secret Mantra,
The ripening does not wait until later; it comes in this [life].

Because other roots of virtue are less powerful,
They are unable to produce strong results, but
One's own yoga and the empowerments of the conquerors
Are incomparable roots of virtue, so they are highly effective.

48. Can the accomplishments be attained without receiving the initiations from a master?

That the great secret hidden by the conquerors of the three times
May be accomplished on one's own, self-produced: such an explanation,
Even after searching all the oceans of teachings without exception,
Will not be found, nor should it be found.

49. Is there danger in someone acting as a teacher without having received the master (*ācārya*) initiation? When such a person is granting initiation, does it help to receive initiation?

Someone who has been appointed to a ministerial rank by a mistaken child
Will never become king and indeed will be diminished.

A vajra-king lacking the good qualities and the power,
Who appoints [others to] the ranks, will destroy himself and others.

50. Is the statement that one should make offerings to the teacher when receiving initiation a fabrication?

For countless eons we have wandered, searching for the long-lost path.
The path to liberation and unsurpassable enlightenment is an unending treasury.
Since it is not exceeded, even by the wealth of ten million rebirths,
What need to speak of some other [offering]? Rely entirely on the secret Tantras.

51. How much of a sin is it to disobey the word of the master?

All the sinful acts of the three realms
Do not compare to even a fraction of the sin of disobeying the teacher's word.
Definite causes for going to hell are accumulated in this way.
The primordially unheard, [however,] remains faultless and utterly virtuous.

This was composed by the master Peljam [*sic* Pelyang]. As may be deduced from the title, the compilations and the Tantras in the Mahāyoga class can disagree from one text to another. Thus the present [work] has been taught in order to clarify any obscure points among the Tantras or doubts that may arise. [Also] regarding its purpose, it was taught for the Nanam (Sna nam) and Dong (Ldong) clans and for the minds of future generations of yogis, with the aim of clarifying any unclear, doubtful, or difficult points. This aim, which is present from beginning to end, has been formulated into fifty-three questions in verse, each in two parts—a question and an answer.

Penned by Phu shi meng hwe'i 'gyog.

—11—

The Six-Phased Yoga of the *Abbreviated Wheel of Time Tantra* (*Laghukālacakratantra*) according to Vajrapāṇi

Vesna A. Wallace

The text translated here is an excerpt taken from the *Summary of the Ultimate Reality* (*Paramārthasaṃgraha*) commentary on the *Condensed Instruction on Initiation* (*Sekoddeśa*), an Indian text belonging to the literary corpus of the *Wheel of Time Tantra* (*Kālacakratantra*). The commentary was composed by Nāropā, the tenth- to eleventh-century Indian bearer of the Kālacakra Tantric tradition. The excerpt included here contains a brief presentation of six-phased yoga as taught by the Indian master Vajrapāṇi, who made use of several canonical sources for this presentation—particularly, the *Tantra of the Esoteric Community* (*Guhyasamājatantra*), *Ḍākinīs' Vajra Cage Tantra* (*Ḍākinīvajrapañjaratantra*), *Net of Illusions Tantra* (*Māyājālatantra*), *Litany of the Names of Mañjuśrī* (*Mañjuśrīnāmasaṅgīti*), and the abbreviated *Wheel of Time Tantra.* All of these sources share certain commonalities, and are relevant for understanding six-phased yoga in the context of the Unexcelled Yoga Tantras.

Six-phased yoga can be found in various Indic traditions. In the Buddhist esoteric context, the practice of six-phased yoga marks the most advanced stage in the path of the Unexcelled (*anuttara*) Yoga Tantras, which is invariably considered as "the stage of completion," the final stage of Tantric practice. As such, it is believed to lead directly to the attainment of supreme and complete awakening (*samyaksaṃbodhi*), also referred to as the highest supramundane accomplishment (*parama-lokottara-siddhi*). Although six-phased yoga is common to all of the Unexcelled Yoga Tantras, the content of the individual phases varies slightly from one Tantra to another.

Vajrapāṇi begins his exposition by providing a brief definition for each of the six successive phases of this yoga, known under the names of retraction (*pratyāhāra*), meditative stabilization (*dhyāna*), breath control (*prāṇāyāma*), retention (*dhāraṇā*), recollection (*anusmṛti*), and *samādhi.* He further offers a condensed teaching on the repeated cultivation of six-phased yoga as practiced in the *Esoteric Community Tantra* and the *Ḍākinīs' Vajra Cage Tantra*. He also explains the hidden meanings of Buddhist Tantric terms as they are related to the four types of successive *sādhana* practices of six-phased yoga, referred to as (1) worship (*sevā*), which is a preliminary to the retraction and meditative stabilization phases of six-phased yoga; (2) subsidiary contemplative practice (*upasādhana*), which is related to the practices of breath control and retention; (3) contemplative practice (*sādhana*), which is related to the practice of the recollection phase; and (4) sublime contemplative practice (*mahāsādhana*), which is relevant for the final phase of the six-phased yoga, namely, the practice of meditative concentration on emptiness. Visualization practices that are a part of the stage of completion are a preparatory phase for the actual practice of six-phased yoga. Through them, the yogi trains his mind in perceiving the triple world—the worlds of desire, form, and formlessness that constitute cyclic existence—and his own body, speech, and mind as manifestations of the indivisible body, speech, and mind *vajra*s of the Buddha. The unhindered and indestructible capacities of the Buddha's body, speech, and mind that are mutually pervasive are here referred to as three indivisible *vajra*s, which are actualized by the yogi at the moment of his spiritual awakening, itself induced by accomplishing the six-phased yoga. However, as in other Buddhist Tantric texts, here too, in the context of yogic sexual practices, the term *vajra* also designates the male sexual organ, whereas the "lotus" designates the female sexual organ. Moreover, as in Buddhist texts, the word "lotus" is also used to respectfully refer to the hands and feet of the Buddha.

In the contemplative practice (*sādhana*) of six-phased yoga, partially described in this text, the yogi engages in a Tantric consort practice characterized by non-emission of semen, which is commonly referred to in Tantric language as the moon and *bodhicitta* ("mind of enlightenment"). The sexual bliss accompanied by seminal non-emission generates heat in the navel, called *caṇḍālī* and the great seal (*mahāmudrā*), or sublime consort. In this particular context, the term "great seal," otherwise known as the yogi's highest achievement—the full and perfect awakening characterized by the gnosis of bliss, beyond which there is nothing else to achieve—denotes a bliss-induced heat in the navel that results from seminal non-emission. Thus, the great seal also refers to the aforementioned *caṇḍālī*, which is said to be the yogi's innate consort facilitating his highest achievement. At the time of the arising of this fire of bliss, the yogi practices two types of yoga in sequence. The first is so-called drop-yoga, during which seminal fluid flows in the form of drops through four bodily *cakra*s—that is, through the forehead, throat, heart, and navel *cakra*s, which are sometimes named after particular Hindu deities considered to be contained within the body, speech, mind, and gnosis of the Buddha and present within the body of the yogi. The second is subtle yoga, characterized by meditative stabilization (*dhyāna*).

Six-phased yoga consists of the different stages of meditation associated with the practice of inner yoga, comprised of the withdrawal of the sense-faculties from the external world; visualization; manipulation and purification of vital energies; generation of bliss that does not involve consort practice and seminal emission; retention of the spontaneously arisen appearance of the Kālacakra deity and his consort in the yogi's heart as his own image; and meditative absorption in which the yogi's mind abides in the non-duality of bliss and emptiness.

In the practice of the retraction phase of six-phased yoga, the yogi's sense-faculties are withdrawn from their external objects and thereby unified. When this takes place, the yogi perceives all phenomena of this world as mere images in a prognostic mirror. In other words, just as images of the future events that are seen in a prognostic mirror are insubstantial and do not reflect any existing things or events outside the mirror, because the future events have not yet come into existence, so the entire phenomenal world is seen by the yogi as a set of mere appearances devoid of any substantiality. Observing future events in a mirror is one of the various means of prognostication utilized in the Indian Tantric tradition; others include the observation of future events in the pupil of one's eye, on the thumbnail, and so on. Prognostication with a mirror requires that a Tantric adept empower the mind of a virgin girl with specific *mantras*, which enable her to observe images of various future events in the mirror.

As a result of the unification of his sense-faculties in the retraction phase, the ten daytime and nighttime signs—such as smoke, a mirage, fireflies, a lamp, a flame, the moon, the sun, the universal form of the Buddha, and a drop—sequentially appear to the yogi's mind. Since these signs are not visualized or conceptualized by the yogi but are spontaneously arisen as reflections of his own mind, they are not regarded as his meditative objects. Therefore, it is said that meditation on them should not be seen as meditation.

In the final section of his condensed presentation, Vajrapāṇi presents the *Wheel of Time Tantra*'s parallel explanation of six-phased yoga. He points to the paramount importance of six-phased yoga as the sole practice that brings about full and perfect awakening within one's lifetime. The text below indicates that this perfect awakening is possessed of diverse aspects—twelve, sixteen, and twenty—and it makes references to this awakening as a supramundane accomplishment (*lokottara-siddhi*), the Gnostic Body (*jñāna-kāya*), a particular type of meditative concentration (*samādhi*), and supreme, imperishable bliss.

The text below also demonstrates that in the Unexcelled Yoga Tantras, the immediate and more distant results of the contemplative practice (*sādhana*) related to six-phased yoga are multiple, manifesting in various mundane and spiritual accomplishments, such as (1) the five extrasensory perceptions: namely, the ability of seeing hidden objects and hearing sounds from a distance, telepathy, recollecting one's past lives, and having paranormal abilities; (2) the attainment of twelve Grounds within a single lifetime, which are otherwise achievable by those following the path of Mahāyāna only after incalculable eons of practices; and (3) the powers of the Buddha. The expedient soteriological efficacy of six-phased yoga itself is seen in its ability to thoroughly transform the constituents of the yogi's mind and body—his psychophysical aggregates; sense-bases consisting of sense-faculties and their sense objects; and the elements of earth, water, fire, wind, and space that make up both his gross physical and subtle bodies. Clusters of these elements, kept in motion by karmic winds, circulate throughout the body in the form of small discs (mandalas) in the form of vital energies (*prāṇa*). The vital energies that constitute the yogi's subtle body are invariably associated with a mind subject to transmigration. For so long as the vital energies that carry the essence of seminal fluid and menstrual blood flow on the left and right sides of the body in the *lalanā* and *rasanā* channels respectively, the yogi's mind remains engaged in conceptualizing and dualistic modes of perception, which are characteristic of the transmigratory mind. Thus, in order to induce non-conceptual and blissful states of mind, which are indispensable for the subsequent dissolution of all karmic winds in the body and resultant spiritual awakening, the yogi must dissolve the two aforementioned channels by bringing them into the central channel, called the *avadhūtī*, by means of breath control. Through sequential progress in the practice of six-phased yoga, the yogi experiences a spontaneously arisen bliss characterized by seminal non-emission. He brings that experience of bliss into the four bodily *cakra*s that contain the four subtle drops (*bindu*), which are the material bases of the four states of the transmigratory mind—namely, the states of waking, dreaming, deep sleep, and sensual bliss. By bringing his seminal drops (*bodhicitta*) into the four *cakra*s in a sustained fashion, the yogi experiences four types of bliss known as joy, supreme joy, extraordinary joy, and innate joy. Since each of these four types of bliss has four aspects—body, speech, mind, and gnosis—the seminal *bodhicitta* that induces these types of bliss within the *cakra*s is said to be complete, with all sixteen of its digits stacked incrementally along the central channel.

Having incinerated the four drops through the power of the heat generated by bliss (called *caṇḍālī*), the yogi now purifies all of the aforementioned constituents of his body and mind of the afflictive and cognitive obscurations that have kept him bound to cyclic existence. A yogic process of the generation of the fire of bliss, or *caṇḍālī*, in the navel, and the incineration of the four drops, is referred to as *caṇḍālī-yoga*. The text further advises the yogi who owing to this yoga perceives emptiness but does not experience the moment of imperishable bliss, to restrain his *prāṇa* by directing it into the central channel by means of *haṭha-yoga* and by retaining his seminal *bodhicitta* within his sexual organ as it rests inside the sexual organ of his consort. During that time, the *prāṇa* that moves outward through the nostrils from the center of the navel (the wind of *prāṇa* carrying the earth-element spreads outward as far as twelve fingerbreadths, and the wind carrying the space-element as far as sixteen fingerbreadths) is brought into the central channel within the navel. Immediately after that, the yogi engages in the so-called *nāda* practice by raising the wind of *apāna* into the central channel within the navel. Having collided in the navel, the winds of *prāṇa* and *apāna* move upward, splitting the *cakra* on the top of the yogi's head.

After describing this yogic process, Vajrapāṇi also sketches out the dissolution of the bodily elements in a sequence through which the elements dissolve into one other at the time of death, a process also visualized during the generation stage in which one imaginatively dissolves oneself before visually generating oneself in the form of the Kālacakra.

As a result of the actual dissolution of the gross and subtle elements, the yogi's new psychophysical aggregates, now purified of all material substances, manifest as empty form, characterized by bliss and emptiness: this is known as the Gnostic Body. Liberated from transmigratory existence and endowed with extraordinary abilities, it has mastery over the three worlds of transmigration.

Vajrapāṇi's comparison of meditative practice in the retraction phase of six-phased yoga with profound meditative concentration on space—or on emptiness, as expounded in the Mahāyāna's *Perfection of Wisdom Sūtra*—shows that he saw the Unexcelled Yoga Tantras as intimately connected to the Mahāyāna's *Perfection of Wisdom* tradition, not only in terms of its teachings on emptiness but also in terms of practices conducive to the realization of emptiness. In both systems, meditation on a cloudless sky or empty space is related to realization of emptiness. As indicated below, in the context of the Unexcelled Yoga Tantras, meditation on the spontaneously arisen sign of a cloudless sky is also called "meditation on the great seal (*mahāmudrā*)," the great seal being in this context another designation for the indestructible, innate bliss and emptiness that characterize the non-conceptual and blissful mind.

In both of these traditions, the term yoga designates a particular state of meditative concentration (*samādhi*). In the context of six-phased yoga, the term refers to different modes of practice and meditative experience as well as to the final result of the practice: nondual, ultimate reality consisting of empty form characterized by bliss. Thus, on the one hand, it denotes temporary states of meditative concentration as characterized by the realization of emptiness and bliss in accordance with the given modes of practice; and on the other, it represents the final state of *samādhi* manifesting in the experience of the gnosis of unchanging bliss arising from the unification of the yogi's mind of bliss with empty form. Hence, yoga here encompasses both a practical method for transforming the body and mind, and the result of that method, or self-cognizing bliss, referred to as full and perfect awakening. Since in the context of the Unexcelled Yoga Tantras, the yogic method and the result of yoga are seen as fundamentally nondual (since both involve the realization of emptiness and compassion), yoga is often referred to in these texts as a "*vajra-yoga* consisting of wisdom and method."

The excerpt translated here is taken from *The Sekoddeśaṭīkā by Nāropā* (*Paramārthasaṃgraha*). Sanskrit text edited by Francesco Sferra with Tibetan text edited by Stefania Merzagora. Serie Orientale Roma, 99 (Rome: Istituto Italiano per l'Africa e l'Oriente, 2006).

Suggestions for Further Reading

Ronald M. Davidson, "The Litany of Names of Mañjuśrī: The Text and Translation of the *Mañjuśrīnāmasaṅgīti*," in *Tantric and Taoist Studies in Honour of R. A. Stein*, edited by Michel Strickman, vol. 1. (Brussels: Institut Belge des Hautes Études Chinoises, 1981), contains an excellent translation of the text, replete with extensive annotations and followed by the original Sanskrit text. "The Litany of Names of Mañjuśrī" gives a description of the Gnostic Body as ultimate reality. Gen Lamrimpa, *Transcending Time: An Explanation of the Kālacakra Six-Session Guru Yoga*, translated by B. Alan Wallace (Boston: Wisdom Publications, 1999), closely follows the *Kālacakra Tantra* and its commentaries in describing the following stages of the Kālacakra practice: initiation preceded by the six-session *guru-yoga*, the *kālacakra-sādhana*, and six-phased yoga.

Günter Grönbold, *The Yoga of Six Limbs: An Introduction to the History of Ṣaḍaṅgayoga* (Santa Fe: Spirit of the Sun Publications, 1996) gives an account of the different variants of six-phased yoga as found in certain Hindu and Buddhist texts, and it compares sequences of their individual phases. See also

Edward Henning, "The Six-Vajra Yogas of Kālacakra," in *As Long as Space Endures: Essays on the Kālacakra Tantra in Honor of H. H. The Dalai Lama*, edited by Edward A. Arnold (Ithaca, NY: Snow Lion Publications, 2009). Khedrup Norsang Gyatso, *Ornament of Stainless Light: An Exposition of the Kālacakra Tantra*, translated by Gavin Kilty, The Library of Tibetan Classics, vol. 14 (Boston: Wisdom Publications, 2004) is an exposition of the five chapters of the *Kālacakra Tantra* as understood in the Tibetan Gelug tradition. Francesco Sferra, ed. and tr., *Ṣaḍaṅgayoga of Anupamarakṣita* (Rome: Istituto Italiano per l'Africa e L'Oriente, 2000) contains the edited Sanskrit text and translation of Anupamarakṣita's exposition of the *Kālacakra Tantra*'s six-phased yoga. Vesna A. Wallace, *The Inner Kālacakratantra: A Buddhist Tantric View of the Individual* (New York: Oxford University Press, 2001) gives an analysis of the *Kālacakra Tantra*'s exposition on the nature and constitution of the individual and his place in the cosmos and society. Its last chapter delineates various stages of practice, including that of six-phased yoga. Vesna A. Wallace, *The Kālacakratantra: The Chapter on Sādhana together with the Vimalaprabhā*, Tanjur Translation Initiative, Treasury of Buddhist Sciences Series (New York: American Institute of Buddhist Studies and Columbia University Center for Buddhist Studies and Tibet House, 2010) is a translation of the stage of generation practice, in which the practice of the *sādhana* of six-phased yoga is included.

Sekoddeśaṭīkā, 3.123–136

This type of six-phased yoga is described by these words of Ārya Vajrapāṇi.

1. Here retraction (*pratyāhāra*) is the non-engagement of the sense-faculties—of the visual sense-faculty and so on, and of the visual consciousness and so forth—with external sense objects, such as form and the like. It is an engagement of the divine visual faculty and so on, and of the divine visual consciousness, etc. with the eternal sense objects. With internal emptiness as a meditative object, the appearance of all phenomena in space is uncontrived, like a virgin's perception of an image in a prognostic mirror. Therefore, the retraction phase is due to the perception of the Buddha's body as the three worlds.

2. Then so-called "meditative stabilization" (*dhyāna*) takes place when all phenomena are perceived as empty. (1) Mental engagement (*citta-pravṛtti*) with these [empty phenomena] is called "wisdom" (*prajñā*). (2) The mind's apprehension of [empty] phenomena is called "ascertainment" (*vitarka*), and (3) the awareness of the perception of [empty] phenomena is called "reflection" (*vicāra*). (4) Fixing the mind on all [empty] phenomena is called "joy" (*rati*), and (5) the attainment of bliss due to all [empty] phenomena is called "immutable bliss" (*acala-sukha*). This is the fivefold phase of meditative stabilization.

3. Thereafter, cessation of the left and right paths of the *lalanā* and *rasanā* is called "breath control" (*prāṇāyāma*). It is a constant flow of the wind of *prāṇa* in the central path of the *avadhūtī*. This is the breath control phase: by means of the yoga of inbreath (*pūraka*), outbreath (*recaka*), and breath retention (*kumbhaka*), with [the silent utterance of] the syllable *oṃ*, the yogi brings breath into the central channel; with the syllable *hūṃ*, he holds it; and with the syllable *ā* he exhales it, in accordance with the natures of the moon, sun, and Rāhu [or semen, uterine blood, and consciousness].

4. Then, so-called "retention" (*dhāraṇā*) is the entrance of the vital energies into the mandalas of Mahendra, Varuṇa, Agni, and Vāyu—that is, into the navel, heart, throat, and forehead—and their exiting [from them]. The retention phase is [also known as] the "entering of vital energies into a drop (*bindu*)."

5. After that, so-called "recollection" (*anusmṛti*) is the appearance of one's own chosen deity, which is like a reflection [in a prognostic mirror] and is free from conceptualizations. Thereafter comes a disc of light, an image that emanates numerous light rays. Then comes the arising of the three worlds as a form manifesting with numerous aspects. This is the recollection phase.

6. Afterward, when the attainment of indestructible bliss takes place as a result of affection (*rāga*) for one's own chosen deity, then there is the so-called "meditative concentration" (*samādhi*), or unification of the mind. A mind that is free from the [duality of the] apprehending subject and the apprehended object is referred to as the "*samādhi* phase" by the Tathāgatas.

Now I will discuss a condensed teaching on the repeated cultivation of six-phased yoga in other Tantras.

[Contained] here in the splendid *Samājottara* (*Esoteric Community Tantra*) are worship, a subsidiary contemplative practice (*upasādhana*), a contemplative practice (*sādhana*) and a great contemplative practice (*mahāsādhana*). The Holy One stated this:

> Having meditated diligently on the image in the sublime crown *cakra* at the time of worship and on the image of the ambrosial *kuṇḍalī* during the subsidiary contemplative practice, one [who is] dedicated to yoga

> should meditate on the image of the deity during the contemplative practice. But during the great contemplative practice, one should meditate on the image of the supreme lord of the Buddhas. (*Esoteric Community Tantra*, 18.172–73)

In terms of the cryptic language [employed] here, one should place the mind-*vajra* on the source of phenomena [or on emptiness] in space; and during worship in the retraction [phase], one first should meditate on the image in the crown *cakra*, or on the image of a Buddha, as the entire three worlds. Then one should stabilize this [image] in the course of the meditative stabilization phase. Here is an assertion of the Holy One:

> Having abandoned all thoughts, one should try it for a day. If evidence does not arise at that time, then these words of mine are false.

In this case, evidence is the sign of smoke and so on and not something else. The evidence will arise for Tantric adepts on the very day in which they meditate on the mantra and the like. Thereafter, having abandoned the conceptions of existence and nonexistence and having made them groundless, the profound evidence that is without sensory support appears in space. That evidence, smoke and so on, should be meditated upon by the yogi. This is a principle of the Tathāgata. Likewise,

> With the sense-faculties joined together, one should meditate on the three worlds.

By means of the sense faculties, [that is,] by means of the visual sense faculty and so on, one should meditate on the three worlds as the Buddha's body. This very instruction should be learnt from the mouth of the *guru*. In that case, in accordance with the *guru*'s instruction, the yogi first sees smoke in the sky and not a mirage. He will know this from his own experience. A mirage will follow this [sign]. These very [signs], smoke and so on, which are devoid of conceptualizations, are similar to an image [perceived] in a prognostic mirror. Thus, the sign of smoke is the first, the sign of a mirage is the second, the sign of fireflies is the third, the sign of a lamp is the fourth, and the sign similar to a cloudless sky is the fifth.

This was stated by the Holy One in the *Esoteric Community Tantra* and in the *Ḍākinīs' Vajra Cage*. In addition to this, the Holy One said [this] in the *Ḍākinīs' Vajra Cage* (4.75):

> This cause of the All-knowing furthers [the yogi on his path] toward accomplishment. Afterward, immediately, in an instant, it has an appearance of an illusion and a dream.

Thus, according to the words of the Holy One, the evidence of meditation on the signs of smoke and the like appears at the beginning. Some will say that it will take place at the time of [the occurrence of] a supernatural ability (*siddhi*), but they all are refuting the assertion of the Holy One. Those revilers of the words of the Holy One say: "Having abandoned all thoughts, one should examine the evidence for one day." The ordinary signs of smoke and so on that appear at the time of [the occurrence of] a [mundane] supernatural power are not similar to an illusion and a dream because an act of the [actual] burning of the flame, smoke, and so on is obvious in this case. Showers of saffron, flowers, gems, and gold are also [expressions of the yogi's supernatural ability]. Thus, the signs of smoke and so on arise on account of six-phased yoga. The Holy One has also stated in the *Ḍākinīs' Vajra Cage* (4.72cd–73ab):

> Therefore, one should repeatedly cultivate six-phased yoga, which is equivalent to self-empowerment. Afterward, one should mark one's own emblems in a successive manner.

In this context, seeing conventional reality by means of the retraction [phase] is called "self empowerment." An appearance similar to clouds and smoke is called an "emblem." This, up to the [fourth sign of the] lamp, is seen first. After that comes the cloudless, stainless sky. In the *Net of Illusion*'s (*Māyājāla*) "Chapter on Samādhi," The Holy One said: "According to the *Tantras* there are six other different signs, beginning with the flame and so on and ending with the drop." For example,

> Arisen from the sky, self-arisen, the fire of gnosis and wisdom, the sublime [Buddha] Vairocana, the great brilliance, the light of gnosis, the sun, a lamp of the world, the torch of gnosis, a luminous sublime luster, the king of spells, the lord of the foremost *mantras*, the king of *mantras*, an accomplisher of the sublime goal. (*Litany of the Names of Mañjuśrī*, 6.20cd–22ab)

With [these] two stanzas and through the [use of] cryptic language, the Holy One described other signs in the *Net of Illusions*. An appearance that arises from the previously mentioned cloudless sky is a "self-arisen" one, which arises in the sky from a mind that is free from all conceptualizations. In this context, the appearance of the flame is the "fire of gnosis and wisdom." The appearance of the moon is "Vairocana, the great brilliance." This very Vairocana is the light of gnosis. The appearance of the sun is "a lamp of the world." The appearance of Rāhu is "the torch of gnosis." The appearance of lightening is "the luminous sublime luster." The appearance of the drop that has the aspect of a blue-colored moon-disc is "the king of spells, the lord of the foremost *mantras*." The king of *mantras*, an "accomplisher of the sublime goal," is the appearance of the phenomena of the three worlds with all their aspects, which the yogi perceives with his visual and other sense-faculties during the retraction [phase] as being similar to an illusion, to a dream, or to an image in a prognostic mirror; subsequently, [he perceives them as such] due to the union [of the sense-faculties] through breath control. With the sense-faculties joined together, he should meditate on the three worlds, characterized by desire, form, and formlessness, as being of a stable and mutable nature. The Holy One stated in the *Ḍākinīs' Vajra Cage* (4.76) that "one arises as the entire three worlds, animate and inanimate, as massive as those possessed of *vajra*-bodies in all world systems . . ." by means of the cultivation of six-phased yoga. This is a principle of the Holy One. Similarly, the Holy One declared in the splendid [*Esoteric*] *Community* [*Tantra*] (2.3):

> In the absence of a phenomenon there is an absence of meditation. Meditation is indeed not meditation. Since a phenomenon is not a phenomenon, no meditation is ascertained.

Meditation on the absence of a phenomenon or on a cloudless sky is the retraction [phase]. This very absence of meditation on a non-phenomenon means that meditation is indeed not meditation. Here, meditation in the retraction [phase]—which is meditation on the absence of a phenomenon, on a cloudless sky—is indeed not meditation on account of the absence of meditation with conceptualizations. Thus, a phenomenon perceived during the retraction [phase] is not a phenomenon owing to the non-conceptualized perception of the absence of past, future, and present phenomena. Hence, meditation with conceptualization is not ascertained in the meditation of the retraction [phase]. This is an assertion of the Holy One.

The Holy One also taught this meditation in the *Perfection of Wisdom* [*Sūtra*]. For example, "Then Śakra, the lord of gods, said this to the Venerable Subhūti: 'Noble Subhūti, whoever attains yoga [meaning here, "meditative concentration"] on this perfection of wisdom: on what does he attain yoga?' Subhūti replied: 'Kauśika, he who attains yoga on the perfection of wisdom attains yoga on space. Kauśika, the one who wishes to obtain yoga on space shall be deemed worthy of instruction in the perfection of wisdom.'" The Holy One said that meditation on the great seal (*mahāmudrā*), which is similar to an image [seen] in a prognostic mirror and to an illusion, is [meditation] on a cloudless sky. Thus I have described the phase of worship, together with retraction and meditative stabilization.

Then, in the cryptic language [of these teachings], "wind" is implied by the designation "a form of the ambrosial *kuṇḍalī*"; and it is of five kinds. The Holy One spoke thus in the *Esoteric Community Tantra* (18.147):

> Having expelled the breath in the shape of a pellet, which consists of the five jewels and is empowered by the five Buddhas, one should meditate on the tip of the *nāsikā*.

Here, the word "jewels" refers to the five elements, earth and so on, which are of the nature of the five mandalas of the right path of the breath. [One should expel] the breath that consists of these [elements], or of the five jewels, in the right nostril. Likewise, the five Buddhas are the five psychophysical aggregates, consciousness and so on, which are of the nature of the mandalas of the left path of the breath. [One should expel] breath empowered by these in the left nostril. "Having expelled it in the shape of a pellet" implies here that the pellet is a unification of the wind of the vital energies of the right and left mandalas in the central channel. Having expelled that wind of the vital energies in the shape of a pellet, one should meditate on the tip of the *nāsikā*. In this context, the pericarp of the lotuses of the navel, heart, throat, forehead, and crown [*cakra*s] is expressed by the word "*nāsikā*." "One should meditate on the tip of the *nāsikā*" means that one should meditate on the tip of that [pericarp], and not on the right and left petals of the lotuses in the center of the pericarp, [which are] away from the [tip of the] pericarp. In this way, *prāṇa* having the shape of a pellet is restrained in the place of the drop. This describes retention of that [*prāṇa*]. Thus, a subsidiary *sādhana*, together with its two phases, is implied by "the image of the ambrosial *kuṇḍalī*." That same subsidiary *sādhana* is called a "*vajra* recitation" (*vajra-jāpa*). It is to be recited by means of the [two] uninterrupted sequences in the central channel: by means of the [two] uninterrupted sequences, *prāṇa* does not flow in the right and left channels. The Tantric adept should practice breath control after an image of the crown *cakra* has been perceived. The *guru*'s instruction is to be understood in accordance with the cryptic language [of these teachings]. The subsidiary *sādhana* of the breath control and retention [phases] has been described.

After this, an image of a deity appears during the *sādhana* [phase]. Here, due to the power of [the practice of] retention, the yogi perceives the *caṇḍālī* blazing in the navel, the great seal, similar to an image in a prognostic mirror and free from all obscurations, emanating multitudes of rays of limitless Buddhas and shining forth as a disc of light. He, [the Holy One] termed this recollection [phase] a "*sādhana*." At the end of the retention [phase], one should meditate on the yoga of *caṇḍālī*. After that, owing to the flame of the gnosis of that [*caṇḍālī*], the incinerated psychophysical aggregates, elements, and sense-bases become unified. Consciousness and so on—as well as the earth and other elements that are of the nature of the mandalas and that are situated in the left and right channels—are brought into the moon-disc in the forehead *cakra*. Afterward, when the flame of the gnosis of the *caṇḍālī* melts the moon [or semen], *bodhicitta* [that is, seminal fluid] in the form of a drop descends into the throat, heart, navel, and secret lotus, being of the nature of bliss, supreme [bliss], and special [bliss]. Then, with the nature of innate bliss, or with the nature of the diverse, ripening, dissolving, and non-characterized [moments], it descends into the *vajra*-jewel [or into the sexual organ]. Thus, when [the *bodhicitta*], complete with sixteen digits, is present in the jewel, then due to the power of meditation it affords a bliss that is similar to the bliss of emission. This is only an analogy; by its nature, perishable bliss that arises from the two [sexual] organs is not worth even a thousand-millionth of the supreme, imperishable bliss. Here, immature yogis are unable to cognize the state of imperishable bliss, which is tantamount to innate bliss as a specific state. Bodhisattvas call [this state] a "*samādhi* on emptiness." However, this [*samādhi*] cannot be developed by mundane people nor can it be cultivated by non-believers.

Hence, it is by means of six-phased yoga that the Buddhahood of yogis is realized.

> Worship is [accomplished] with the five ambrosias and the like, the four *vajras*, the recitation of mantras, and so on. The subsidiary *sādhana* is [accomplished] with the retraction [phase] and so on, and with the nectar produced in the *vajra* and in the [woman's] lotus. This *sādhana* is a meditation that is of the same essence as the three *vajras* and the lotus due to joy (*ānanda*) and so on. The non-emission [of semen] in union with the wisdom [consort] is [called] the great *sādhana* because of subtle yoga. (*Abridged Tantra of the Wheel of Time*, 4.113)

Here, the beginner should first worship in the manner of *sādhana*. Worship is [accomplished] with the five ambrosias and so on. In the external [practice], the five ambrosias are feces and the like. Beef, dog [meat], and such like are implied by the phrase "and the like." Worship with these ingested ambrosias is [carried out] for the sake of gratifying deities. In terms of the individual, the five ambrosias are the five psychophysical aggregates. The five sense-faculties, or the five lamps are implied by the phrase "and the like." [Here,] worship is a disregard for these, a renunciation of craving for the body and material objects. Deities become propitious by virtue of this worship, and not due to the ingestion of feces and the like.

Worship with the four *vajras* is disregard for the pleasures of the body, the pleasures of speech, the pleasures of the mind, and the bliss of emission. In other words, it is control over body, speech, and mind, and [the practice of] celibacy. Deities become propitious by virtue of this [worship], and not due to yearning for the pleasures of cyclic existence. [Worship] also entails recitations of mantras and so on. Here, breath control is called the "recitation of mantras." Due to the phrase "and so on," worship always [entails] the yoga of outbreath (*recaka*), inbreath (*pūraka*), and breath retention (*kumbhaka*). Owing to this [yoga], as opposed to the unrestrained breath released through speech, deities become propitious. This is a definitive meaning. Moreover, in terms of its provisional meaning, one should engage in recitation with a rosary and the like, for the sake of mundane *siddhis*.

Now, beginning with "retraction" and so on, he, [the Holy One,] discussed the subsidiary *sādhana*. In this context, it is the retraction [phase]. Here, the apprehension of sense objects such as form and the like—by means of the sense-faculties such as the visual faculty and so on—is the grasping of transmigrating beings. Renunciation of this [grasping] is called "retraction." With regard to the form of emptiness, the apprehension of different sense objects, form and so on—by means of the different visual and other sense-faculties, which are distinct from the physical [sense-faculties]—constitutes the subsidiary *sādhana*. Meditative stabilization, breath control, and [the] retention [phase are also included in the subsidiary *sādhana*]. In terms of the definitive meaning, the subsidiary *sādhana* is accomplished through the non-emission of [seminal] ambrosia that is produced in the sexual organs [during intercourse]. In terms of the provisional meaning, the accomplishment of this subsidiary *sādhana* is a result of the external emanation of the deities [in the visualized *kālacakra-mandala*].

Now, [in the passage] beginning with [the word] "bliss" and so on, the *sādhana* [phase] is discussed. Here, with regard to bliss, there are three *vajras*—the drops of body, speech, and mind. This *sādhana* is a meditation that is of the same nature as the lotus. This means that the drops remain in the heart, navel, and secret [*cakras*]. Such is the *sādhana*.

"Next, the great *sādhana* [is discussed]. When imperishable bliss arises during union with the wisdom [consort], this is [known as] the great *sādhana* due to subtle yoga. In terms of the definitive meaning, this is called the "great *sādhana*" because of the confluence of semen above the central channel. In terms of the provisional meaning, it is a white mustard seed and the like on the tip of the *nāsikā* of the source of phenomena [or the vulva] of the wisdom [consort]. This is a principle. The great *sādhana* takes place in this way" (*Stainless Light* commentary on the *Abridged Tantra of the Wheel of Time,* 4.113).

Now, [in the passage] beginning with "delicate" [or "a child"] and so forth, he [the Holy One] described the worship [phase] and so on.

> Indeed, at first, there is an awareness of emptiness, then a seizing of the drops of the moon [or semen]. After that comes a generation of [the deity's] bodily image. Then comes the placing of syllables in accordance with the six most excellent families. There is this ordinary worship with four *vajras* and the middle *sādhana* [or the completion of the meditative generation of vital energies]. Here, the method [male consort] is of four kinds: it is delicate and strong [in the subsidiary *sādhana*], and it is also such in the *sādhana* phase. (*Abridged Tantra of the Wheel of Time*, 4.114)

Here, in the stage of generation [of oneself in the form of the deity] there is an awakening to emptiness. The interval between the abandoning of the psychophysical aggregates at the death of living beings and their acquiring of [new] psychophysical aggregates that partake in birth is a single moment of [the awareness of] emptiness, which is said to see the three worlds as empty [of inherent existence]. "Indeed," means "certainly." Then, after that moment, there is the seizing of the [seminal] drops of the moon. Here, the repository consciousness's *(ālaya-vijñāna)* appropriation of seminal drops in the mother's womb is called "seizing." Due to the seizing of semen and the like, within seven months, a completion in the womb takes place, i.e., there is a completion of the body, which is called the "origination of a bodily image." Afterwards comes the placing of syllables of the eye and the like—that is, there comes the engagement with the sense objects, with form and so on, in accordance with the six most excellent families, or in accordance with the six psychophysical aggregates. Likewise, in the *sādhana* of the deities, the beginner should meditate on that which is of an imaginary nature. There is the ordinary worship (*sāmānya-sevā*) with the four *vajras*, or with the generated *vajras* of the body, speech, mind, and gnosis; and there is the middle *sādhana*, the origination of the vital energies. Here, in the worship [phase], the method [consort] is of four kinds, and in the subsidiary *sādhana*, it is delicate and strong. Likewise, in the *sādhana* phase, [the method consort] is [a boy] up to the age of sixteen. This is a principle. In this context, "delicate" refers to a newborn child. After the fall of the [first] teeth, one is a youth. After the growth of the new teeth, one is an adult because one begets sons and daughters.

Thus, the yogi should meditate on the fourth phase with regard to all the deities. This is a principle of mundane reality.

Now, the generation of the Buddha's body is discussed in terms of ultimate reality. In this context, there is an awakening to emptiness; that is, in darkness, one should not think of anything whatsoever. After that comes retention of the drop of the moon, an apprehension of the signs beginning with smoke and ending with the drop. Afterward comes the origination of the body, meaning that after that drop there is the arising of clairvoyance and the origination of a bodily image. In accordance with the most excellent families, or in accordance with the psychophysical aggregates that are free from obscurations, there follows the placing of letters. [In other words,] the cessation of the localized psychophysical aggregates, elements, and sense-bases takes place. Thus, in accordance with the attainment of the [twelve Bodhisattva] Grounds, there is the classification of the delicate and other [phases of life], until one becomes a master of the twelve Grounds. Hence,

> He is a referent of the truth having twelve aspects; he knows reality with sixteen aspects; he has full awakening with twenty aspects; he is fully awakened, omniscient, and supreme. (*Litany of the Names of Mañjuśrī,* 9.15)

Now, the results of the retraction and other [phases] are discussed:

> The yogi [who has been] freed from the sense objects due to the retraction [phase] is empowered with mantras. Purified by means of the yoga of meditative stabilization, O king, he has the five extrasensory perceptions. Purified by means of breath control, free from the sun and the moon, he is honored by Bodhisattvas. By the power of the retention [phase], he attains the ten powers and the annihilation of the Māras and mental afflictions. (*Abridged Tantra of the Wheel of Time,* 4.118)

> Completely purified by means of the recollection [phase], he is a stainless disc on account of his gnostic form. Thereafter, purified in the *samādhi* [phase], he is the Gnostic Body [which is] achieved after several days. If this accomplishment desired by Tantric adepts is not attained by means of the retraction and other phases, then one could achieve it after the *nāda* practice accompanied by *haṭha* [yoga], and after preserving drops in the *vajra*-jewel within the lotus. (*Abridged Tantra of the Wheel of Time*, 4.119)

Here, when the yogi becomes purified by means of the retraction [phase], he is empowered with all the *mantras* by [means of] a stabilized image, and he offers boon-granting and the like with his speech. Purified by the yoga of meditative stabilization, O king, he becomes endowed with five extrasensory perceptions. Here, when the eyes are fixed, the divine eye comes forth. Similarly, the divine ear becomes purified by means of meditative stabilization. It becomes purified by means of breath control. When the yogi becomes free from the paths of the sun and the moon and when there is a constant flow [of *prāṇa*] in the central channel, then, purified through breath control, he is honored. This means [that] he is praised by Bodhisattvas. He attains the ten powers and the annihilation of the Māras and mental afflictions. By the power of the retention [phase], he achieves the form of emptiness, the apprehending-and-apprehended mind. Due to the destruction of past and future vital energies, he becomes unified.

Here [in the phrase], "purified by means of the recollection [phase]," recollection is an embracing of the mind's image, the mind's freedom from conceptualization. Therefore, when he is purified, he becomes a stainless disc of light. Moreover, on account of the word "and," [it is implied that] the five lights emanating from the pores of his skin come forth from the gnostic form or from the empty form. Afterward, he is purified in *samādhi*.

Here, the imperishable bliss that arises due to the unification of the apprehending-and-apprehended mind is called "*samādhi*." Therefore, purified through this, purified through *samādhi*, [and] contained in stainlessness, within several days (or within three years and three fortnights) he succeeds as a Gnostic Body. He becomes a Bodhisattva who has attained mastery over the ten powers, and so on. This is a principle of the retraction [phase].

Now, *haṭha-yoga* is described. Here, if, due to *prāṇa* being unrestrained, the moment of imperishable [bliss] does not arise when the image is perceived through the retraction and other phases, then, having conveyed *prāṇa* into the central channel through *nāda* practice and *haṭha* [*yoga*], one should give rise to imperishable bliss by preserving the drops of [the seminal] *bodhicitta* in the *vajra*-jewel present in the lotus of a wisdom [consort], without vibration. This is *haṭha-yoga*. The *nāda* practice is described here:

> The *śakti* [or the power of *prāṇas*] that moves from the center of the navel [through the nostrils] to another place [outside the body] as far as twelve [finger-breadths] and as far as sixteen [finger-breadths], is obstructed in the navel. It is similar to a flash of lightning and is arisen in the shape of a stick. Stirred in the central channel, it has a subtle and playful motion from the [navel] *cakra* to another *cakra*, until, like a needle, it forcefully reaches the aperture of the *uṣṇīṣa* and the outer skin. (*Abridged Tantra of the Wheel of Time,* 4.196; 2.120)

> At that time, with utmost force, one should direct the downward wind (*apāna*) into the upward course. When the pair of winds is obstructed, having split the crown *cakra*, it reaches another abode. Thus, due to awakening the *vajra* in the mind, which is with an object, he obtains the

> power of flight. Moreover, this [power] of the yogis is Viśvamātā, who is of the nature of the five extrasensory perceptions. (*Abridged Tantra of the Wheel of Time,* 4.197; 2.121)

> Wisdom and gnosis become the mind and its tenfold appearance. Initiation is an immersion into this [appearance], which is similar to an image in a prognostic mirror and resembles the stainless moon. He for whom the face of the Buddha appears in the heart and in the mouth is a glorious *guru*. (*Abridged Tantra of the Wheel of Time,* 5.114)

Here, wisdom and gnosis respectively are the apprehending mind and the tenfold apprehended, mirror-like appearance of that apprehending mind, smoke and so on, which is like an image in a prognostic mirror. This means that this very gnosis is the apprehended mind. Wisdom and gnosis are [related] in this manner: one's own eye is apprehended like a reflection of one's own eye in a mirror. Initiation, which is an immersion into this [apprehended mind], means this: here, the entering of the apprehending mind into this apprehended mind is a non-engagement with the external sense objects. In six-phased yoga, the immersion is called "retraction, meditative stabilization, breath control, and retention." After this immersion, the felicity of *nirvāṇa*, the non-emitted, innate, and imperishable, fourth bliss—which is a desideratum for youths, adults and the elderly, and which transcends resemblance to the world—is described according to the convention of the three worlds [and not from the standpoint of the inexpressible ultimate truth]. This is the meaning.

It is free from laughing, gazing, touching, embracing, hand-holding, and coupling. It is devoid of an actual consort and an imagined consort as its causes, and it has the characteristic of the appearance of all aspects of emptiness. This means: a preceptor who at all times has the face of the Buddha, the face of gnosis, present in his heart, or cultivated and personally experienced, and who has it in his mouth for the sake of imparting it to disciples, is a glorious *guru*, a *vajra*-holder.

Now, a summary of the yoga is discussed.

> There is the entering of *prāṇa* into the central [channel], the unification of the paths of the sun and the moon in the right and left [channels], the mind that has entered supreme bliss in union with a consort, the *vajra*'s awakening, or a sound of the *vajra* in a lotus, agitating [one's *vajra*] with one's lotus-hands for the sake of bliss, the non-release of semen, and a bliss that removes the fear of death, which is the face of the glorious *guru*. (*Abridged Tantra of the Wheel of Time,* 5.121)

Here, the yogi must first bring the *prāṇa* into the central channel, by means of which he perceives a sign in the central channel, which is said to be the face or the body-*vajra* of the Buddha, the glorious *guru*. After that comes the uniting of the *prāṇa*'s left path, the path of the moon, together with its right path, the path of the sun. This is a principle. Breath control is the second, the speech-*vajra*. The mind [that is] fond of a bodily form in union with the consort, or a melted [seminal] *bodhicitta*, is the third. This is the mind-*vajra* abiding in supreme bliss, and the *vajra*'s awakening. If bliss does not arise due to a bodily form, then one should slowly create a sound of the *vajra* in the lotus. If one does not acquire a woman, he should agitate [his *vajra*] with his lotus-hands for the sake of bliss, not for the sake of emission. His non-release of semen thereby becomes that bliss, which removes the fear of death, and which is the face of the glorious *guru*, the fourth face of gnosis. This is a principle of the practice of yoga.

Now, the destruction of the five *mandalas* is discussed.

> The earth [-*mandala*] enters the water, the water enters the fire, the fire enters the wind, the wind enters the space, the space enters the ten signs, and the ten signs enter the supreme, indestructible bliss, the "unstruck" (*anāhata*), the Gnostic Body having all aspects. Due to gnosis, O king, the supernatural power becomes a human accomplishment here, in this life. (*Abridged Tantra of the Wheel of Time*, 5.122)

This is implied here: when the yogi has his eyes open and his mind located in space with the gaze of a fierce deity, then the earth [mandala] is either on the left and or on the right. This is a method when the yogi meditates during the flow of the earth [mandala] on the right, but not during its flow in the left channel due to the sequence of the space-mandala and so on. Therefore, the mandala that *prāṇa* carries in the left or in the right is named after that very mandala due to its being of the nature of that [mandala]. Hence, the *prāṇa* in the earth-mandala within the right channel enters into the water-mandala. The same [process continues] up to the gnosis-mandala. In the left channel, it enters into the space and other mandalas. Thus, it dissolves into space, or into the ten signs, smoke and so on [in space]; the signs dissolve into the form [of Kālacakra and Viśvamātā] having all aspects; and form dissolves into imperishable bliss. That very gnosis is of the perfection of wisdom. Due to gnosis, the supernormal powers (*ṛddhi*s) and supernatural abilities such as sky-walking and so on, O king, demonstrate men's [yogis'] mastery over the three worlds right here, in this life. This is the principle of entering the path.

—12—

Eroticism and Cosmic Transformation as Yoga: The *Ātmatattva* of the Vaiṣṇava Sahajiyās of Bengal

Glen Alexander Hayes

The composition of the *Ātmatattva*, an anonymous text written mostly in Bengali (with some Sanskrit verses), has been dated by Edward C. Dimock, Jr. to the early seventeenth century CE. The title of this northeastern Indian yoga text may be translated as either "The Cosmic Principles (*tattva*) of the Self (*ātma*)" or "The Metaphysics of the Self." The version used for this translation runs to only two printed pages in a Bengali anthology, and it has many similarities to a number of other short manuscript texts also dated to the early seventeenth century. Dating is imprecise, however, and the text may be from as late as the eighteenth century. Although it is relatively short, the text reflects many diverse sources of Hindu traditions. These were brought together by a lineage of Tantric yogic gurus who collectively formed what recent scholars have called the "Vaiṣṇava Sahajiyā" traditions of Bengal. Although the term "Vaiṣṇava" literally refers to followers of the god Viṣṇu, in greater Bengal (modern West Bengal and Assam in India, as well as portions of Bangladesh) the term more often indicates the devotional worship of the playful and majestic cowherd god Kṛṣṇa, who is eternally present along with his lover Rādhā in the heavenly realm of Vṛndāvana. These devotees of Kṛṣṇa and Rādhā are called Bengali or "Gauḍīya" Vaiṣṇavas, and they have been a dominant branch of Hinduism in the region since at least the time of the ecstatic god-man Kṛṣṇa Caitanya (ca. 1486–1533 CE). Caitanya's activities and intense devotionalism led to the growth of the Bengali school, centering upon singing, chanting, and dancing out of devotional love (*bhakti*) for Kṛṣṇa. These activities—themselves an ideal form of "devotional" or "emotional" yoga—were adapted by contemporary Tantric Hindu *gurus*, who integrated them into their own form of rituals and worship in order to realize *sahaja*. *Sahaja* may be translated as "the Innate," "Co-eval," "Natural," or "Together-born" (*saha-ja*), a blissful state of cosmic consciousness in which all dualities are merged—into a perfect yogic "union." These later, post-Caitanya Tantrics came to be known as "Vaiṣṇava Sahajiyās," and although they continued at least into the early twentieth century, some of their modern-day descendants are the Bāuls ("mad men"), wandering musical mystics who sing of blissful inner states and practice ritual sexual intercourse.

The Sahajiyās, as Tantrics, used ritualized sexual intercourse to realize the God and his divine consort within; as Kṛṣṇa, the inner masculine principle in all men; and Rādhā as the inner feminine principle in all women. Their activities and interpretations shocked and outraged the orthodox Bengali Vaiṣṇavas back in the seventeenth century (as they continue to do today). So, in summary, this small, complicated yoga text comes from a blending of both devotional *bhakti* yoga and Tantric yoga, and also brings together other fascinating South Asian traditions (for example: the creation process of Sāṃkhya philosophy, the system of vital breaths and meditation from classical yoga, and the erotic and emotional categories from Sanskrit and Bengali Vaiṣṇava religious aesthetics and dramaturgy). The *Ātmatattva* for all its brevity is complex.

The broader social, cultural, and religious context of the *Ātmatattva* is seventeenth- to nineteenth-century Bengal, with its many forms of Hinduism, as well as Islam. Bengal was the seat of British colonialism at the time, centered in Calcutta (now Kolkata). For many centuries prior to the rise of British colonial power in Bengal in the late seventeenth and early eighteenth centuries, the area had been largely under the control of Muslim sultans, and Sufi Islam had thrived. The region also had many Hindu followers of the god Śiva and different aspects of the Great Goddess, especially as Durgā and Kālī. Prior to the Muslims, many other famous Hindu as well as Buddhist rulers had governed Bengal. In sum, the context, culture, and history of Bengal of the time of this text were rich and diverse.

An Introduction to the Text

The text begins with traditional opening praises of Bengali Vaiṣṇavism: "Glory to holy Rādhā and Kṛṣṇa! Glory to the holy *guru*!" This is a classic offertory verse which links the text and its readers not only to the surrounding Vaiṣṇava traditions, but also to lineages of the realized masters (*gurus*), who would guide the adepts as they traveled the yogic journey outlined in the subsequent passages. The printed version of the *Ātmatattva* is divided into six sections (to which I have added section numbers for reference), although these may have been added by a later editor. The sections are: (1) on the nature of the individual Being (*jīva*); (2) on the Vital Breaths (*prāṇa*) (a classical yogic concern); (3) on the "Flower Arrows" of the god of Desire, Kāmadeva (identified here with Kṛṣṇa); (4) on the divinities; (5) on creation and its metaphysics (*tattva*); and (6) on powerful Sanskrit incantations (*mantras*) and "seed-syllables" (*bīja*). Most of the analysis in the text arranges things into groups of five, or pentads, and we find this technique used throughout the sections. Interestingly, a pentadic worldview and organizing technique is quite ancient in South Asia; for example, the *Taittirīya Upaniṣad* (ca. fifth- to fourth-century BCE) not only makes the important yogic and ritual connections between the body as microcosm and the physical universe as macrocosm, but it also employs pentads to help explain the details of these correspondences. Thus, although separated by many centuries, both the *Ātmatattva* and the *Taittirīya Upaniṣad* articulate a pentadic cosmology replete with secret correspondences and connections, and then reveal the knowledge and rituals by which the adept can master this structured cosmos and thereby gain liberation. It is similar to a complex modern computer game, which requires mastery of the levels in order to "win" the game. Seen this way, the *Ātmatattva* in some ways is simply continuing an organizing and relational theme found many centuries earlier in the Vedas and Upaniṣads, while also adding further dimensions of theism, eroticism, and ritual sexual intercourse. It is a most interesting version of yoga.

On the Different Levels of "Being" (*jīva*)

One of the basic goals of any yoga is to realize the nature of one's body and through that of one's inner being as reflected in its states of consciousness. Then, depending upon the type of yoga, the adept "joins" these aspects with the fundamental reality of the cosmos—which is not different from the self or from the divine being—forging a synthetic realization of the nature of reality. As this volume illustrates, there are indeed many understandings of what "yoga" is. The first section of the *Ātmatattva* is concerned with the different kinds of *jīva* (which I translate by the noun "Being" or adjective "Living"), how they are connected to the universe, which powers they have, and—importantly—how the adept may learn to control these levels of being through *sādhana*, that is, the system of yogic practices and rituals. There are, following the pentadic structure, five levels of Being: the "gross" (*sthūla*), the "indifferent" (*taṭastha*), the "bound" (*baddha*), the "liberated" (*mukta*), and the "subtle" (*sūkṣma*). The "gross Being" refers to the most basic physical entity, which arises from the sexual fluids at conception but lacks fully developed human form. The "indifferent Being" is like a detached observer; it uses the senses but lacks focus or intention. The "bound Being" is tied up with worldly life and obligations, "like a father tied to his son." Reflecting the traditional tension in classical Hinduism between obligatory life in the world (*dharma*) versus asceticism and giving up worldly attachments (*saṃnyāsa*), the next Being is called "liberated" (*mukta*), because one has now "become a servant of the *guru*" and "renounced all worldly pleasures." This might seem to be the highest, but that in fact is called the "subtle" (*sūkṣma*) Being, which is said to enjoy an existence of loving and serving Kṛṣṇa in a celestial realm. In Bengali Vaiṣṇavism, a loving relationship with Kṛṣṇa (or, with Sahajiyās, realizing one's own inner nature *as* Kṛṣṇa) is far superior to the classical Hindu philosophical state of pure nondual "liberation" (*mukti*), which, as is the case in this text, is generally admired but relegated to a lower level.

Having briefly presented the five levels of Being, the text now goes deeper into the cosmic structure and discusses the five types of "*ātmā*," an ancient Sanskrit term (a reflexive noun) which is typically translated as "Soul" or "Self." The first is called the "Living Self" (*jīvātmā*), and it is said to reside in an unexplained type of inner yogic "vessel" (*bhāṇḍa*), which itself is generated out of the basic building blocks of the cosmos, the fundament of reality (*tattvavastu*). The Self is said to be composed of the five basic cosmic elements (*bhūta*s) of earth, water, fire, air, and space. Yet in other Sahajiyā texts studied by this author (see Further Reading), these basic units of reality (*vastu*) can also be generated out of the sexual fluids collected during ritual sexual intercourse. The yogic body, then, is generated through the yogic manipulation or "reversal" of the sexual fluids. While the natural mingling of sexual fluids may result in the birth of a physical baby, the yogic blending of sexual fluids issues in the "birth" of the yogic "body" or "vessel" *within* the physical body. Thus, the "Living Self" commences its pursuit of the higher yogic realms using this inner vessel/body. All Sahajiyā journeys thus require a yogic body to make the trip. This powerful "Living Self" can be "brought under control" by mastering everything from the basest "greed" (*lobha*) up to the pinnacle of "liberation" (*mukti*)—no small feat for most people.

The next level is called the "Elemental Self" (*bhūtātmā*), which seems to obtain when consciousness has mastered the five elements. The text states that it may be controlled by two types of *sādhana* developed by Bengali Vaiṣṇavas: "the moods and experiences of a young maiden" (*sakhī-bhāva-āśraya*) and through the use of a powerful Sanskrit incantation (*mantra*) called the "Verse of the Seed-syllable of Desire" (*kāma-bīja gāyatrī*). As David Haberman has shown, a powerful way for a Bengali Vaiṣṇava devotee (male or female) to participate in the divine "love-play" (*līlā*) of Rādhā and Kṛṣṇa is to ritually and emotionally "construct" the situations, mood, and even the "body" (*śrī-rūpa*) of a young "maiden" from the stories of Kṛṣṇa, who beholds the celestial trysts of the divine couple in the eternal, heavenly realm of Vṛndāvana. This has the effect of projecting the adept into higher cosmic regions and gaining even greater yogic powers. The use of *mantras* further enhances this transformative and salvific process, as we shall see.

Although it often comprises the highest level of consciousness in many other yogic traditions, the next level of Self, the "Supreme Self" (*paramātmā*), is only the third level for the *Ātmatattva*. (As we will see, the higher two levels express Vaiṣṇava Sahajiyā ideals of aesthetics and eroticism.) The Supreme Self can be controlled by chanting the names of Kṛṣṇa and by using *mantras* and seed-syllables. The fourth level is the "Delight in Knowing the Self" (*ātmārāma*), a theological and aesthetic term from Bengali Vaiṣṇavism that refers to the necessary role of desire by all created beings for Kṛṣṇa in the yogic process. Although Vaiṣṇava texts equate the *ātmārāma* with the Vedantic knowledge of the Self (which is thus a lower form of spiritual knowledge), it is also reinterpreted in terms of the desire or delight experienced in knowing Kṛṣṇa. And it is here we can see a major difference between the *Ātmatattva* and many other yogic texts: the necessity of really using—as opposed to renouncing—desire and erotic sexuality to gain liberation. This also reflects the Tantric heritage of the Sahajiyās. However, the means of controlling the "Delight in Knowing the Self" is "deep meditation" (*dhyāna*), one of the eight "limbs" or stages of Pantañjali's classical tradition of yoga. The *Ātmatattva* implies a complex series of rituals here, as this *sādhana* involves food, sleep, cognition, music, thought, worship, infatuation, and modesty. Alas, no further details are provided (they would likely have been taught orally by the *guru*). But this is not simply a matter of lust or desire (*kāma*); the correct attitude requires that desire be transformed into the purest, most selfless kind of spiritual love (*prema*) and directed to Kṛṣṇa, if the yoga is to succeed. Very briefly, the text also mentions the yogic experiences of "moods" (*bhāva*), which must be elevated to that of heightened rapture (*rasa*), through the "pursuit of desire" (*kāmānugā*) and "eroticism" (*śṛṅgāra*). In Sanskrit and Bengali Vaiṣṇava aesthetics, one identifies fundamental emotions (*bhāva*), the experience of which in ritual becomes a pure state of religious rapture known as *rasa* (literally, the "sap" or "juice," and by extension the "distilled essence of an experience"). The Sahajiyās achieve this sublime state through ritualized sexual intercourse wherein they regard the sexual fluids as the physical analogues of *rasa*. Hence *rasa* might be translated as "Divine Essence," which, either as a sweet experience or a sexual fluid, "flows" as a result of *sādhana*. No details are provided about this process by the text, but it refers to the Sahajiyā adaptation of Bengali Vaiṣṇava rituals of devotion and the young maiden, and to the practices of Tantric ritual sexual intercourse, mentioned above.

The fifth and highest level of Self (mentioned a bit further along in the first section), also adapted from Bengali Vaiṣṇavism, is the "Lord Who Delights in Knowing the Self" (*ātmārāmeśvara*), and has been interpreted by Dimock to mean "Kṛṣṇa, containing Rādhā within himself." What this means is that the cosmic male principle, as Kṛṣṇa, has been lovingly united with the cosmic feminine, as Rādhā. The result, for Bengali Vaiṣṇavas, is an overwhelming intense cosmic delight (*hlādinī*) experienced by both Kṛṣṇa and Rādhā (and indirectly appreciated by devotees). For the Sahajiyās who used this text, this condition, given a Tantric interpretation, joined the cosmic male and female powers in the experience of *Sahaja*, which was their goal.

The text then moves on to provide the "locations" of the different Selves in the yogic body. The "Living Self" is placed in a four-petaled lotus (*padma*) in the "hidden land" (*guhyadeśa*), which refers to the anal region. The "Elemental Self" resides in a six-petaled lotus at the base of the penis (*liṅga*), while the "Supreme Self" exists in the place of "the coiled one" (*kuṇḍalī*), amidst a complex lotus of ten petals, each of which is comprised of twelve petals! Omitting the location of the "Delight in Knowing the Self" (possibly a scribal error?), the "Lord Who Delights in Knowing the Self" is placed in a "blazing" (*ujjvala*) lotus, each petal of which has sixteen petals. This incomplete and vague description of the lotuses and petals, at any rate, is clearly different from the best-known model of the six "wheels" (*cakras*) and the uppermost thousand-petalled lotus, although the "coiled one" is similar to the "coiled serpent power" (*kuṇḍalinī-śakti*) of other yogic and Tantric systems. It bears recalling that the "yogic body" in fact varies in its segments and structure even among Vaiṣṇava Sahajiyā texts; while there are five lotuses implied here, other Sahajiyā texts envision only four (see Further Reading).

The first section of the text concludes by filling out the pentadic structure a bit more, providing each level of Self with a symbolic color, a sustaining element, and a function (*karma*). The "Living Self" is blood red, is sustained by water, and bears burdens. The "Elemental Self" is bright yellow, sustained by copious amounts of food, and helps to understand the six vices that impede realization: lust, anger, greed, infatuation, intoxication, and malice. The "Supreme Self" is the color of lightning, is sustained by the wind, and functions to control the various mental states. The "Delight in Knowing the Self" is the color of the moon, sustained by the sweetness of the stories of Kṛṣṇa, and serves to keep joyful speech foremost in one's mind. The "Lord Who Delights in Knowing the Self" is the color of the sun, sustained by the nectar of the stories of Kṛṣṇa, and has the tasks of Kṛṣṇa-worship, perception (*buddhi*), strength, knowledge, and the "tasting" (*āsvādana*) of *rasa. Rasa*, especially in Sahajiyā texts like the *Ātmatattva*, again has the dual meaning of heightened religious rapture as well as sexual fluids.

A Brief Mention of the Yogic "Vital Breaths" (*prāṇas*)

The second section is the briefest of the *Ātmatattva*, running to but five verses. It addresses the five basic types of "Vital Breath" (*prāṇa*) that are standard to most yoga systems: *apāna* ("Breathing In"), located in the anus; *prāṇa* ("Breathing Out"), located in the heart lotus; *samāna* ("Equalizing Breath"), centered in the navel; *udāna* ("Upward Breath"), found in the throat; and *vyāna* ("Traversing Breath"), found throughout the body. The brief treatment of the Vital Breaths, which are seldom given much attention in other Sahajiyā texts, assumes a basic knowledge of the Patañjalian traditions of yoga.

On the Erotic Arrows, Cosmic Development, Senses, and Organs

The third section brings us to the erotic dimensions, as well as to the Sahajiyā adaptation of Sāṃkhya cosmogony for the manifestation of the universe, the mind, and the sensory organs. To know through direct experience the power of desires and emotions, as well as their place and function in the cosmological structure, is to gain control over them and to reach liberation. Drawing upon the much earlier traditions of Sanskrit aesthetics and dramaturgy, the idea is that the god of love and sexual desire, Kāma-deva, is actually just another manifestation of the also-playful Kṛṣṇa. In many Sanskrit plays, Kāma-deva has a quiver of "Flower Arrows" (*bāṇa*), which he "shoots" into the hearts of characters (after the fashion of Cupid in Greco-Roman cultures). Once a person has been shot in this way, he or she develops passion and desire for another. Intriguing exploits and romantic trysts may then take place, and there are many interesting incidents of such in South Asian literature and plays. Following the classical model, the five arrows mentioned in the *Ātmatattva* are *Madana* ("delight in love"); *Mādana* ("intoxication in love"); *Śoṣaṇa* ("absorption in love"); *Stambhana* ("suspension of all sensation but that of love"); and *Mohana* ("complete bliss"). But, the reader might ask: "How is this yogic?" The arrows create passions and energies that are to be enacted, realized, mastered, and unified into *Sahaja*, the final union of male and female principles. The *Ātmatattva* may be alluding to Sanskrit plays, which some may have seen, but this more likely refers to the preliminaries and foreplay of the Sahajiyā ritual sexual intercourse, in which the "hero" (*nāyaka*) develops desire (*kāma*) for the "heroine" (*nāyikā*). In fact, the text locates each of the arrows in a region of the lover's (usually the woman's) face, which in Indian literature itself is often compared to a lotus flower. Thus the Madana is located in the left corner of the left eye, Mādana in the right corner of the right eye, Śoṣaṇa in the lower lip, Stambhana in passionate sexual union (*śṛṅgāra*), and Mohana in a sultry, side-long glance. In other words, this is a yoga not only of uniting lower and higher consciousness, but of uniting male and female sexual energies and fluids, and of harnessing and transforming the erotic into the spiritual.

The final portion of the third section then takes a turn away from eroticism, and presents a basic Sahajiyā interpretation of the classical dualism of Sāṃkhya. But it does so by remaining on the topic of male and female union, observing that the *prakṛti* (female matter) and *puruṣa* (male consciousness) unite to create both the most fundamental Cosmic Reality (*mahā-tattva*) and creation itself (*utpatti*). This is important, for the text is using Sāṃkhya cosmology to support an underlying Tantric yogic worldview: that the cosmos is gendered, and that ritual sexual intercourse and eroticism are tools for gaining mastery over the entire universe. What follows is a neat parallel to the unfolding of creation as described in Sāṃkhya: the emergence from the ultimate Cosmic Reality of the three basic levels of ego-sense (*ahaṃkāra*) and qualities (*guṇa*): activity (*rājas*), inertia/darkness (*tamas*), and purity/light (*sattva*). The connections between the microcosmic body and the macrocosmic universe are also maintained, as the five elements are said to emerge from the "awareness of activity" (*rājasa ahaṃkāra*). Each cosmic element is connected to a bodily sense; for example, the earth quality is located in the nose, involves the sense of smell, and is pearly-white in color. Each of the other four elements/senses/locations/colors is similarly detailed in the text. After all five are mentioned, an important claim is made: "If one can know these five principles, the Being (*jīva*) will become liberated (*mukta*) and even the body will become eternal (*nitya*)." This is a not uncommon trope in many other forms of yoga, for all forms seek to master the cosmic reality through the exploration of interior landscapes. But the Sahajiyās are also claiming here that one can create, via ritual, an "eternal yogic body" (*nitya-deha*) made out of the reversed sexual fluids (*vastu*) of the ritual sexual intercourse. It is this "body" (comparable to the "maiden" body mentioned earlier) that the adept will eventually inhabit in the celestial abode of Rādhā and Kṛṣṇa in the realm of Vṛndāvana.

While the five cosmic elements are said to evolve from the "awareness of activity," the "awareness of inertia" (*tamasa ahaṃkāra*) is said to be the source for the ten sensory organs (*indriya*), including the five organs of knowing (*jñānendriyas*: the nose, tongue, eyes, skin, and ears) and the five organs of action (*karmendriyas*: the mouth, hands, feet, anus, and genitals). Working yet again with pentads, the text makes basic observations on what each of these senses or organs do; for example, the eye perceives gradations of light and darkness, while the genitals excrete sexual fluids, urine, and such. Again, all of these are mentioned, as the adept must gain yogic mastery over each sense and organ. By "knowing" where they emerge from, one is enabled in the pursuit of liberation. Thus concludes the third section.

How the Divinities Emerge from "Pure Awareness"

The fourth section of the *Ātmatattva* continues the analysis of Sāṃkhya cosmology from a Sahajiyā perspective, as it discusses the emergence of the various divinities (*devatās*) from the "awareness of purity" (*sāttvika ahaṃkāra*). There are two sets of five divinities, and each is correlated to the previous pentads of senses of knowledge (*jñāna*) and of action (*karma*). As for the senses of knowledge, the *Dikpālas* (the guardians of the directions) are located in the ears; *Vāyu* (the god of winds) is in the skin; *Arka* (the sun god) is in the eyes; *Prochetā* (god of waters) is in the tongue; and *Aśvinīkumār* (the twin gods) are in the nose. With regard to organs of action, *Vahni* (the Vedic god of fire) is connected with the mouth; *Indra* (warrior god of the Vedas) is linked with the hands; *Upendra* (Viṣṇu, as brother of Indra) with the feet; *Mitra* (the Vedic god of cosmic order) with the anus; and *Prajāpati Brahmā* (the creator god) with the genitals (*liṅgamūla*, literally "base of the penis"). Again, the *Ātmatattva* version of yoga suggests that even the mightiest of the Vedic and other Hindu gods (who were often worshipped as independent and major deities in other Hindu traditions) can also be understood and internalized by the adept of this yoga. This is but another example of how this version of Tantric yoga, while acknowledging the relative merits and powers of *bhakti* yoga and theism, ultimately places all cosmic powers within the superhuman bodies and minds of the Sahajiyā adepts. Perhaps as a mnemonic for memorizing these many senses, organs, and deities, this section concludes with a bit of numerological "compression," wherein all of the previous cosmic truths are added up to a memorable number. Thus, the three levels of qualities and awarenesses (activity, inertia, and purity) are three in number. To these are added ten divinities and ten organs—making twenty-three—with the final addition of the single basic body in which these are all internalized, bringing the total to twenty-four, which encompasses and serves as a means for recalling these many aspects of the structured body-cosmos that the Sahajiyā adept must master. This might be called yoga "by the numbers," and a parallel to the system of the Sāṃkhya products of evolution.

On the Metaphysics of the Cosmic Principles (*tattva*) and Their Control by Yoga

The penultimate section of the *Ātmatattva* builds further upon the Sahajiyā interpretation of Sāṃkhya creation (*utpatti*), once again deriving the five sensory capacities from the five cosmic elements. All of the phenomenal universe, however, is said to emerge from a single point or "seed" (*bindu*). From this single point space arises, followed by wind, fire/sun, water, and earth. It is an "unfolding" from simplicity to complexity, from the timeless to time. Each of these then generates its specific sense: sound, touch, form, taste, and smell. By controlling each of the senses, the Sahajiyā practitioner extends control to its correlative cosmic principle. All aspects of the universe may thus be controlled through Sahajiyā practices. The process begins with the grace of the *guru*, as secret initiation (*dīkṣā*) by a *guru* is a necessary gateway to the yoga. Other Sahajiyā texts state that another master, a "teaching master" (*śikṣā-guru*; often a woman), is the one to teach the actual practices. These include the communal singing of devotional songs to Kṛṣṇa and Rādhā (*nāmasaṃkīrtana*), contemplation (*bhāvanā*), deep meditation (*dhyāna*), and above all, ritual sexual intercourse with a female partner (*nāyikā-sādhana*). The text notes that space and the *bindu* may be controlled through this sexual ritual, and the implication here is that the actions of the male and female Tantric practitioners are paralleled to the principles of Sāṃkhya: the *puruṣa* (male consciousness) and *prakṛti* (female matter). This is the way to establish connections between the human microcosm and the larger macrocosm, using the knowledge of the underlying cosmic principles or metaphysics (*tattva*s) of both. The text observes that the *sādhana* of the five elements of the universe involves both the Kāmagāyatrī *mantra* and the Kāmabīja seed-syllable, indicating the centrality of the power of the erotic in the cosmic and soteriological process. The section concludes with a Sanskrit version of the Kāmagāyatrī: "We meditate on the god of love, whose arrows are flowers, so that the bodiless one may compel it." As we have seen, the god of love, Kāmadeva, is identified with Kṛṣṇa, and his Flower Arrows are essential to the transformative erotic yoga. Although Bengali Vaiṣṇavas and Sahajiyās may conflate Kāmadeva and Kṛṣṇa, earlier classical Hindu scriptures such as the *Mahābhārata* and the *Purāṇas* depict Kāmadeva as a quite independent and mischievous god. In one cycle of tales, he is burnt to ashes by the god Śiva after attempting to distract the ascetic meditating god by shooting him with one of his tempting arrows. Although Śiva later revives Kāmadeva, he gains the epithet "bodiless one" (*anaṅga*), which is used in the Kāmagāyatrī.

The Meaning of the "Seed-syllables" (*bīja*s)

The final complete section of the *Ātmatattva* (there are also four closing couplets) is the most technical, and is a good example of how this Tantric yogic tradition has made extensive use of the "compression" of many meanings into Sanskrit syllables, vowels, and consonants. It is an excellent example of the power of sacred language and phonemes in the yogic process. This is also pentadic in nature, as the basic Kāmabīja "seed-syllable" is the mysterious "empowered" word of *klīṁ*, which is broken down into the three letters (k, l, ī): the fourth element is the nasal sound (*candra-bindu*) over the final –m, and the fifth is the superscripted *bindu*-dot (·). The section begins with a Sanskrit verse connecting the dot to the five sounds regarded as "ornaments" (*alaṃkāra*): "Joined with the five ornaments, the seed-syllable is most beautiful." This *mantra* compresses the entire universe to the sound and vision of a solitary dot. The sound is to be heard, the vibrations felt, and the actual Sanskrit syllables of *klīṁ* should be visualized. The five cosmic elements are homologized, as well as the features of the celestial Vṛndāvana realm in which Rādhā and Kṛṣṇa engage in their "amorous sporting" (*vilāsa*). These include Kṛṣṇa (who is "in" the "k"), Rādhā ("in" the "l"), their conjugal bliss ("in" the "ī"), the inner maiden-body (*śrī-rūpa*, "in" the nasal sound), and Vṛndāvana "in" the *bindu*-dot itself. The maiden-body is used to serve as an inner yogic body that Bengali Vaiṣṇavas seek to discover as their real identity in order to participate in the joyful play of Rādhā and Kṛṣṇa. Thus, the entirety of the physical and divine universes can be "compressed" into the potent "seed-syllable" of *klīṁ*. This technique is similar to many other versions found in other yogic and Tantric texts. It is important to Buddhist yoga traditions as well. This cosmic power of the Sanskrit language continues into modern times in many contemporary yogic traditions.

The sixth and final section of the *Ātmatattva* explains the "inner meaning" of the Kāmagāyatrī *mantra* cited above, concerning the god of Desire, the Flower Arrows, and the bodiless state of Kāmadeva. This *mantra* is used during ritual sexual intercourse (*vilāsa*), when the erotic sentiment (*śṛṅgāra*) is experienced at its highest, and during which the sexual fluids are yogically collected (*praptivastu*, literally "acquired substance"), and the states of *rasa* (as rapture and fluid) and *prema* are experienced. The text then states: "What happens from the tasting of that Divine Essence? The *guru* appears in the heart in the form of Caitanya!" Caitanya, the famous god-man who launched the Bengali Vaiṣṇava movement, was himself regarded as the androgynous incarnation of both Kṛṣṇa and Rādhā, mysteriously fused. So to realize in the heart the *prema* of the *guru*, which is the same *prema* as that of Caitanya, is to attain the goal of cosmic bliss. The five Flower Arrows are each matched to a special erotic power: generation of heat, burning, agitation, fascination, and attraction—all of which are important cognitive and physiological markers of the sexual joining of the male and female adepts. The final portion of the exposition offers a unique interpretation of the Kāmagāyatrī *mantra*, arguing that the adept must know the full range of sexual partners and activities to realize the truth.

The *Ātmatattva* concludes with four summative couplets (a different format than the preceding paragraph-style), extolling the value and power of the *mantras* and the seed-syllable, and stating that, "The Vedas and the Tantra speak of these as 'joined phrases' (*yugala mantra*), i.e. *mantras* for coupling." It also implies that the verse and seed-syllable should be used together in *sādhana*, as "mantras for coupling" that enable and empower the ritual sexual intercourse. The final couplet makes several more extensive claims with regard to yoga: "Each and every Kṛṣṇa *mantra* is replete with all the cosmic powers (*śakti*s). By establishing such a state of emotional awareness (*bhāva*), the *siddhis* are spontaneously realized." This is notable, as it not only refers to the mystical powers (*siddhi*s) so well known to pan-Asian cultures, but also extols the ability of the Kṛṣṇa *mantra* to evoke all cosmic powers. Acquisition of *siddhis*, if not their egotistic display, is a highly regarded sign of progress in many yogic traditions, while awakening the immense cosmic powers of *sakti* is the means to highest attainment. In sum, the *Ātmatattva* tries to be a yogic text for many different people of diverse traditions, including Bengali Vaiṣṇavas, Vaiṣṇava Sahajiyās, other Tantric and yogic practitioners, and followers of the Goddess. It does this by drawing upon an astonishing range of earlier material, in an ingenious way, and in just a few pages. It is a superb example of a local variant of yoga, adapted to the vernacular traditions of Bengal.

The printed Bengali and Sanskrit text used for this translation may be found in the anthology *Vaiṣṇava-granthāvalī*, edited by Satyendranath Basu (Calcutta: Basumati sāhitya mandir, 1342 BS/1936 CE), pp. 151–52. Although there are no line numberings, each of the six major sections is opened by a Sanskrit phrase describing the basic subject of each section, which I have translated as a section title. For the convenience of readers, I have added numerals to each of these six sections, all of which are composed in paragraph format. Only the four concluding Bengali couplets are composed in end-rhymed verse format. In his classic study of the Vaiṣṇava Sahajiyās, *The Place of the Hidden Moon: Erotic Mysticism in the Vaiṣṇava-sahajiyā Cult of Bengal* (Chicago: University of Chicago Press, 1966; Phoenix Press, 1989), pp. 170–71, the late Edward C. Dimock, Jr., noted that the great Bengali scholars Sukumar Sen and S. K. De studied a number of early seventeenth-century manuscripts with lines similar to the *Ātmatattva*, and Dimock agreed with the dating. The author would like to thank Tony K. Stewart, Bruce M. Sullivan, and Julie Hayes for their assistance with earlier drafts of this work.

Suggestions for Further Reading

The study by Edward Dimock, noted above, remains the best general overview of the Vaiṣṇava Sahajiyās and their relationship to Bengali Vaiṣṇavism. He examines portions of the first section of the *Ātmatattva* on pp. 170–74. A new study of Bengali Vaiṣṇavism that includes discussion of the Sahajiyās may be found in Tony K. Stewart, *The Final Word: The Caitanya Caritāmṛta and the Grammar of Religious Tradition* (New York: Oxford University Press, 2009). Recent translations of other Sahajiyā texts by the author of this chapter are Glen A. Hayes, "*The Necklace of Immortality*: A Seventeenth-Century Vaiṣṇava Sahajiyā Text," in *Tantra in Practice*, edited by David Gordon White (Princeton, NJ: Princeton University Press, 2000), pp. 308–25. This excerpted text deals in greater detail with the structure and process of the yogic body, as well as the sexual rituals and visualization practices. A variety of other Sahajiyā texts, including short lyrical poems and excerpts from longer manuals and Sahajiyā interpretations of Bengali Vaiṣṇavism, may be found in Glen A. Hayes, "The Vaiṣṇava Sahajiyā Traditions of Medieval Bengal," in *Religions of India in Practice*, edited by Donald S. Lopez, Jr. (Princeton, NJ: Princeton University Press, 1995), pp. 333–51. For a detailed study of Bengali Vaiṣṇava visualization and devotional practices involving the "maiden" and other techniques, see David L. Haberman, *Acting as a Way of Salvation: A Study of Rāgānugā Bhakti Sādhana* (New York: Oxford University Press, 1988) and his *Journey through the Twelve Forests* (New York: Oxford University Press, 1994). Earlier useful works on the Vaiṣṇava Sahajiyās now available in reprinted editions are: Manindra Mohan Bose, *The Post Caitanya Sahajiā* [sic] *Cult of Bengal* (reprint, Delhi: Gian Publishing House, 1986) and Shashibhushan Dasgupta, *Obscure Religious Cults* (reprint of third edition, Calcutta: Firma KLM, 1976). Bose tends to focus on the connections between the Sahajiyās and Bengali Vaiṣṇavism, while Dasgupta argues for influences from earlier Tantric Buddhism.

Dasgupta also examines other contemporary Bengali Tantric traditions, including the Bāuls and Nāths. For an interesting study and translations of Bāul materials, see Carol Salomon, "Baul Songs," in Lopez, *Religions of India in Practice*, pp. 187–208. For a study of another group which continued some medieval Sahajiyā practices, the Kartābhajās, see Hugh B. Urban, *The Economics of Ecstasy: Tantra, Secrecy, and Power in Colonial Bengal* (New York: Oxford University Press, 2001). For a useful essay discussing the great variety of structures and numbers of *cakras* in the yogic body, see David Gordon White, "Yoga in Early Hindu Tantra," in *Yoga: The Indian Tradition*, edited by Ian Whicher and David Carpenter (London: RoutledgeCurzon, 2003), pp. 143–61. For the definitive study of the alchemical traditions of yoga and Tantra, which served as an influence on the later Sahajiyās, also see David Gordon White, *The Alchemical Body: Siddha Traditions in Medieval India* (Chicago: University of Chicago Press, 1996). Finally, a thorough analysis of Tantric ritual intercourse may be found in White's *Kiss of the Yogini: "Tantric Sex" in Its South Asian Contexts* (Chicago: University of Chicago Press, 2003).

Ātmatattva ("The Cosmic Principles of the Self")

Glory to the holy Rādhā and Kṛṣṇa! Glory to the holy *guru*!

1. *Now for a metaphysical discourse regarding the nature of Being (jīva).* How many Beings (*jīvas*) are there? There are five Beings. What kinds are they? There are the Gross (*sthula*) Being, the Indifferent (*taṭastha*) Being, the Bound (*baddha*) Being, the Liberated (*mukta*) Being, and the Subtle (*sūkṣma*) Being—these are the five Beings. What is called the Gross Being? It is that gross mass (*sthulākāra*) arising from the union of female seed and male semen (*rajobīrja*), which is to say, it is not fully formed. What is that called the Indifferent Being? That Being which controls the ten senses (*indriyas*), but [is focused on] no distinct qualities (*guṇas*). What is that called the Bound Being? Like a father who is tied to his son, it is the Being subject to karma and such. What is that called the Liberated Being? One who has become a servant of the guru, and who has renounced all worldly pleasures. What is that called the Subtle Being? One who is the servant of Kṛṣṇa. Where does the Living Self (*jīvātmā*) reside? In the yogic vessel (*bhāṇḍa*). How does this yogic vessel come to be? It develops from the basic building blocks of the universe (*tattvavastu*). What, then, are these building blocks? Five elements (*bhūta*) constitute the Self (*ātmā*). What are these five elements that make up the Self called? The five are earth (*pṛthivī*), water (*āpa*), fire (*teja*), air (*vāyu*), and space (*ākāśa*). How might the Living Self be brought under control? [By experienc-

ing] everything from greed (*lobha*) to liberation (*mukti*). How might the Elemental Self (*bhūtātmā*) be brought under control? By *sādhana*! And what is the *sādhana*? Adopting the moods and experiences of a young maiden (*sakhī-bhāva-āśraya*). The most fundamental *sādhana* hinges initially on the foundation of the Verses of the Seed-Syllable of Desire (*kāma-bīja gāyatrī*). How is the Supreme Self (*paramātmā*) to be brought under control? Through *sādhana*s involving the names of Kṛṣṇa (*nāma*) and by *mantras*. If one combines the names with their corresponding seed-syllables (*bīja*s), the Supreme Self can be brought under control. How may the Delight in Knowing the Self (*ātmārāma*) be controlled? By deep meditation (*dhyāna*). What is the *sādhana* of the Delight in Knowing the Self? It includes eight things: food (*āhāra*), sleep (*nidrā*), cognition (*cintā*), music (*saṅgīta*), thought (*manana*), worship (*bhajana*), infatuation (*mohana*), and modesty (*lajjā*). What is the *sādhana* that gives voice (*svara*) to the Delight in Knowing the Self? The qualities of the Pure Love (*prema*) for Kṛṣṇa. By pursuing lust (*kāmānugā*), one tastes the ultimate experience of love, starting with eroticism (*śṛṅgāra*), and the rest. Where does the Living Self reside? It dwells in a four-petaled lotus in the "hidden land" near the anus (*guhyadeśa*). Where does the Elemental Self reside? It dwells at the base of the penis (*liṅga*), in a six-petaled lotus. Where does the Supreme Self reside? In a ten-petaled lotus, which is in the place of the Coiled One (*kuṇḍalī*). Each petal of that lotus in turn has twelve petals. Where does the Lord Who Delights in Knowing the Self (*ātmārāmeśvara*) reside? In the place of the blazing (*ujjvala*) lotus. Each petal there has sixteen petals. Such are the locations of these five lotuses. What is the nature of these five Selves in the five lotuses, and what functions (*karmas*) do they perform? Furthermore, what is their appearance (*ākāra*) and what sustains (*āhāra*) them? What is the appearance of the Living Self? It is blood-red (*raktavarṇa*) in color, and it is sustained by water (*jala*). Its function is the bearing of burdens (*bhāravahana*). What is the appearance of the Elemental Self? It is bright yellow (*haritālvarṇa*) in color, and it is sustained by great quantities of food (*āhāra bahu bakṣaṇa*). Its function is bringing about the understanding (*buddhikaraṇa*) of the six vices (*ripu*). What are the names of these six vices? They are desire (*kāma*), anger (*krodha*), greed (*lobha*), infatuation (*moha*), intoxication (*mada*), and malice (*mātsarya*)—these are the six vices. How do these six vices function? They animate (*cetana*) the senses (*indriya*). What is the appearance of the Supreme Self? It is of the color of lightning (*vidyūt*), and it is sustained by the wind (*vāyu*). What is its function? Its function is the controlling of the various mental states (*cinta*). What is the appearance of the Delight in Knowing the Self? It is the color of the moon, and it is sustained by the nectar of the stories of Kṛṣṇa. Its function is joyful speech, and always keeping it foremost in one's mind. What is the appearance of the Lord Who

Delights in Knowing the Self? It has the form of the sun. It is sustained by the nectar of the sacred stories (*kathāmṛta*). Its tasks (*kārya*) are the worship (*bhajana*) of Kṛṣṇa, as well as cognition (*buddhi*), strength (*bala*), knowledge (*jñāna*), and the tasting of the Divine Essence (*rasa āsvādana*). These are all of the functions of the five Selves.

2. *Now for matters concerning the five types of Vital Breaths (prāṇa).* What are the five Vital Breaths (*prāṇas*)? They are "Breathing In" (*apāna*), "Breathing Out" (*prāṇa*), "Equalizing the Breath" (*samāna*), "Upward Breath" (*udāna*), and "Traversing Breath" (*vyāna*)—these are the five Vital Breaths. Where do they reside? "Breathing In" dwells in the anal region; "Breathing Out" is in the lotus of the heart; "Equalizing the Breath" is in the navel; "Upward Breath" is in the throat; and "Traversing Breath" is found throughout the body. The five Vital Breaths are located in all of these regions.

3. *Now for matters concerning the five Flower Arrows of Desire (bāṇa).* What are the five Flower Arrows of Desire (*bāṇa*)? They are *Madana* ("delight in love"); *Mādana* ("intoxication in love"); *Śoṣaṇa* ("absorption in love"); *Stambhana* ("suspension of all sensation but that of love"); and *Mohana* ("complete bliss"). These are the five Flower Arrows [of the god of desire, Kāmadeva]. Where are they located? And in whom? *Madana* is located in the left corner of the left eye. *Mādana* is located in the right corner of the right eye. *Śoṣaṇa* is located in the lower lip. *Stambhana* is located in passionate sexual union (*śṛṅgāra*). *Mohana* is found in a sultry sidelong glance. These five aspects reside in these five places. From the union of the cosmic feminine matter (*prakṛti*) and the cosmic male consciousness (*puruṣa*) comes the birth of the most fundamental Cosmic Reality (*Mahā-tattva*); that is, creation (*utpatti*). From the fundamental Cosmic Reality arise the "awareness of activity" (*rājasa ahaṃkāra*), "awareness of inertia" (*tamasa ahaṃkāra*), and "awareness of purity" (*sāttvika ahaṃkāra*)—these three arise. From the "awareness of activity" arise the five material elements (*bhūtas*). What are these five material elements called? They are earth (*pṛthivī*), water (*āp*), fire (*teja*), air (*vāyu*), and space (*ākāśa*). These are the five. Who has these qualities (*guṇa*), and where are they located? What are the qualities of earth? It involves the sense of smell (*gandha*), and is pearly-white (*śukla*) in color. It is located in the nose. What about the qualities of water? It involves the qualities of taste, is somewhat golden (*gaura*) in color, and is located in the tongue. What are the qualities of air? It has the quality of touch (*sparśa*), is dark-colored (*syama*), and is found in the eyes. What about the qualities of space? It has the attributes of sound (*śabda*), is dark purple (*dhūmra*) in color, and is located in the ear. If one can know these five principles, the Being will become liberated (*mukta*), and even the body will become immortal (*nitya*). From the "awareness of inertia" come the ten sensory organs

(*indriya*s). What are these? The five organs of knowledge (*jñanendriya*s) and the five organs of action (*karmendriya*s)—these are the ten. First of all, what are the five organs of knowing? These are the five: the nose (*nāsikā*), tongue (*jihvā*), eyes (*cakṣu*), skin (*carma*), and ear (*karṇa*). How is it possible for one to feel the sensations of these diverse sensory organs? The nose senses a sweet-smelling fragrance; the tongue tastes that which is bitter or sweet; the eye perceives the many gradations of light and dark; the skin feels the cold and the heat; and the ear detects sounds and such. These are the attributes of the five [organs of knowing]. There are five organs of action (*karmendriya*s). What are they? The five organs are the mouth (*vākya*), hands (*pāṇi*), feet (*pada*), anus (*pāyu*), and the genitals (*upastha*). What are the qualities of these organs? The organ of speech produces utterances both good and bad; the hand is namely the hand's ability to grasp various articles; the feet provide a means of coming and going; the anus excretes fecal matter; while the genitals secrete sexual fluids, urine, and so forth (*śukramūtrādi*). These are the qualities of the five [organs of action].

4. *Now for matters concerning the divinities.*
From the "awareness of purity," the ten divinities (*devatā*s) are born. There are five organs of knowledge, and for each of these there is a presiding divinity. What are these? *Dikpāla* (the guardians of the directions), *Vāyu* (the god of winds), *Arka* (the sun god), *Prochetā* (god of waters), and *Aśvinīkumār* (the twin gods)—these are the five [divinities]. Where do each of these divinities reside? The *Aśvin* twins are in the nose, *Prochetā* is in the tongue, *Arka* is in the eyes, *Vāyu* is in the skin, and the *Dikpālas* are in the ears—these are the five [locations]. And as for the five organs of action, there are also five divinities that preside over them. Who are they? *Vahni* (the Vedic god of fire), *Indra* (warrior god of the Vedas), *Upendra* (the god Viṣṇu, as brother of Indra), *Mitra* (Vedic god of cosmic order), and *Prajāpati* (god of creation). Which organ is each divinity associated with? *Vahni* is associated with speech; *Indra* with the hands; *Upendra* with the feet; *Mitra* with the anus; and *Prajāpati Brahmā* with the genitals. These are the five [associations]. Thus there are ten: nose, tongue, eyes, skin, and ear; speech, hands, feet, anus, and genitals. And thus there are ten presiding divinities as well. Who are they? *Dikpāla*, *Vāyu*, *Arka*, *Prochetā*, *Vahni*, *Aśvinīkumār*, *Indra*, *Upendra*, *Mitra*, and *Prajāpati*. [Including the ten organs over which they preside,] there are twenty. Adding "awareness of activity," "awareness of inertia," and "awareness of purity," these three make for twenty-four, meaning that you should know the body (*śarīra*) [counting it as one] amongst the twenty-four Cosmic Principles (*tattva*s).

5. *Now for matters regarding the emergence of the Cosmic Principles (tattvas).*
Wind emerges from space, the sun emerges from wind, out of the sun emerges

water, and from water emerges earth. Yet the origin of space is the "Single Point" (*bindu*). It has the qualities of sound vibrations (*śabda*). Wind arises from space; it has the qualities of sound and touch. From wind arises fire; it has the qualities of sound, touch, and form (*rūpa*). Water arises from fire; it has the qualities of sound, touch, form, and taste (*rasa*). Earth emerges from water; it has the qualities of sound, touch, form, taste, and smell. These are the five. How can the earth element be controlled? Through the power of the mercy of the *guru*. How can water be controlled? By the communal singing of the names of Kṛṣṇa (*nāmasaṃkīrtana*). How may fire be controlled? By deep contemplation (*bhāvanā*). By what means is the wind controlled? Through deep meditation (*dhyāna*). How is space to be controlled? Through *sādhana* with a female partner (*nāyikā*). What is the *sādhana* of these five elements (*bhūta*s)? It consists of the "Verse on Desire" (*Kāmagāyatrī*) and the "Seed-syllable of Desire" (*Kāmabīja*). [The "Verse on Desire" is:] "We meditate on the god of love, whose arrows are flowers, so that the bodiless one may compel it." (Sanskrit: *kāmadevaya vidmahe puṣpabāṇāya dhīmahi tan no'naṅgaḥ pracodayāt*)

6. *Now for the meaning of the "Seed-syllable" (bīja).*
"Joined with the five ornaments, the seed-syllable is most beautiful" (Sanskrit: *pañcālaṃkārasaṅgyuktam bījang taṅg paramādbhūtam*). Thus is the "Seed-syllable of the Five Ornaments." What are the "Five Ornaments" called? [1] *kaḥ*, [2] *laḥ*, [3] *ī*, [4] *candra-bindu*, and [5] *bindu*. These "Five Ornaments" may be realized through the five elements. The earth element is in the sound of the "*kaḥ*." The water element is in the sound of the "*laḥ*." The fire element is in the sound of the "*ī*." The wind element is in the nasal sound of the *candra-bindu*. The element of space is found in the sound of the *bindu* dot. These are the five. The five may be obtained. Kṛṣṇa resides in the "*kaḥ*." Rādhā resides in the "*laḥ*." Joyful bliss (*hlādinī*) resides in the "ī." *Śrī-Rūpa* [the inner damsel] resides in the nasal sound. Vṛndāvana [Kṛṣṇa's abode of play] resides in the *bindu* dot. These are the five. That same Vṛndāvana is the unmanifested abode (*dhāma*) of God, Nārāyaṇa, the Philosopher's Stone (*cintāmaṇi*). Now for the meaning of the Verses. Who is the erotic player in the mind (*manaso vilāsā*)? It is the god of Desire (*Kāmadeva*); the embodiment of desire (*kāmarūpa*) is Kṛṣṇa. What is Kṛṣṇa's own erotic dalliance (*vilāsa*) called? It is the tasting of the Divine Essence, the ultimate experience (*rasa*) of erotic love (*sṛṅgāra*) in all of its forms. That Divine Essence, the juice of love, born of the act of love, what is it called? It is called "acquired substance" (*praptivastu*), which then generates pure love (*prema*). What happens from the tasting of that Divine Essence? The *guru* appears in the heart in the form of Caitanya! What are the

Flower Arrows called? The Flower Arrows are the weapons of one's own self. "Hail the flower-arrows of the god of Desire" (Sanskrit: *asau puṣpabāṇaḥ kāmadevaḥ*). What are the Flower Arrows? They are five flowers! *Āmra* blossoms, *aśoka* blossoms, *mallikā* blossoms, *mādhavī* blossoms, and *vakula* blossoms—these are the five. There are five duties (*dharma*) that go with these. What are they? These are the five: *tāpana* (generation of heat), *dāhana* (the act of burning), *ucāñana* (agitation), *manomohana* (fascination), and *ākarṣaṇa* (attraction). Specific duties go with each flower. Generation of heat is the duty of the *āmra* blossom. The act of burning goes with the *aśoka* blossom. For the *mallikā* blossom the duty is agitation. The duty of the *mādhavī* blossom is fascination. Attraction is the duty of the *vakula* blossom. These are the five duties. Now you may grasp the real meaning of the [words of the *kāmagāyatrī*], *dhīmahi*, etc. To be truly knowledgeable [is to know that] there are three types of [female partners (*nāyikās*)]: the patient and stable, the impatient and anxious, and those who are both. And [the Sanskrit phrase] "*tanno'naṅgaḥ*" means: "O, the Bodiless One is found within ourselves by means of another and her body." To what does "another" refer? Endless lovemaking (*vilāsa*) with the physical body.

In this fashion, the meanings of all of the Verses (*mantras*) are collected.

Knowing this, be happy, and make yourself pure-hearted!

The Kṛṣṇa *mantras*, such as the Seed-syllable of Desire and the rest;

The Vedas and Tantras speak of these as "joined phrases" (*yugala mantra*), the *mantras* of coupling.

Equivalent to the Wish-fulfilling Cow, the Wish-fulfilling Tree, the Philosopher's Stone, and the Lord Nārāyaṇa.

As the apex, these contain the meanings of all the *mantras*.

Each and every Kṛṣṇa *mantra* is replete with all cosmic powers (*śakti*).

By establishing such a state of emotional awareness (*bhāva*), the mystical

powers (*siddhis*) are spontaneously realized.

—13—

The Transport of the Haṃsas: A Śākta Rāsalīlā as Rājayoga in Eighteenth-Century Benares

Somadeva Vasudeva

Origins

The term *rājayoga* or "royal yoga," commonly applied as a retronym—at least since the publication of Swami Vivekananda's Rāja Yoga—to Patañjali's system of *aṣṭāṅgayoga*, designates in many medieval and pre-colonial works on yoga something quite different. In the *Haṃsavilāsa*, or "Transport of the Haṃsas," the work translated here, *rājayoga* is an ecstatic sensual rapture, a Śākta form of the *rāsalīlā*. The Haṃsa bird, commonly identified as the bar-headed goose (Anser indicus), has a long and complex history in Indian literature as a mantra or as a metaphor, symbol, or allegory for the liberated soul. In the present context "Haṃsa" designates more specifically the esoteric identity of the work's authors, and "Haṃsa (masc.)" or "Haṃsī (fem.)" is also the general title of any initiate into the religion taught in the "Transport of the Haṃsas." Chapter 34 stipulates that initiates may not use their "worldly" name in the collective *rāsalīlā* gathering. Women are to use the name "Rasikā," "Haṃsī," or "Śakti," and men "Rasika," "Haṃsa," or "Śiva," and there is a recurring metaphorical dichotomy between the initiated and self-aware Haṃsa or Haṃsī on the one hand and uninitiated and animalistic "other birds" (mostly crows) on the other. From the context it is evident that we should understand Haṃsa- in the title as a "single-remainder compound" (*ekaśeṣa*) standing for "Haṃsa and Haṃsī," the two main speakers in the work. The introductory passage explicitly acknowledges the revelation of this "royal yoga" as the telos for the composition of the work:

> Now, desiring to make known, right here, the "royal yoga," the esoterium of the yogins, to couples of women and men whose minds are eager to taste bliss, who are seekers of liberation primed by Paramaśiva, I am setting forth the "Transport of the Haṃsas" in a dialogue with my wife.

This "Transport of the Haṃsas" is a complex and unusual work composed in Sanskrit by a *smārta* brahmin named Miṭṭhu (or Miṭṭha) Śukla who was born in 1737 CE in the western Indian state of Gujarat. Calqued on the established scriptural genre of the tantric dialogue between Śiva and Śakti, the text is in part a spiritual autobiography, in part a learned doxography of competing soteriologies, in part an acute philosophical polemic and invective against contemporary strands of moralizing reformist Hinduism, in part a mantra and ritual manual, in part a text on the fine arts, musicology, aesthetics, and erotics, and above all an outspoken work of Śākta or Kaula apologetics.

So far, the autobiographical sections of the "Transport of the Haṃsas" are the only sources that have come to light that allow us to locate Miṭṭhu Śukla as an historical agent in eighteenth-century Benares and Gujarat. His work can be further contextualized by its richness of citations, refutations, and allusions. We may provisionally sketch Miṭṭhu's spiritual career as follows.

In 1742 CE, when Miṭṭhu was in his fifth year, he received his Vedic *upanayana* initiation. Since this is the earliest possible age for a brahmin to undergo this rite of passage we might assume either that he was especially gifted, or that his parents were very ambitious for him. Thereafter Miṭṭha Śukla tells us that he mastered the Śrīvidyā system of Śākta Tantra with ease. This Kaula system called the Śrīvidyā had originated in love-magic and was once a rival religion to the brahminic religions that denied the validity of any religion not grounded in the authority of its own corpus of Vedic revelation and secondary texts. In Miṭṭhu's writings we can perceive a syncretic Kaula system that actively seeks accommodation with this brahminic mainstream. In his twelfth year he married Bhūlī and lived as a householder with her until his sixteenth year, "frolicking like a crow" as he himself puts it.

In 1754 CE, when Miṭṭhu Śukla was still a teenager, he ran away from his home and his teenage bride Bhūlī in Gujarat because he was overcome by a sudden and inexplicable dispassion. Miṭṭhu was drawn to Benares, which under the rule of the Bhūmihāra brahmin Balwant Singh (reg. 1740–1770 CE) had become a rapidly growing boomtown. There he spent some time studying Upanishadic and Tantric scriptures, but he found no solace in these, and finally left for the Vindhyācala temple in Mirzapur to commit ritual suicide and thereby attain liberation, or at least a pleasant sojourn in a paradise world. At this moment of spiritual crisis a chance meeting with a Paramahaṃsa mendicant who imparted secret teachings changed everything for Miṭṭhu: in a sudden awakening he remembered the esoteric secret of who he really was and the sequence of events that had brought him to incarnate in our world. Miṭṭhu's hidden identity was Haṃsa, the beloved attendant of Śiva, and his wife was Haṃsī, his consort. It is with the voices of this Haṃsa and this Haṃsī that Miṭṭhu and Bhūlī speak in their "Transport of the Haṃsas." Their true home is described as being "on the other side" of our universe, beyond our ontological referents of space and time in a place called Śrīnagara, the "City of Glory." At the same time, the terminology Miṭṭhu uses is instantly recognizable as descriptive of the Śrīcakra, the central mandala of the cult of the Goddess Tripurasundarī. There, the inexplicably manifested androgynous Ardhanārīśvara had procreated the universe through cosmic sensual revelry. As a consequence of their androgyne origin, all souls are created with a counterpart with which they need to unite before they can return to the "City of Glory." After impressing Śiva with their devotion, the curious Haṃsa and Haṃsī ask for permission to visit our universe, a perishable counterpart of their home. This wish is granted and they incarnate for a single human life with the mission of saving a few souls who are ready to benefit from their teachings. After receiving this realization, Haṃsa rushes back to his wife and reveals the secret of their identity. They then spend the rest of their lives engaged in sensual Kaula revelry that is identified as the highest kind of yoga, and they also write a work, called the "Transport of the Haṃsas," for a small circle of initiates.

Royal Yoga

It is not Patañjali's *aṣṭāṅgayoga* that is designated "royal yoga" in the "Transport of the Haṃsas." That form of yoga is elaborated in the ninth chapter of the "Transport of the Haṃsas" as part of a longer doxographical section that first summarizes and then rejects various soteriologies and systems of philosophy. Haṃsa conflates Patañjali's yoga with *haṭhayoga*, treating a number of disparate yogic traditions as subsystems of each other. This chapter, while of great interest for eighteenth-century perceptions of Patañjali's yoga, is not explored any further here, for Haṃsa ultimately dismisses Pātañjala yoga quite brusquely:

> My dear! Pātañjala yoga is nonsense since there is no spontaneity when something is mastered through force. An effortless, holistic royal yoga has been taught by the wise.

The Haṃsas proceed to teach a fourfold yoga of which this "royal yoga" is the culmination. Capacity for one or more of these is determined by the intensity of the descent of the power of divine grace, followed by one of three kinds of initiation: initiation for ritualists, initiation for renouncers, and combined initiation for those eligible for royal yoga. The first yoga is *karmayoga*, defined as ritualistic *mantrayoga* and elaborated in chapters 34–35. The second is *bhaktiyoga* or devotionalism. The third is *jñānayoga* or gnostic yoga. The highest yoga is *rājayoga*, which is none other than the *rāsa* or *rāsalīlā* celebration, other forms of which had been popularized by Vaiṣṇava *bhakti* traditions such as the Puṣṭimārga of Vallabhācārya, already well established in eighteenth-century Gujarat. The Haṃsas betray an intimate familiarity with Vaiṣṇava texts such as the *Bhāgavatapurāṇa* and its commentarial traditions. However, the Haṃsas' *rāsa* is not the *rāsalīlā* familiar from devotional Vaiṣṇava self-representation. Rather, they openly advocate and defend the kind of sexual practices with which the Vallabhācāryas were to be charged in the notorious "Maharaja Libel Case" of 1862, and the Haṃsa's *rāsa* is here translated as "sensual rapture," for it involves above all sexual intercourse. The "Transport of the Haṃsas" is explicit and detailed about this, amplifying its Kaula Śrīvidyā ritualism with material drawn from texts on aesthetics, musicology, and *kāmaśāstra*, the science of erotics. At the beginning of chapter 49, Haṃsī complains that Kṛṣṇa Dvaipāyana and his followers had only revealed *rāsa*s that were "incomplete, external raptures." This prompts Haṃsa to reveal the esoteric sensual rapture, the *rahasyarāsa*. Chapters 49 and 50 derive substantial amounts of material from the *Anaṅgaraṅga* of Kalyāṇamalla, a sixteenth-century Sanskrit manual on erotics. The passage translated below picks up immediately after these detailed practical instructions. It theorizes a tripartite classification of esoteric sensual rapture, using the three categories of the divine, material, and spiritual.

The sexual rapture of the Haṃsas is not one that transcends the boundaries of caste. The Haṃsas accept the *smārta* stipulation that caste status is entirely dependent on initiation with the Gāyatrī mantra and as such available only to brahmins, *kṣatriya*s and *vaiśya*s: "Only those initiated into the Gāyatrī mantra are twice-born, those that are not are *śūdra*s and others." He explicitly rejects the more radically transgressive *nirmaryāda* ("boundary-less") forms of the Kaula religion that denounce such strictures. This is a conspicuous instance where the Haṃsas eschew the more universal or even confrontational voice of earlier Kaulism and revert to the mores of their parochial Gujarati *smārta* brahmin upbringing. A major paradigm in the "Transport of the Haṃsas" is the attempt to show the functional equivalence of Vedic practices and Kaula practices: thus the consumption of soma in Vedic ritual is equated with the consumption of wine in Kaula ritual. Whether this is intended as ecumenism, reconciliation, corroboration, co-validation, or something quite different altogether is a complex issue that requires more careful analysis than is possible here. For now we may note that the end product, a syncretic religion that advocates feasting, drinking alcoholic cocktails, and sexual congress with one's own spouse is hardly shockingly antinomian. The very foundations of this syncretic system were evidently laid in Haṃsa and Haṃsī's early childhood: reverence for the Gāyatrī mantra as the essence of Vedic revelation, and the esoteric view of this mantra as equivalent to the essence of Śrīvidyā.

The Text

Despite being published already in 1937 in Gaekwad's Oriental Series (GOS) by Swami Trivikrama Tirtha, a collaborator of John Woodroffe, and Mahamahopadhyaya Hathibhai Shastri of Jamnagar, an early voice calling for the reconversion to Hinduism, the "Transport of the Haṃsas" has suffered a nearly total scholarly neglect. I was only able to find a few very brief notices at all, and none touching on the main subject of the work.

The work's deliberate homologization of Śākta ritual, non-dualist doctrine, erotics, and a Kṛṣṇabhakti-derived Kaula *rāsalīlā* in the "esoteric sensual rapture" is in some respects reminiscent of some aspects of what was later to evolve into modern "new age Tantra." The hitherto unstudied textual history of the "Transport of the Haṃsas" might contain clues to the still far from clear dynamics that shaped this new religious movement. Unfortunately, the text-critical value of the 1937 edition is so poor that it must be treated like a conflated manuscript. The editors consulted two manuscripts but decided to use only one because the other was faulty. I have silently corrected the haphazard word separation and some spelling errors for my translation. The text can be improved further by tracing its numerous citations and paraphrases. Important Kaula sources for *Haṃsamiṭṭhu* are, among others, the *Kulārṇavatantra*, a version of the *Rudrayāmala*, the *Samayācāra*, and the *Kulapradīpa* of Śivānandācārya (alias Sevānandācārya, son of the Gauḍa author Jagannivāsa).

I hope that the following passage will give an idea of Haṃsamiṭṭhu's original and lively style of writing. The "Transport of the Haṃsas" is a complex and learned work that can give us valuable insights into the religious milieu of Gujarat and Benares in a period crucial to the formation of modern Hinduism.

The edition translated here is the *Haṃsavilāsa of Haṃsamiṭṭhu*, Gaekwad's Oriental Series 81, Baroda 1937, edited by Swami Trivikrama and Mahamahopadhyaya Hathibhai Shastri of Jamnagar Tirtha.

Suggestions for Further Reading

On the Śrīvidyā system in general, see André Padoux, *Le coeur de la Yoginī "Yoginīhṛdaya" avec le commentaire "Dīpikā" d'Amṛtānanda*, Publications de l'Institut de Civilisation Indienne (Paris: DeBoccard, 1994). See also Douglas Renfrew Brooks, *Auspicious Wisdom: the Texts and Traditions of Śrīvidyā Śākta Tantrism in South India* (Albany: State University of New York Press, 1992), and also Madhu Khanna, "The Concept and Liturgy of the Śrīcakra Based on Śivānanda's Trilogy," Ph.D. Dissertation, Oxford University, 1986. On the origins of the Tripurā cult and for more details of the Śrīvidyā, see Alexis Sanderson, "The Śaiva Age: The Rise and Dominance of Śaivism During the Early Medieval Period" in Shingo Einoo, ed., *Genesis and Development of Tantrism*, Institute of Oriental Culture Special Series, 23 (Tokyo: University of Tokyo, Institute of Oriental Culture, 2009), pp. 47–49. On the history of the Śrīvidyā in Kashmir, see Alexis Sanderson, "The Śaiva Exegesis of Kashmir," in Dominic Goodall and André Padoux, eds., *Mélanges tantriques à la mémoire d'Hélène Brunner* (Pondicherry: Institut Français de Pondichéry, 2007), especially pp. 383–85, 409–11.

Euphoria 51

[p. 306] Śrīhaṃsa:

My beloved! What can I say if even the sacred texts censure sex?

> The *Chāndogyopaniṣad* teaches:
> "May I not go to the pink and toothless, to the toothless, pink, and slimy!"
> "Toothless" means "devoid of teeth," "slimy" means "slippery," the "pink" is the female sexual organ. In the *Bhāgavatapurāṇa* also:
> "To those who take refuge in you, the omni-delightful soul,
> of what use are one's own people, sons, one's own wife,
> wealth, home, land, or fair chariots?
> For those who, not realizing this truth, make love in couples,
> what can give pleasure in this inherently-condemned world,
> inherently deprived of happiness?"

This is how the scriptures rebuke even devotees who are married couples.
Then, O good lady! what opportunity can there be for sex?
Therefore one should take the revelation of the *Śrīparāgamarahasya* to

heart: "It is not at all sinful." Beautiful woman! The abhorrence for sex that is found in the Vedas and so forth can be understood by God alone, not by simpletons. So even if sex can be blameworthy, nevertheless, it is only praiseworthy to the glorious Rasikas. As it is stated in the *Śivarahasya*:

> When the vulva is remembered there is merit, so also when the vulva is seen.
> When the vulva is worshipped there is merit, so also in intercourse with the vulva.
> O Goddess, the bliss I experience in intercourse with the vulva,
> is unlike that of mantra repetitions, fire sacrifices, charitable giving, or penance.
> The merit that accrues in this world by sex cannot be equaled,
> O Goddess, bathing in tens of millions of sacred fords.
> Engaging in mantra repetition, charitable giving,
> and religious ceremonies such as initiation and sacrifice and so on
> are not worth the sixteenth part of the deeds of the devotee of sex.
> My dear! After her thirteenth year up to the age of twenty-five years
> a woman is worthy of sex, especially if she has borne no children.
> O great Goddess, especially a woman who has borne no children,
> but also a woman who has borne children but only a few,
> must definitely engage in sexual intercourse according to her capacity.

Such statements, intended as praise of sex, are found thousand-fold in esoteric scriptures such as the *Samayācāra*. Of what use are false teachings? Enough of them!

Divine Sensual Rapture

If God incites his own devotees to enact sexual union then what could be suspect about Śaiva sensual rapture? He himself enjoys the bliss of consummated sexual union that is the source of all happiness, so no real doubt need be entertained. For in Viṣṇu's heaven Vaikuṇṭha, Lakṣmī and Viṣṇu engage in love-sport. On Mt. Kailāsa, Gaurī is intimate with Rudra. In the celestial palace of Brahmā, Sarasvatī with Brahmā. In the celestial palace of Indra, Śacī and Indra make love. And how many women did the Sun-god not make love to? The Moon-god has intercourse with the stars headed by Rohiṇī etc., Manu Svāyambhuva with Śatarūpā. Vasiṣṭha revels with Arundhatī. Agastya has sex with Lopāmudrā. The illustrious Rāma enjoys sexual union with Sītā, and Kṛṣṇa with Rādhā. How many passionate women has Kṛṣṇa not enjoyed? If sexual union is sinful then why did these gods, who were able to do, not do, or do differently, uphold the duty of sexual union with their beloveds?

On the one hand they censure sex in order to criticize those addicted to external objects of sense and to encourage introspection. But ultimately the pleasure of sex is the final truth. My beloved! In this way, supreme Śiva, who is not separate from the revered Śakti, revels in Śrīnagara in glorious sensual rapture with hundreds of thousands of Śaktis by day and night in private and in public. Who can find words for the greatness of the magnificent supreme Śakti? Every now and again Śrīnagara's king, the illustrious supreme Śiva, wearied by sensual rapture, falls asleep with the Queen, supreme Śakti who ever enjoys conjugal felicity, on a pleasure-couch. Then Śrīnagara's learned citizens, embodiments of the revealed scriptures, stand below the illustrious Hall of Plenitude and awaken the Lord and Lady with sweet music produced by flutes and lutes and the like, playing various musical modes such as the wonderful Bhairavarāga and so forth, informed by hymns of praise embracing the truth of revealed scripture. The chief Queen awakens first, and then the supreme Lord wakes up. Then, realizing that the revered Lord and Lady of the sensual rapture are awake, many citizens, female companions and male servants rush there to be of assistance.

This concludes the description of divine sensuality.

Material Sensual Rapture

Whatever is appropriate to the seasonal raptures is acceptable. The honorable revelers should indulge themselves while staying within bounds. All of the four kinds of beings are devoted to the rapture of sensuality. But because of their subjection they do not realize this: that constitutes for them a net of suffering including birth, death and so on. Therefore a person should first become a Haṃsa through obedience to the teacher who has incarnated as the illustrious Haṃsa, and then adhere to the marvelous doctrine of sensuality. Striving with singing and music in unison with the circle of the glorious Haṃsa, severing the eight bonds of dislike, doubt, fear, shame, repulsion, family-ties, decorum, and status by birth, one should joyfully observe the rapture of sensuality. He should make love to only a Haṃsī, and not to any other bird. A woman of his own caste is best. If a Haṃsī happens to be of a different caste then he should not make love to her. A Haṃsī also should not make love to other birds. The boundaries must be respected. If there is not at least one couple it is not sensual rapture. If it is only Haṃsas or Haṃsīs it is not auspicious. In divine sensuality a solitary Śiva carouses with countless Śaktis, but here in this world, because things perish in an instant, because bodies abound in filth, urine, and phlegm, and because of a lack of capacity, there can be only revelry with one's own wife. A woman is obliged to make love with her own Śiva. With the permission of one's own spouse sexual relations with others are also permitted. One may not have sex with a woman after lustfully forcing oneself upon her, or after seducing her with money or stories. Otherwise there is peril in this world and in the next world. All the rest corresponds to divine sensuality. In India only, this rapture of worship is auspicious, because other raptures are inapplicable and not permitted.

This concludes the description of material sensuality.

Spiritual Sensual Rapture

After attaining one's pure true nature through the grace of a good teacher, one should, by means of creative contemplation, engage in sensual revelry with one's own awakened intellect as a consort together with its various emanations of power such as faith, wisdom, memory, fortitude, devotion, and so on as companions. Such spiritual rapture is insipid in contrast to the aforementioned material kind which is delectable. A single woman, or a man who is separated from his Haṃsī, should sing the praises of this rapture or even better of divine sensual rapture. But a woman and a man who are together must always engage in material sensual rapture, considering it to be divine sensual rapture, interpreting it as spiritual sensual rapture. As the maxim says: "The efficacy of an action is grounded in the power of the great, not in what is done." Is hunger and thirst removed by talk of food and water? Therefore, a living being, if he has personally experienced that "I am Haṃsa," should always avail himself of material sensual rapture while still conforming to mundane existence. If that experience has not taken place, divine sensual rapture should simply be eulogized. But it is obligatory to conceive of sensual rapture with a spiritual vision. The animalistic revelry of the bound leads to rebirth, but there is no danger of adversity in Paramahaṃsic sensual rapture. The Esoterium of Revelation states:

> Yogis, drunk with alcohol, fall upon the bosoms of women;
> the *yoginīs*, reeling with liquor, fall upon the chests of men.
> They fully sate each other's desires, their hearts are transformed,
> —euphoria arises.

Material sensual rapture is celebrated in scripture with abundant statements such as these. Divine sensual rapture should be viewed as the goal. The esoteric interpretation of spiritual rapture should be understood to add a sense of wonder. But ultimately it is universal fusion that is the goal. The bounds of the world are great, therefore one should to a certain degree respect them and ever remain in the euphoria of ecstatic fusion (*sāmarasya*). One should not do anything blameworthy. In the glorious sensual rapture there is nothing blameworthy. All exist only within a glorious sensual rapture of cosmic proportions. Because they are bound souls they do not realize this, and out of wickedness they criticize it.

[There follow two long sections defending the validity of, and establishing the rules governing, the consumption of alcohol, cannabis, sweets and meat. Then the topic of sensual rapture is taken up again]:

Euphoria 52

[p. 318, line 14] Sexual intercourse is not disagreeable to anyone. All embodied beings, beginning with Brahmā, Viṣṇu and Rudra, enjoy the pleasure of the sexual organs. Why should we be inhibited about it? The generative organ has come into being as the organ of pleasure, ecstasy is its domain, not urine, and so on. "The form of brahman is bliss," and this can only be experienced in the sexual organ through fusion. Haṃsī! Are you listening? Only at the time of sexual union is one freed from all inhibiting bonds etc., nowhere else is there such liberation.

[Haṃsī] But surely cattle and so on are always untrammeled by such inhibitions, so how come they are bound? As the scripture says: "Constrained by inhibitions one is called "bound"; freed from inhibitions one is Sadāśiva."

[Haṃsa] True. Even though the [eight] inhibiting bonds headed by dislike and so forth are sometimes seen to be absent in animals such as cattle even without sexual union taking place, nevertheless, because they lack any direct experience of the bliss of the self, neither they nor human beings can be anything other than bound souls without engaging in sexual union. Haṃsas, on the other hand, proceed through transmigration observing social constraints and appear to be bound, like elephants fettered with lotus fibers. Does this make them bound souls? Some beings appear to be spontaneously freed from bondage at times other than love-making, but are they really liberated? To the contrary! Only those who have had a direct experience of the bliss of the self, whether they exhibit the inhibiting bonds or are free from them, are truly liberated, not others. At the time of love-making all are freed from the inhibiting bonds, but subsequently, the euphoria of luxuriating in the aftertaste of that bliss arises only for Rasikas, and not for others who have had no direct experience of the self.

[Objection] But surely, does not cannabis, consumed even without prior acquaintance, produce euphoria? Similarly, the euphoric aftertaste of the pleasure of love-making is experienced by all beings, regardless of whether they have had a direct experience of the self, and not only by Rasikas. If not, why engage in it at all?

[Reply] Granted. Even though all beings experience the pleasure of love-making there is nevertheless a difference between Haṃsa birds and crows. A male bird does not know its own true form, nor the form of the female, nor the truth of its generative organs, nor the transport of the androgyne Ardhanārīśvara taught in the sacred scriptures, nor liberation, nor the inhibiting bonds, nor the rapture. It experiences pleasure merely through the ejaculation of semen in consequence of "the itch." But a glorious Haṃsa makes love after discerning everything beginning with the true nature of the self. Why say more? There is a vast gulf between the lovemaking of Haṃsa birds and crows. The pleasure that connoisseurs with cultivated palates derive from various intoxicating cocktails made from cannabis, *phuka*, "poison," liquor and so on, is unlike that of ignoramuses.

The goal is simply euphoria. But of what use are utterly false conjectures and denials for those who have realized the truth? For those who have realized the truth, love-making taught in Śaiva scriptures is the ultimate truth: we Rasikas do not care for all of the contrary, false truths propounded by those that doubt. It is a bad day, I aver, when there is no union with doe-eyed women. The Kaula esoterium teaches: "Let there be uniting with the fifth every day." Here the fifth means love-making. "Homage! Homage to the servants and the leaders, who are intent on making love to new lovers!" Many such statements, preoccupied with love-making, are found in the Śaiva esoteric scriptures, [so] why should we be anxious? If a category, well discerned, properly experienced, being the essence of the Upaniṣads, taught in esoteric Śaiva scriptures, should be blameworthy, then so are all other categories taught in the Vedānta etc. This is simply atheism! Are you listening, woman with gracefully parted hair?

What are we saying? In divine sensual rapture an indescribable nectar is to be drunk. Food cooked to one's taste is to be eaten. And I insist that love-making involves the deliberate ejaculation of semen. In material sensual rapture people such as I should drink the aforementioned milk and so forth, while considering it to be nectar. One should eat milk-rice, cakes, sweetmeats and bread etc., and make love to a woman prescribed in the scriptures. There should be singing etc. of various kinds. In spiritual sensual rapture one should drink water acquired without effort, and food of a similar kind. Love-making consists merely of singing.

There are others whose hearts are greedy for paranormal powers, who drink liquor etc., [p. 320] and eat meat etc. Their love-making serves to obtain this-worldly pleasure or to produce the commingled sexual fluids. They also perform mantra repetition, worship and recitation. Yet other clerical communities drink wine etc. whenever they want and eat meat and so on. At a whim they make love to women of their own caste or another caste, to their own wives or the wives of others, but they are denizens of hell. Because they are condemned by the scriptures, and because they are bound souls, they are doomed to the great misery of dying and being born.

Some cowards, eunuchs, weaklings, valetudinarians, dotards, washouts, and bums revile lovemaking, the essence of all, on the basis of other scriptures. But if one has no such prejudice yet is in some manner incapacitated, then, one should sing its praises every moment until one dies.

And another thing, Haṃsī. Those who despise lovemaking in the sensual rapture are themselves despised. After realizing, in a gradual progression, the esoterium of the Śaiva scriptures, the apotheosis of revealed scriptures, from the lineage of a true teacher, can that which is so praiseworthy be called blameworthy? If one does so censure it, then the reward is disaster. How amazing is it that even those who engage in lovemaking censure it! Have they no shame? This is the delusory power of the glorious Tiraskāriṇī, that even those who engage in drinking, eating and sleeping decry these activities. What can we say about this?

Ecstatic woman! Look at the world. What credibility does people's gossip have? Like a jaundiced eye it perceives what is pure as impure. Even though it knows what is right, thinking itself wise, it enviously denounces it as wrong. How much worse than this is it with people who are imbeciles! Why even bother in debating with lies? The great sages revealed many doctrines, and there are many contradictions among them. Who is to say whose opinion is right and whose is not? Therefore we illustrious Haṃsas accept only the Śaiva teachings as authoritative in all instances. One should observe the teachings of a tradition to the extent that one is drawn to that tradition. All are under the sway of maturing karma, we are not so free that we all should follow the same modes of behavior. Because of such subordination there is diversity everywhere. But once one has realized the goal of the lineage of a true guru one should do as one wishes, but even then one should in no way censure it.

Those who have faith in this teaching,
Let them now proceed in it for their own benefit.
Those who do not have such faith,
Let them follow a different teaching.
But vilification is not called for.

Yoga of the Nāth Yogīs

—14—

The Original *Gorakṣaśataka*

James Mallinson

The *Gorakṣaśataka* or "Hundred Verses of Gorakṣa" contains some of the earliest teachings on *haṭha yoga* to be found in Sanskrit texts. It is the first text to describe complex methods of *prāṇāyāma*, breath control, and the first to teach the esoteric *sarasvatīcālana*, "the stimulation of Sarasvatī," a technique for arousing Kuṇḍalinī, the coiled serpent goddess who lies dormant at the base of the spine in the unenlightened. Most of the varieties of yoga practiced around the world today derive from *haṭha yoga*. The first texts to teach its techniques appeared soon after the beginning of the second millennium.

What unites these early texts and sets them apart from other works on yoga are the physical techniques known as *bandha*s and *mudrā*s, which are used to control the breath and raise Kuṇḍalinī. Much of *haṭha yoga*'s development can be seen as a reaction against the exclusivity and complexity of Tantric cults and practices. The esoteric physiology of Tantra is taken as the template for the human body, but the means of accessing and controlling the energies and substances within has become purely physical. The only external aid necessary is a guru qualified to teach *haṭha yoga*'s practices. There is no need for Tantra's elaborate initiations, nor the secret mandalas and mantras passed down within occult Tantric lineages, nor elaborate ritual paraphernalia, including the infamous *pañcamakāra* or "five Ms": *madya* ("wine"), *māṃsa* ("meat"), *matsya* ("fish"), *mudrā* ("hand gestures"), and *maithuna* ("sex"). As is made clear in the last verse of the *Gorakṣaśataka*, alternatives for these can be found within the body of the yogi. The techniques may differ, but the results of *haṭha yoga* are the same as those of Tantric rituals and yoga: supernatural powers (*siddhi*s) and liberation (*mukti*). In contrast to the usual conceptions of Tantric liberation, however, the latter can be achieved while alive, in a body immortalized by means of *haṭha yoga*.

Mukti, liberation, is the goal of the yoga of the *Gorakṣaśataka*. As is made clear in its first verse, its teachings are aimed at ascetics, men who have renounced worldly existence and devoted their lives to becoming liberated. Some other texts on *haṭha yoga*, such as the *Śivasaṃhitā*, teach that householders can benefit from its practice, and there are occasional hints in such works that women also used its techniques, but the male renouncer is the usual intended audience of texts on *haṭha yoga*.

The Yoga of the *Gorakṣaśataka*

The theory and method of the *Gorakṣaśataka*'s path to liberation are relatively clear, unlike those found in many other works on *haṭha yoga*. For the yogi to be liberated, his mind must be controlled. The mind and the breath are connected, so to control his mind the yogi should control his breath. Three methods should be used simultaneously to master the breath: eating a controlled diet, assuming a particular posture, and stimulating Kuṇḍalinī.

The ingredients of a controlled diet are not identified in the text; the yogi's food is simply required to be such that it "is unctuous and sweet, leaves a quarter [of the stomach] empty and is eaten in order to please Śiva."

"Posture" is *āsana*. Only two *āsana*s are recommended in the *Gorakṣaśataka*: *padmāsana*, the lotus posture, and *vajrāsana*, the diamond posture. The *Gorakṣaśataka*'s *vajrāsana* is known in other texts as *siddhāsana*. Both *padmāsana* and *vajrāsana* are relatively simple seated postures. *Haṭha yoga* later became associated with the practice of more complex *āsana*s, but they are absent from its early texts. They first appear in the thirteenth-century *Vasiṣṭhasaṃhitā*, whose yoga is not *haṭha yoga* but rather an attempt to accommodate Tantric Kuṇḍalinī yoga within an orthodox Vedic soteriology. The *Vasiṣṭhasaṃhitā*'s verses on *āsana* were used in the fifteenth-century *Haṭhapradīpikā* (or *Haṭhayogapradīpikā*), the first work in which complex *āsana*s are included among the techniques of *haṭha yoga*.

Kuṇḍalinī can be made to move either by *sarasvatīcālana*, stimulating Sarasvatī, or by *prāṇarodha*, restraining the breath. Sarasvatī is the goddess of speech; her home in the body is the tongue. The yogi is to move his tongue by wrapping it in a cloth and pulling it from side to side. The tongue is connected to the Suṣumnā *nāḍī*, the central and most important of the 72,000 *nāḍī*s or channels in the body. Pulling the tongue lifts the base of the Suṣumnā at the bottom of the spine, which is where Kuṇḍalinī sleeps, thereby stirring the dormant Kuṇḍalinī into action and allowing her, assisted by the associated rush of *prāṇa*, the vital breath, to enter the Suṣumnā.

This esoteric technique was misunderstood by most later commentators and anthologists because the text does not state explicitly where the cloth is to be applied. Kuṇḍalinī resides at the base of the spine, and stimulating her is said in the text to free the yogi from various diseases that might afflict the abdominal region, so the practice has been misunderstood as being performed in the lower part of the upper body. A variant of the *Gorakṣaśataka*'s verse describing the cloth is found, without any instructions as to what should be done with it, in the context of *śakticālana*, "stimulating the goddess," in two other early works on *haṭha yoga*—the *Yogabīja* and *Haṭhapradīpikā*. The Hindi translation of the Gorakhpur edition of the *Yogabīja* supplies *nābhi*, the navel, as the location at which the cloth is to be applied. Brahmānanda, who wrote a commentary on the *Haṭhapradīpikā* in 1843 CE, understands the verse to be describing the *kanda*, a bulb in the region of the navel from which all the body's *nāḍī*s are said to arise (to make sense of the verse he adds that the *kanda* appears as if wrapped in a cloth). The *Yogakuṇḍalyupaniṣad*, a late Yoga Upaniṣad, includes most of the *Gorakṣaśataka* in its first chapter.

Upaniṣadbrahmayogin, who wrote commentaries on a corpus of 108 Upaniṣads, makes no attempt to explain *sarasvatīcālana* in his commentary on the *Yogakuṇḍalyupaniṣad*. In his translation of the *Yogakuṇḍalyupaniṣad*, T. R. Srinivasa Ayyangar, who translated all the Yoga Upaniṣads for the Adyar Library, ingeniously turns the practice into a variant of *śāmbhavīmudrā*, a meditation technique in which the fingers are used to block the orifices of the head. The dimensions of the cloth are taken to refer to the distance that the breath is "elongated" to surround the Suṣumnā. In the description of *śakticālana* found in the *Gheraṇḍasaṃhitā*, which probably dates to the early part of the eighteenth century, the cloth is said to be wrapped around the *nābhi*, the navel. *Śakticālana* is not mentioned in most modern manuals of yoga, such as B.K.S. Iyengar's otherwise encyclopedic *Light on Yoga*. In his translation of the *Haṭhapradīpikā*, the present-day guru Satyananda Sarasvati says that *nauli*, churning of the stomach, is to be used to stimulate the goddess. There are two later Sanskrit texts which incorporate the *Gorakṣaśataka*'s verses on *sarasvatīcālana* and understand them correctly: the *Bṛhatkhecarīprakāśa*, a commentary on the *Khecarīvidyā* probably written in the first half of the eighteenth century, and the *Haṭharatnāvalī*, which was compiled in the seventeenth century. The latter borrows from the *Gorakṣaśataka* wholesale but substitutes *jihvām*, "the tongue," for the original's *tannāḍīm*, "her channel," as the location of where to wrap the cloth. Here lies the crux of the passage's misinterpretation elsewhere: as mentioned above, the location of Sarasvatī's *nāḍī* or "channel" is not made clear in the text of the *Gorakṣaśataka*. In some texts—the Sanskrit *Amṛtasiddhi*, *Brahmajñāna*, and *Haṭhatattvakaumudī*, and the Hindi *Gorakhbāṇī*—Sarasvatī is said to be a synonym of either Kuṇḍalinī or Suṣumnā. Both identifications make sense because of the different possible referents of

Sarasvatī. Kuṇḍalinī and Sarasvatī are both manifestations of Śakti, the feminine principle of the universe; Sarasvatī is also the name of the now mythical river said to meet the Ganges and Yamuna in a triple confluence at Allahabad which is paralleled in the body by the confluence of the Iḍā, Piṅgalā, and Suṣumnā *nāḍī*s. Both analogues only serve to obscure, however, the location of Sarasvatī in the body. In other texts—the Sanskrit *Matsyendrasaṃhitā*, *Śārṅgadharapaddhati*, and *Siddhasiddhāntapaddhati*; and the Hindi *Prāṇ Saṃkalī*—Sarasvatī is neither Kuṇḍalinī nor Suṣumnā but a separate *nāḍī*, all or one end of which is located in the tongue. In the *Khecarīvidyā*, the tongue is frequently called Vāgīśī, "Goddess of Speech," a synonym of Sarasvatī. It is this identification of the Sarasvatī *nāḍī* that makes sense of the compound *sarasvatīcālana*.

Cālana, "stimulation" or "causing to move," is part of the practice of *khecarīmudrā*, an important haṭhayogic technique in which the tongue is loosened and lengthened so that it can be turned backwards and inserted above the soft palate in order that the yogi might taste the *amṛta*, the nectar of immortality dripping from the moon in the head. *Khecarīmudrā* is not taught in the *Gorakṣaśataka* but is described in some other early Sanskrit works on *haṭha yoga*, including the *Dattātreyayogaśāstra*, the *Vivekamārtaṇḍa*, and the *Khecarīvidyā*. In the latter, *cālana* is a means of loosening the tongue (by wrapping it in a cloth and pulling on it) in order that *khecarīmudrā* may be performed. Many of the traditional practitioners of *haṭha yoga* whom I have met in India have demonstrated this technique to me. Theos Bernard also reports, in his account of a traditional training in *haṭha yoga* (*Hatha Yoga*, London: Rider, 1950), that he was told to practice it. *Cālana* as a preliminary to the practice of *khecarīmudrā* is not in itself said to stimulate Kuṇḍalinī, but *khecarīmudrā* is. Ballāla says in the *Bṛhatkhecarīprakāśa* that Kuṇḍalinī is to be awakened "by means of *āsana*, breath-retention, moving the tongue, *mudrā* etc." In this way, a quintessentially haṭhayogic technique consisting of the crude manipulation of the body, leads to the awakening of Kuṇḍalinī and thence to liberation. While *sarasvatīcālana* was an important component of *haṭha yoga* at its inception, it appears—if one takes Sanskrit texts on *haṭha yoga* as one's yardstick—to have fairly quickly fallen into obscurity, understood by only a handful of later practitioners or scholars. Within vernacular texts and the oral tradition, however, the idea of a connection between the tongue and Kuṇḍalinī, or at least the region in which she is said to lie sleeping, has survived. Thus, various medieval and later Hindi works—for example, the *Gorakh Bāṇī*, *Pañc Mātrā*, and *Mahādev Jī Kī Sabdī*—mention a link between the tongue and the penis (the yogi must restrain both), as does the eighteenth-century *Jogpradīpakā*, in which a single channel, identified with the Suṣumṇā, is said to join the tongue and the penis. The *Jogpradīpakā* passage associates the lengthening of the tongue with *laghutā*, "lightness" ("flaccidness"?), of the penis, the overcoming of sexual urges, and the awakening of Kuṇḍalinī. In 1996, at the Yoga Centre of Benares Hindu University, I met Dr. K. M. Tripathi, who demonstrated a technique in which the tip of the tongue is pressed against the front teeth and held there while the mouth is repeatedly opened wide and closed again. It is to be done at least a thousand times a day, he said, and the technique tugs on the *merudaṇḍa*, the spinal column, causing Kuṇḍalinī to rise. Dr. Tripathi told me that he had to give up this technique when he was married: householder practices that pull on the lower end of the *merudaṇḍa* are incompatible with the yogi's practice of tugging at the top.

The second method for stimulating Kuṇḍalinī taught in the *Gorakṣaśataka* is restraining the breath. Some later texts, which do not teach *sarasvatīcālana*—such as the *Śivasaṃhitā* and *Yuktabhavadeva*—say that Kuṇḍalinī should be stimulated by manipulating *apāna*, the lower breath. Holding the breath is called *kumbhaka* in the *Gorakṣaśataka*. *Kumbhaka*, which means "pot," can be unassisted, i.e., spontaneous and unstructured, or it can be assisted and take one of four forms. The former is superior. The latter is described in the *Gorakṣaśataka* in verses that are also found in the *Haṭhapradīpikā* and which are the earliest descriptions of complex breath control (*prāṇāyāma*) to be found in any Sanskrit text. The four varieties of *kumbhaka* are Sūryā, Ujjāyī, Śītalī, and Bhastrī. Each involves inhaling and exhaling in a different way. Sūryā is performed by inhaling through the right nostril and exhaling through the left. For Ujjāyī the yogi is to make a rasping noise in the lower part of the throat as he inhales. In Śītalī he is to inhale through his rolled tongue. For Bhastrī he is to pump the breath in and out as if working a pair of bellows. These *kumbhaka*s have various physical effects, ranging from the elimination of diseases to the awakening of Kuṇḍalinī. To achieve mastery of the breath and assist the stimulation of Kuṇḍalinī, there are three further practices that the yogi should undertake: the three *bandha*s or locks. These archetypal haṭhayogic practices are *mūla bandha*, in which the perineum is contracted; *uḍḍiyāna bandha*, in which the stomach is drawn up toward the abdomen; and *jālandhara bandha*, in which the chin is held down on the chest.

The *Gorakṣaśataka*'s yoga is summarized in its description of the best way to *samādhi*, the ultimate stage of all yogas. The yogi is to sit in a correct posture, stimulate Sarasvatī, and control his breath with the four *kumbhaka*s in conjunction with the three *bandha*s. *Samādhi* will ensue. In a subsequent passage which is likely to be a later addition to the core of the text, Kuṇḍalinī's ascent up the Suṣumnā is described. Heated by the inner fire and stimulated by the breath, she enters the Suṣumnā and climbs in staccato steps as she pierces the knots of Brahmā, Viṣṇu, and Rudra. Finally she reaches the *cakra* of the moon, which she melts into an ambrosial fluid. As a result of her drinking this, the yogi's mind becomes inured to external pleasures and hence controlled. Kuṇḍalinī then unites with Śiva before disappearing.

The Text

The *Gorakṣaśataka* has not been critically edited, published, or translated before. The translation below is of the text as found in a single manuscript, MS R 7874 in the collection of the Government Oriental Manuscripts Library (Madras), a xerox copy of which was kindly provided to me by Christian Bouy. There are catalogue references to four more manuscripts, which may also be of this *Gorakṣaśataka*, but I have been unable to consult any of them. There are nearly one hundred catalogue references to manuscripts of another text called the *Gorakṣaśataka*. This, however, is quite different from the work translated here, and much better known: several recensions of it have been published and translated. This latter *Gorakṣaśataka* was originally known as the *Vivekamārtaṇḍa*, and for simplicity's sake that is what I shall call it here. It seems likely that the *Vivekamārtaṇḍa* became known as the *Gorakṣaśataka* through confusion with the text translated here. The earliest recension of the *Vivekamārtaṇḍa*—which is found in a manuscript written in 1477 CE and predates that text's being called the *Gorakṣaśataka* by nearly two hundred years—has 173 verses; the *Gorakṣaśataka* has approximately 100, a more suitable number for a *śataka* or "century." (There is one late manuscript of the *Vivekamārtaṇḍa*-as-*Gorakṣaśataka* that consists of one hundred verses, but it is almost certainly a *précis* composed to make sense of the name.)

The oldest catalogued manuscript of the *Gorakṣaśataka* was written in 1795 CE. Barring the mention of Gorakṣa in its opening verse, which is likely to be a later addition to the text's central core, there is no internal evidence in the *Gorakṣaśataka* that can be used to date its composition. The only method of doing so at our disposal is to identify borrowings from it in works which can be dated. Unlike many other texts on *haṭha yoga*, the *Gorakṣaśataka* presents a coherent unit (at least in its central core: vv. 7–64), and is unlikely to include verses borrowed from elsewhere. It is from this central core that all of the borrowings from it found in other texts are taken (apart from those in the relatively late *Yogakuṇḍalyupaniṣad*). The *Haṭhapradīpikā*, the best known Sanskrit work on *haṭha yoga*, was compiled in the fifteenth century and includes twenty-eight verses from the *Gorakṣaśataka*. The *Yogabīja*, another early work on *haṭha yoga* and the likely source of five verses in the *Haṭhapradīpikā*, borrows nine verses from the *Gorakṣaśataka*. The *Śārṅgadharapaddhati*, an encyclopedic compendium of verses on a wide range of subjects including an extensive final section on *haṭha yoga*, was compiled in 1363 CE, but does not contain any verses from the *Gorakṣaśataka*. We may therefore tentatively conclude that the central core of the *Gorakṣaśataka* was composed (or at least became well known) in about 1400 CE. As the *Vivekamārtaṇḍa* gained in popularity under the name *Gorakṣaśataka*, the original *Gorakṣaśataka* fell into obscurity, whence the relative paucity of its manuscripts. In the eighteenth century, verses from the *Gorakṣaśataka* were used to compile the encyclopedic *Haṭhatattvakaumudī*. These verses are said to be *granthāntare*, "in another book": the *Gorakṣaśataka* is not named, perhaps to avoid confusion with the *Vivekamārtaṇḍa*, which by then was already widely known as the *Gorakṣaśataka* and which is frequently cited in the *Haṭhatattvakaumudī*. It is likely that the text was not originally a complete *śataka*. In addition to the central core consisting of verses 7–64, the introductory material at verses 2–6 may also be original, as may verses 65–74, which teach the sequence in which the techniques presented earlier in the text are to be used in order to attain *samādhi*, and which describe the obstacles that may impede the practitioner. Verses 75–88 are somewhat tautological in the light of what precedes them, and the non-dual Vedantic philosophy espoused in verses 88–100 is similarly incongruous, suggesting that these passages were added to the text to make it a *śataka*.

It is also highly unlikely that the text was originally associated with or attributed to Gorakṣa, let alone composed by him. The earliest datable references to Gorakṣa are found in two texts written in the early part of the thirteenth century. They are from opposite ends of the subcontinent and refer to him as a master of yoga, suggesting that his reputation was already well established. As we have seen above, the *Gorakṣaśataka* was probably composed around 1400 CE, long after Gorakṣa's time. During the fifteenth or sixteenth centuries, Gorakṣa was credited with having founded an order of yogis. (This order is nowadays widely referred to as that of the "Nāths" or "Nāth Siddhas," but there is no evidence for the use of the name "Nāth" to denote an order of yogis until the eighteenth century. Prior to that time the word *nātha/nāth*, when used in Sanskrit and Hindi works in the context of *haṭha yoga* and yogis, always refers to the supreme deity.) It is in the fifteenth century, when the yogi order that was to become the Nāths was seeking to become established and to distinguish itself from the other orders of yogis also beginning to coalesce at that time, that Sanskrit and Hindi works were first attributed to Gorakṣa. Some verses in the *Haṭhapradīpikā* are attributed to him, but these do not include any of the twenty-eight verses taken from the *Gorakṣaśataka*. The only mention of Gorakṣa within the *Gorakṣaśataka* is at the beginning of the text.

Whether or not this is a later addition to the central core of the text, Gorakṣa cannot have composed the *Gorakṣaśataka* for reasons other than chronology: the text's author distinguishes himself and his guru from Gorakṣa. In the second verse he says that he is describing Gorakṣa's method of yoga, which he has experienced thanks to his guru's teaching. His guru's teaching may or may not have been a direct oral transmission from that of Gorakṣa, but the text itself is clearly not comprised of the words of Gorakṣa.

Verses from the *Gorakṣaśataka* have been used to compile a variety of later works including, as mentioned above, the *Yogabīja*, *Haṭhapradīpikā*, *Haṭharatnāvalī*, *Haṭhatattvakaumudī*, and the *Yogakuṇḍalyupaniṣad*. The first eighty verses of the last text's first chapter are all taken from the *Gorakṣaśataka*. Verses from the *Gorakṣaśataka* are found in later recensions of the *Vivekamārtaṇḍa*, having perhaps first been incorporated as glosses. Through careful examination of these shared verses, combined with textual criticism and observation of the interplay between text and practice, subtle developments in the practice and terminology of yoga become apparent. The confusion over the positioning of the cloth used to perform *sarasvatīcālana* outlined above has resulted in considerable innovation in the techniques employed for the raising of Kuṇḍalinī, exemplified by Swami Satyananda Saraswati's recommendation for that purpose of *nauli* (abdominal churning), among whose many benefits listed in Sanskrit works the raising of Kuṇḍalinī is never found.

The *Gorakṣaśataka* is the first text to teach the *prāṇāyāma* technique now widely known as *sūryabhedana*, "the piercing of the sun." In the *Gorakṣaśataka* it is called the *sūryā bheda*, i.e., the "solar variety" of *kumbhaka*. The passage teaching it ends with the quarter-verse *sūryābhedam udāhṛtam*, "[this] is known as the *sūryā* variety (*bheda*) [of *kumbhaka*]." The same quarter verse is found in the *Haṭhapradīpikā* as *sūryabhedanam uttamam*, "the excellent piercing of the sun." The subsequent popularity of the *Haṭhapradīpikā* made it such that its new name for the technique became definitive. A corollary technique—called *candrabhedana*, "the piercing of the moon," in which the left or lunar channel is used for inhalation—is taught by some modern schools of yoga.

A close reading of the corpus of Sanskrit texts on *haṭha yoga* may provide insights into some of the nuances of its practices. However, the confusion of the names of the *sūryā/sūryabhedana kumbhaka* and the misunderstanding of *sarasvatīcālana* are indications that the primary purpose of such texts, particularly of anthologies such as the *Haṭhapradīpikā*, was not always the elucidation of the techniques of yoga. Rather, Sanskrit works on *haṭha yoga* served to endorse and lend authority to its practices and schools, perhaps under the auspices of a patron devoted to a yogi preceptor. Their terse teachings are not comprehensive enough to serve as foundations for practice and could never replace oral instruction from a qualified guru. Nor are they likely to have been used as mnemonics by the aspiring yogi: no traditional yogi that I have met in India has ever used them in this way. Svātmārāma, the compiler of the *Haṭhapradīpikā*, left other inaccuracies and contradictions in his work, for which he was castigated by later authors such as Śrīnivāsa in his *Haṭharatnāvalī*. These remind us that our view of the practice of *haṭha yoga* in its formative period is little better than that of the proverbial frog's view of the sky from the bottom of a well. There would have been a vast range of experimentation in the new field of *haṭha yoga* during the first four centuries of its development, involving yogis, both male and female, of every stripe, the majority of whom would not have known Sanskrit. There are no historical reports of details of the practice of *haṭha yoga* until Islamic interpretations begin to appear in the fifteenth century and modern-day oral traditions, while they provide some clues, are an unreliable window onto antiquity. All we have to go on is half a dozen short Sanskrit works (and the Marathi *Jñāneśvarī*) written or compiled by scholars who in some cases may not have practiced the techniques they describe.

As stated by Svātmārāma at the beginning of the *Haṭhapradīpikā*, early *haṭha yoga* was a befuddling "darkness of many doctrines." Svātmārāma valiantly tried to create a lamp (*pradīpikā*) to lighten this darkness by synthesizing into one coherent whole the doctrines in the texts he had at his disposal, but their incompatibility made this an ultimately impossible task. By making the *Haṭhapradīpikā* a compilation, however, he has unwittingly left us with a means of identifying the texts that taught those early doctrines, a small number of which do present coherent methods of yoga. One such text is the *Gorakṣaśataka*.

There are many difficulties with the text of the *Gorakṣaśataka* as found in the single manuscript (Government Oriental Manuscripts Library, Madras, MS R 7874) used for the present translation. At several places I have made conjectural emendations; at several others I have emended it using readings found in works which borrow from it, the *Haṭhapradīpikā* and *Yogakuṇḍalyupaniṣad* in particular. Some parts of the text have remained unclear to me despite my best efforts at emendation. These passages are marked with cruxes († . . . †); sometimes I attempt a translation, but where I am completely stumped I leave an ellipsis (. . .). The verse division of the manuscript is also problematic. It is unnumbered but gives single *daṇḍa*s (vertical lines) to mark the end of half-verses and double *daṇḍa*s to mark the end of verses. There are 107 double *daṇḍa*s, but if each pair of half-verses is numbered without regard to the manuscript's punctuation we get a total of 101 verses, the usual number for a *śataka*.

This does, however, result in several infelicitous verse divisions. I have thus decided to leave the translation unnumbered.

Suggestions for Further Reading

Of early (pre-*Haṭhapradīpikā*) texts on *haṭha yoga*, only the following have been edited and translated into English: the *Khecarīvidyā*, ed. James Mallinson (London: Routledge, 2007), and the *Śivasaṃhitā* (various editions, including James Mallinson [New York: YogaVidya.com, 2007]). The best edition and translation of the *Haṭhapradīpikā* is that of Svami Digambarji and Dr. Pitambar Jha (Lonavla: Kaivalyadham S.M.Y.M. Samiti, 1970). There is no English translation of any of the longer recensions of the *Vivekamārtaṇḍa*, but it has been edited and translated into German by Fausta Nowotny (*Das Gorakṣaśataka* [Köln: Richard Schwartzbold, 1976]). Its hundred-verse *précis* has been edited and translated into English by Svami Kuvalayananda and S. A. Shukla (*Gorakṣaśatakam* [Lonavla: Kaivalyadham S.M.Y.M. Samiti, 1958]).

English translations of later works on *haṭha yoga* include the *Yoga-Upaniṣads,* tr. T. R. Śrīnivāsa Ayyangar (Madras: Adyar Library, 1938); the *Haṭharatnāvalī*, ed. M. L. Gharote, P. Devnath, and V. K. Jha (Lonavla Yoga Institute, 2002), the *Haṭhatattvakaumudī*, ed. M. L. Gharote, P. Devnath, and V. K. Jha (Lonavla Yoga Institute, 2007); and the *Gheraṇḍasaṃhitā*, ed. and tr. James Mallinson (New York: YogaVidya.com, 2004).

On Sanskrit texts on *haṭha yoga* and in particular their relationship with the Yoga Upaniṣads, see Christian Bouy, *Les Nātha-Yogin et les Upaniṣads* (Paris: Diffusion de Boccard, 1994). On Tantric precedents of *haṭha yoga*, see Somadeva Vasudeva, *The Yoga of the Mālinīvijayottaratantra* (Pondicherry: Institut Français de Pondichéry, 2004).

On early texts on *haṭha yoga*, see the introduction to the *Khecarīvidyā* (Mallinson 2007). On yogic and alchemical traditions, see David Gordon White, *The Alchemical Body* (Chicago: University of Chicago Press, 1996).

The Hundred Verses of Goraksa

So that renouncers whose essence is consciousness might attain perfection, I shall now duly proclaim the method of yoga which was made public by Gorakṣa, the king of the siddhas, and which gives signs of success in but a few days, for I have personally experienced it thanks to my guru's oral teaching.

The wise man does not fall into rebirth; through the science of sexual pleasure people are mutually ruined. By taking instruction, he who has been made to fall becomes perfect; he who does not take instruction does not. It is according to his actions that a man has a good or bad destiny: the builder of walls goes up, the builder of wells down. Therefore one must initially make an effort in order to be liberated from existence, and through devotion in body, speech and mind, obtain an excellent guru. One should always turn to a guru whose sight, mind and breath do not depend on form for support †. . . †

He is truly liberated whose mind is neither asleep nor awake, neither remembers nor forgets, and neither stops nor starts. He is without doubt liberated whose breath goes neither in nor out, neither in the left nostril nor the right, and neither up nor down. The mind has two impulses: past impressions and the breath. On one of them being destroyed, both are destroyed. Of these two, it is the breath which you must first conquer (on being allowed to do so [by your guru]), in order that you might become a liberated man †. . . †.

[The Conquest of the Breath] There is said to be a triad of methods best for bringing about the conquest of the breath: a controlled diet, posture and the third, stimulation of the goddess. Their characteristics shall now duly be described in turn.

[Measured Diet] Food that is unctuous and sweet, leaves a quarter [of the stomach] empty and is eaten in order to please Śiva is called a measured diet.

[Posture] Posture is said to have two varieties: *padmāsana* and *vajrāsana*.

[*Padmāsana*] If one puts the soles of both feet on the thighs, that is *padmāsana*, the lotus posture, which duly destroys all sins.

[*Vajrāsana*] If one puts the left heel under the bulb and the other one above it, and holds one's neck, head and body straight, it is called *vajrāsana*, the thunderbolt posture.

[The Stimulation of the goddess] Now I shall briefly teach the stimulation of the goddess. The goddess is coiled. Making her move in stages from her home to the place between the eyebrows is called the stimulation of the goddess. There are two chief ways of accomplishing this: the stimulation of Sarasvatī and the restraint of the breath. Through practice, Kuṇḍalinī becomes straight.

[The Stimulation of Sarasvatī] Of the two [methods], I shall first teach you the stimulation of Sarasvatī. Knowers of antiquity call Sarasvatī Arundhatī. By making her move Kuṇḍalinī moves automatically. With the vital breath moving in Iḍā [the left channel], the wise man should sit steadily in *padmāsana*, spread out a cloth twelve fingers long and four fingers broad, wrap it around

[Sarasvatī's] *nāḍī* and hold it firmly with the thumbs and index fingers of both hands. For two *muhūrta*s (one hour and thirty-six minutes) he should fearlessly move it left and right over and over again as much as he can. He should draw [the part of] the Suṣumnā which is at [the level of] Kuṇḍalinī slightly upwards so that Kuṇḍalinī can enter the Suṣumnā's mouth. *Prāṇa* leaves that place and automatically enters the Suṣumnā. [The yogi] should stretch his stomach and, having contracted his throat, he should fill himself up with air through the solar [right] channel: the wind travels up from the chest. Therefore one should regularly stimulate Sarasvatī, she who contains sound. By stimulating her, the yogi is freed from diseases such as inflammation of the spleen, dropsy, splenitis and other [ills] that affect the stomach. All of those diseases are sure to be destroyed by the stimulation of the goddess.

[The Restraint of the Breath] Now I shall teach in brief the restraint of the breath. The vital breath (*prāṇa*) is wind produced in the body. [Its] restraint (*āyāma*) is known as *kumbhaka*. *Kumbhaka* is said to be of two kinds: assisted (*sahita*) and unassisted (*kevala*). [The yogi] should practice assisted *kumbhaka* until unassisted *kumbhaka* is mastered. Sūryā, Ujjāyī, and Śītalī [are the first three] and Bhastrī [is] the fourth: when *kumbhaka* has these variations it is assisted *kumbhaka*. I shall now duly teach in brief [their] characteristics.

[Sūryā *kumbhaka*] In a clean place clear of people and mosquitoes and so forth, as long as a bow and free from cold, fire and water, [and] on a seat that is clean—neither too high nor too low, agreeable and comfortable—[the yogi] should assume *padmāsana*, stimulate Sarasvatī, gently draw in external air through the right channel, fill himself with as much air as is comfortable and then expel it through Iḍā [the left channel]. (Alternatively the wise man should expel the breath once the skull is purified.) This destroys the four diseases of the *vāta* humor and problems with worms. This [*kumbhaka*], which is called the Sūryā or solar variety, should be practiced repeatedly.

[Ujjāyī *kumbhaka*] [The yogi] should close the mouth and gently draw in air through the two channels so that it comes into contact with [the region extending] from the throat to the heart, making a sound. In the same way as before he should hold his breath and then expel it through Iḍā. [This] *kumbhaka*, which is called Ujjāyī, ("the victorious"), should be performed when [the yogi is] walking or at rest. It destroys the fire that arises in the head; it completely removes phlegm from the throat; it increases the fire of the body and it rids the body of edema in the channels and imbalances in its constituent parts.

[Śītalī *kumbhaka*] The sage should draw in air through the tongue and then, after holding the breath as before, gently exhale it through his nostrils. Inflammation of the spleen and other diseases are destroyed, as is fever caused by an excess of *pitta*, the bilious humor. This *kumbhaka* called Śītalī, "she who is cool," destroys poisons.

[Bhastrī *kumbhaka*] Then the sage should assume *padmāsana* and, holding his neck and stomach straight, close his mouth and forcefully exhale through his nostrils in such a way that his breath makes contact with his throat, producing a sound in his skull. He should then quickly draw in a small amount of air as far as his heart lotus. Then he should exhale and inhale as before, repeating the process over and over again. The wise man should pump the air that is in his body in the same way that one might quickly pump a blacksmith's bellows. When the body becomes tired, he should gently inhale by way of the sun until the abdomen becomes full of air. Holding the middle of the nose firmly, without using the index fingers, he should perform *kumbhaka* as before and then exhale through Iḍā. This adamantine [*kumbhaka*] purges the throat of bile; it increases the fire of the body; it awakens Kuṇḍalinī; it frees from sin, and is auspicious [and] pleasant. It destroys the bolt made of substances such as phlegm which is situated inside the opening of the Brahmā *nāḍī* [and] it pierces the three knots that are born from the three *guṇa*s. This *kumbhaka*, called Bhastrī ("the bellows"), is to be practiced above all others.

[The Three *Bandha*s] Now I shall briefly teach the three *bandha*s. Once the four varieties of *kumbhaka* have been learnt and are being practiced regularly, [the yogi] should achieve mastery of the breath. He must perform the three *bandha*s, which I shall now describe. The first is *mūla bandha*, the second is *uḍḍiyāna bandha*, and the third is *jālandhara* [*bandha*]. Their characteristics are as follows:

[Mūla bandha] [The yogi] forces the downward-moving *apāna* breath to move upwards by means of contraction. Yogis call this *mūla bandha*, "the root lock." When *apāna* has turned upwards and reached the orb of fire, then the flame, fanned by the wind, rises high. As a result, fire and *apāna* reach *prāṇa*, which is hot by nature. The overheated *prāṇa* creates a blaze in the body, which heats the sleeping Kuṇḍalinī and wakes her up. Like a snake struck by a stick, she hisses and straightens herself. As if entering a snake-hole, she enters the Brahmā *nāḍī*. Therefore, yogis should maintain the regular practice of *mūla bandha*.

[Uḍḍiyāna bandha] *Uḍḍiyāna* is to be performed at the end of *kumbhaka* and the beginning of exhalation. It is the *bandha* by means of which the breath flies up (*uḍḍīyate*) into the Suṣumṇa, which is why yogis call it *uḍḍiyāna*. Sitting in *vajrāsana*, [the yogi] should hold his feet firmly with his hands and press the bulb there in the region of his ankles. He should very gently pull back his stomach, heart and throat, so that his breath does not reach his belly. Once gastric imbalances have been overcome, [*uḍḍiyāna*] is to be carefully performed at regular intervals.

[Jālandhara bandha] The *bandha* called *jālandhara* is to be performed after inhalation. It involves constricting the neck, and blocks the movement of the breath. Once the neck is constricted, by means of contraction and stretching the abdomen backwards [i.e., by the *mūla* and *uḍḍiyāna bandha*s], the breath quickly enters the Brahmā *nāḍī*.

[Samādhi] Now I shall teach the best way to *samādhi*, an enjoyable method which conquers death and always brings about the bliss of [absorption in] *brahman*. Correctly assuming a posture in exactly the same way as was taught earlier, [the yogi] should stimulate Sarasvatī and control his breath. On the first day he should perform the four *kumbhaka*s, [holding] each of them ten times. On the second day [he should increase] that by five. Adding five each day, on the third day he should do twenty, which is enough. *Kumbhaka* should always be performed in conjunction with the three *bandha*s.

[Obstacles to the Practice of Yoga] Sleeping by day because of staying awake and having too much sex at night; over-agitation due to constant restraint of urine and feces; [and] problems with imbalanced posture on account of worrying about one's breath while exerting oneself: these cause disease to arise quickly. If the ascetic were to stop [his practice], saying "I have become ill from practicing yoga," and then abandon his practice altogether, that is said to be the first obstacle. The second is doubt and the third is negligence. The fourth is sloth and the fifth is sleep. The sixth is stopping one's practice and the seventh is said to be delusion. Irregularity is the eighth and the ninth is known as that with no name. Not attaining the essence of yoga is said by the wise to be the tenth. By reflecting [on them] the wise man should renounce these ten obstacles.

[The Ascent of Kuṇḍalinī] Then the wise man who is established in the true reality should regularly practice [control of] the breath. The mind is absorbed into the Suṣumnā and the breath does not rush forth. As a result of his secretions being dried up, the yogi's journey is begun. He should force the downward moving *apāna* breath to move upwards by means of contraction. Yogis call this *mūla bandha*. When the *apāna* has become upward moving and goes together with fire to the place of *prāṇa*, then—with fire, *prāṇa* and *apāna* having quickly come together—the coiled, sleeping Kuṇḍalinī, heated by that fire and stimulated by the breath, makes her body enter the mouth of the Suṣumnā. Then, having pierced the knot of Brahmā, which is born of the *rajas guṇa*, she quickly flashes like a streak of lightning in the mouth of the Suṣumnā. She hurries up to the knot of Viṣṇu and, after stopping at the heart, she swiftly moves on, having pierced the knot of Viṣṇu. [She then] goes to where the knot of Rudra is found, between the eyebrows, and, having pierced that, she goes to the orb of the moon, the *cakra* called *anāhata* which has sixteen petals. Once there she automatically dries up the fluid produced from the moon. When the sun has been moved from its abode to the place of blood and bile by the force of *prāṇa*, Kuṇḍalinī, having gone to where the *cakra* of the moon (which consists of the white fluid of phlegm) is found, consumes there the heated phlegm that has been discharged and is by nature cold. In the same way the white [fluid] in the shape of the moon is heated forcefully; agitated, Kuṇḍalinī moves upwards and thus [the fluid] flows even more. As a result of tasting this, the mind is beyond the objects of the senses. Having enjoyed the best of what is inside him, the young man [becomes] intent on the self. Kuṇḍalinī goes to †the place whose form is that of the eight constituents of nature.† Having embraced it she moves on to Śiva. After embracing him she disappears. In the same way, the red (*rajas*) from below and the white (*śukla*) from above dissolve in Śiva. Thereafter, the breath similarly joins with the twins *prāṇa* and *apāna*.

[Realization of the Truth] †With the gross element diminished and the speaker [becoming] greater†, the breath] increases and makes all the [bodily] winds flow like gold [heated] in a crucible. With the physical body [absorbed] into the spiritual one, the body becomes extremely pure. I shall now describe this to you clearly. Free of the condition of being insentient, undefiled, with consciousness as its essence, that subtle body is the most important of all [bodies] and contains [the notion of] "I." Freedom from the condition of being insentient [and] the mistaken understanding of that which takes the appearance of time: notions such as these—which have their own form, like that of the rope and the snake—sow doubt about the form of reality. The condition arises of considering their cause to be time. This elemental [universe] is as real as water in a mirage. Beheld by the temporal body, the earth and its other parts are indeed produced from the elements. Like the hare's horn, it is real neither in the meaning of its name nor in its own form. †A bad dream arises in the meantime whose proof is produced. Is that man [i.e., the dreamer] deluded, like the [wild] gaze of a rutting elephant?† It is incorrect [to say] that everything comes into being and it is incorrect [to say] that it disappears, just as it is out of error that a man or a woman thinks mother-of-pearl to be silver.

Knowledge from a dream cannot be called the body even if it might appear real. Thus, after being mistaken, [the truth should be] established by means of careful investigation. In the same way, this body, through thorough introspection, clearly reveals itself to be insentient because it is formed from the elements. Thus, in the same way, just as through lack of thought, the process of the practice of [controlling] the breath comes to an end †. . . †, it is not a thing. Thus are the seven levels, from arising in that which is produced by knowledge. One should attain perpetual happiness in conditions such as that called "being without fire."

We drink the dripping liquid called *bindu*, the drop, not wine; we consume the rejection of the objects of the five senses, not meat; we do not embrace a beloved but rather the Suṣumnā *nāḍī*, her body curved like *kuśa* grass; if we must have intercourse, it takes place in a mind dissolved in the void, not in a vagina.

Thus ends *The Hundred Verses of Gorakṣa.*

—15—

Nāth Yogīs, Akbar, and the "Bālnāth Ṭillā"

William R. Pinch

In early March 1581, the Mughal emperor Akbar visited a major Nāth Yogī center, known as the "Bālnāth Ṭillā." He visited the site at least one other time in later years, and yogis from the "Ṭillā" are said to have visited the Mughal capital on occasion. The "Ṭillā," or "crag," has been known by a variety of names over the centuries, including "Ṭillā Jogiān," "Gorakshanāth Ṭillā," and "Lakṣman Ṭillā." This chapter presents a selection of texts that describe this site and Akbar's visit to it, as well as different ways that Nāth Yogīs gravitated toward or interacted with the Mughal emperor and other sovereign powers in the region. Two of the texts were composed in Persian, one in Portuguese, one in Latin, and the rest in Hindi. The Persian, Latin, and Portuguese texts were committed to writing in the sixteenth century, fairly soon after the events described occurred; the remainder, in Hindi, come from oral tradition passed down over generations, only to be published in written form in the twentieth century.

The contemporary accounts of Akbar's visit to the Ṭillā were composed by two very different men: one was the emperor's close friend and prominent court intellectual, Abu'l Fazl; the other was a European visitor to the Mughal court and a member of the relatively young Society of Jesus (or "Jesuit" order), Antonio Monserrate. Abu'l Fazl, whose Persian account comes from his massive eulogistic biography of Akbar, assumed that the reader possessed a degree of familiarity with India and Mughal political and religious culture; he generally wrote sympathetically about Indian religious practices and tended to cast things in a quasi-Sufi devotionalist light. Thus, as he puts it in a later passage from volume three of the *Ā'īn-i-Akbarī* (pp. 197–98), although yogic claims of superhuman power "may seem incredible in the eyes of those affected by the taint of narrow custom, those who acknowledge the wonderful power of God will find in it no cause of astonishment." By contrast, Monserrate, who wrote in Latin for Europeans (primarily his Jesuit superiors and brothers), assumed very little knowledge about India on the part of his readers; consequently his account contained much more in the way of ordinary details left out of Abu'l Faẓl's chronological narrative. And whereas Abu'l Faẓl saw yogis and their abilities as a reflection of God's marvelous power, Monserrate tended to regard their religious understandings and practices as absurd.

The two supplementary sixteenth-century accounts of Akbar's encounters with yogis were written by analogous figures at the Mughal court. Abdu-l Q̣ādir Badāūnī, to whom we are indebted for his description of Akbar's late night meetings with yogis and his adoption of many of their practices and understandings, was a prominent court intellectual like his rival, Abu'l Faẓl. In the 1580s, overcome with bitterness and hatred due to the political ascent of the latter, Badāūnī began compiling a secret history that expressed his displeasure at the liberal attitudes that came to characterize Akbar's reign. Not surprisingly, therefore, his description of Akbar's visits to the yogis, while full of interesting detail, is laced with invective. Badāūnī's account is supplemented in turn by an unusual (and heretofore untranslated) description by Jerome Xavier, the grand nephew of the celebrated—though not yet canonized—Francis Xavier. A member of the Society of Jesus like Monserrate, Xavier belonged to the much longer-lived "third mission to Mogor." He lived at or near the court in Agra and Lahore for almost twenty years, finally leaving to return to Goa on India's west coast (and the headquarters of Portugal's "Estado da India") during the reign of Akbar's son, Salīm (or "Jahāngīr"), in 1615. His account of a Nāth Yogī gathering on the banks of the Ravi near the palace at Lahore in 1596, not long after his arrival in north India, was part of a long and detailed Portuguese letter that he wrote as a report to his superiors in Goa and Rome. It is informed by the same Counter-Reformation sensibilities that animated Monserrate's account and likewise provides a fascinating level of detail.

Interspersed amid these sixteenth-century accounts are, finally, stories popular among Nāth Yogīs that have been handed down over generations and today constitute a part of the traditional lore of the Ṭillā and its followers. These were recorded during the latter half of the twentieth century and published in Hindi in 1983 by Krishna Kumar Bali. In choosing from the many legends popular among Nāth Yogīs, I have sought material that elaborates details or themes introduced in the sixteenth-century accounts. Whether or not "the legends cloak a near historical fact," as suggested by B. N. Goswamy and J. S. Grewal in their introduction to a collection of Persian documents concerning the "Jogis of Jakhbar," they do afford a glimpse of yogi self-understandings concerning the features of their existence and practices that outside observers deemed worthy of inclusion in their descriptive accounts. In addition, the pairing of the legendary with the more traditional "primary source" accounts affords a sense of how the meanings associated with events, persons, and places from the late sixteenth century have percolated within the Nāth Yogī community over time (more on this point below).

Akbar's visit to the Bālnāth Ṭillā occurred in the wake of the bringing to heel of Mirzā Ḥakīm, the emperor's half brother, resident in Kabul. Akbar's victory over Mirzā Ḥakīm signaled the defeat of the "orthodox" Muslim party in Mughal politics and thus opened a new phase in the half-century long reign of Akbar, who was now free to experiment more liberally with various forms of religious eclecticism. It is in the wake of Mirzā Ḥakīm's defeat that we begin to see the more open expression of interest by the emperor in heterodox groups like Nāth Yogīs. At the same time, Akbar recognized the need to leave a more firm "Akbarī" imprint on the Punjab, a region that had been the scene of much dissension, by engaging in wide-ranging hunting expeditions, building bridges, constructing forts, and laying out gardens. In the wake of military exercises, these construction projects were a way to reshape the north Indian environment according to Mughal self-understandings. The act of visiting, engaging with, and becoming the major patron of the Nāth Yogīs of the Punjab and Jammu-Kashmir hills, whose craggy haunts were difficult to access and inhospitable even for local inhabitants, was also for the Mughal emperor a way to take possession of that geo-strategic territory. But from the Nāth Yogī point of view, it is not at all clear who was possessing whom. Certainly Akbar was making the Himalayan frontier more Mughal, but in the process the Nāth Yogīs were making Akbar more yogic. In other words, yogis and Mughals seemed to be domesticating each other. Indeed, this is precisely how empire works, when it works: as a dual process of incorporation (or projection and possession), from above and below.

The Bālnāth Ṭillā is today located in Jhelum District, Pakistan. During Partition in 1947, many of the Nāth Yogīs connected to the Ṭillā, including the head of the monastery, shifted to Ambala on the Indian side of the Punjab. Not surprisingly, many of the legendary vignettes related in Bali's 1983 work reflect the more recent post-Mughal history of the subcontinent, particularly the challenges posed by the emergence of regional eighteenth-century states, the rise of British power, and the crystallization of Hindu and Muslim religious-nationalism. Even those tales that purport to describe events in Akbar's day seem colored by more recent sensibilities and anxieties, particularly religious anxieties that are produced by modern communalism.

While few if any original Mughal-era documents connected to the Ṭillā have come to light, or have been subject to scholarly scrutiny, it was reported in the 1904 *Jhelum District Gazetteer* (a kind of administrative handbook) that the monastery was in possession of a "sanad" from Akbar confirming "an ancient grant" of a *jāgīr* or tax-free estate owned by the Ṭillā. By contrast, Mughal records concerning a related Nāth Yogī institution, at Jakhbar, located on the Indian side of the Punjab, have benefited from painstaking historiographical investigation by B. N. Goswamy and J. S. Grewal. From these documents it is clear that Jakhbar was established during the reign of Akbar, and with Mughal support. The founder, who was known both as Bhau Nāth and Udwant Nāth, is said to have impressed Akbar with his feats of yogic prowess, which included the power of flight. According to a legend from Jakhbar, Udwant Nāth regularly flew from Jakhbar to the Ganga to fetch water for his guru's bath. Stories of such supernormal powers are, as demonstrated below, a commonplace of Nāth Yogī lore. And indeed there is a similar story (also included here) concerning a differently named Nāth Yogī of the Ṭillā who was contemporaneous with Akbar, suggesting that these were—or at least are remembered as—one and the same individual, and (more importantly, from the Ṭillā point of view) that Jakhbar is subordinate to the Ṭillā in the Nāth Yogī hierarchy.

Though today—especially in the West—yoga is associated with physical postures and breathing exercises and the good health that is thought to follow from such practices, many of the actual primary source descriptions of yogis from the early modern era suggest—and sometimes make explicitly clear—that the "yoga" of Nāth Yogīs was principally about the cultivation of supernormal power. Of particular importance was power over the natural world—whether in the form of climate, gravity, flora, or fauna—and indeed over death itself. As David Gordon White has argued, the Nāth Yogī's ability to project himself onto, and into, other beings—to quite literally take bodily possession of both living and inanimate things around him and, in some cases, render himself deathless—was central to what it meant to be a yogi. In fact, a Nāth Yogī's ability to project himself and take possession—to yoke the world to his will—determined his status as a "siddha" or "perfected being," the highest rank among yogis. Quite naturally, then, the Nāth Yogīs and their "siddha" gurus were of immense interest to wielders of political power, whose business it was, also, to project force and take possession—of territory, people, animals, and plants. And the feeling was, evidently, mutual. Siddhas and sovereigns were, in a sense, rivals, but this meant they could also be allies—for so long as the terms of their relationship could be properly calibrated. No doubt this calibration had much to do with Akbar's visit to and his patronage of the shrine, as well as the Nāth Yogī gravitation toward Akbar in later years. But as the case of Akbar seems to suggest, Nāth Yogīs were also useful in other, more intimate ways.

The legends from Krishna Kumar Bali, *Ṭillā Gorakṣanāth* (Haridwar: Pir Kala Nath Prakashan, 1983), are translated from Hindi by me. For the passages by Abu'l Faẓl, Badāūnī, and Monserrate, I have used the translations done around the turn of the twentieth century by H. Beveridge (Abu'l Faẓl), George Ranking (Badāūnī), and John S. Hoyland and S. N. Bannerjee (Monserrate): see the passages for bibliographic details. My translation of the Xavier letter was corrected and enhanced by Dr. Javier Castro-Ibaseta, to whom I am grateful.

Suggestions for Further Reading

The most detailed examination of Mughal and post-Mughal land-grant documents concerning a Nāth Yogī shrine is B. N. Goswamy and J. S. Grewal, *The Mughals and the Jogis of Jakhbar: Some Madad-i Ma'ash and Other Documents* (Simla: Indian Institute of Advanced Study, 1967). Munis D. Faruqui, "The Forgotten Prince: Mirza Hakim and the Formation of the Mughal Empire in India," *Journal of the Economic and Social History of the Orient* 48: 4 (December 2005): 487–523, provides a cogent investigation of the internal politics governing Akbar's religious development. Abu'l Faẓl makes reference, in the excerpt below, to his discussion of the "Patanjali Canon" in the final volume. This discussion can be found in his *A'in-i Akbari*, vol. 3, trans. H. S. Jarret, corrected and annotated by Jadunath Sarkar (Calcutta: Royal Asiatic Society, 1927–1949), pp. 187–98. There are many other Mughal-era passages that describe yogis: among the most entertaining is a description by the traveler Maḥmūd Walī Balkhī (from Balkh, in northern Afghanistan) in 1625–31, recently revisited in Muzaffar Alam and Sanjay Subrahmanyam, *Indo-Persian Travels and the Age of Discoveries, 1400–1800* (Cambridge: Cambridge University Press, 2007), pp. 131–74. On powerful ascetics (including yogis) and the implications for Mughal and British imperialism and Indian nationalism, see William R. Pinch, *Warrior Ascetics and Indian Empires* (Cambridge: Cambridge University Press, 2006). On possession and projection in early modern and modern India, see David Gordon White, *Sinister Yogis* (Chicago: University of Chicago Press, 2009), especially chapter 6.

Akbar's visit to the Bālnāth Tillā

(From Abu'l Faẓl, *Akbarnāma*, vol. 3, trans. H. Beveridge (Calcutta: Asiatic Society of Bengal, 1897–1918), pp. 513–14.)

Also at this time [March 1581] he visited the shrine of Bālnāth Tillāh. It is loftily situated and near Rohtās. It is so old that its beginning is not known. It is regarded as the prayer-spot of Bālnāth Jogī, and is held in veneration, and visited by many people. In the extensive country of India there are various ways of obtaining deliverance (*āzādī*). One set are called Jogīs. Their tenets are according to the Pātanjal Canon, of which some account has been given in the final volume.

They place eternal existence in the kingdom of annihilation, and act, in many respects, contrary to customs. Many are distinguished for contentment and innocence, and, one by one, attain to enlightenment. Bālnāth was at the head of these enthusiasts. They say he was the younger brother of Rām Cand, and it is commonly said that he became an ascetic, and that he chose this place in order to mortify his passions. In short, the world's lord [Akbar] did not regard his own spiritual beauty, and searched for servants of God, and always offered up supplications to God with every body of men who seemed to have attained the truth, or wherever men offered up prayer. With this view he went to that retreat of worshippers of God. The company of ascetics in that neighbourhood obtained enlightenment from the glory of the presence of the world's lord.

Akbar and Zindā Pīr

(From Bali, *Ṭillā Gorakṣanāth*, pp. 18, 33–34.)

In emperor Akbar's time a yogi named "Zindā Pīr" was the head of the Ṭillā. Zindā Pīr was also considered a perfect "siddha" and there are many stories told in connection with him. Some people believe that Zindā Pīr never really died but that he simply disappeared. Indeed, because of this he is called Zindā Pīr [the "still living" Pīr]. In his time the emperor Akbar came to the Ṭillā. The meeting with him [Zindā Pīr] had a profound effect and he [Akbar] bestowed nine villages on the Ṭillā monastery in the form of a jāgīr. In addition he began the construction of a fort at the Ṭillā.

When Akbar's soldiers began building the defensive works for the fort, the yogi inhabitants (who were lovers of solitude) began to complain. In addition, some of the Mughal officials traveled with their harems, that is, their wives. This the yogis could not tolerate and they appealed to the Pīr to cause them [the Mughals] to retreat. Zindā Pīr also opposed the fort construction. But the Mughal officials didn't listen to his request and continued working on the fort. At this, Zindā Pīr by his own power caused the walls of the fort to collapse. [In addition] the heads and torsos of those who were working on the walls began to disappear. When those soldiers and laborers saw each other headless they were terrified and fled. When word of this reached the emperor Akbar, he immediately gave the order to halt construction. And he begged forgiveness from Pīr Zindā Pīr. Afterwards many other rajahs tried to build forts there, but due to the influence of the yogis not one was successful. Even during the English government, the English tried to build a "rest house" there.

In those days the head of the monastery was Kalā Nāth. Some old servant-devotees [of the Ṭillā] informed the author that every time the walls of the "rest house" were built they would collapse. In the end the English government built a "dak bungalow" at the foot of the Ṭillā, which still exists today. On the Ṭillā itself, in addition to the Gorakṣanāth and Śiva temples there is only the monastery where the yogis live and the cowshed etc. There are no government buildings whatsoever . . .

Many stories about the pīrs of the Ṭillā were told to the author by old yogis and servant-devotees. Some have already been related earlier. Many tales are connected to Zindā Pīr. Zindā Pīr is thought to have been a contemporary of Akbar. Every year in his [Zindā Pīr's] name, on the fifteenth day of Āṣāḍh [late June to early July], "daliyā" [a kind of soup or gruel] is distributed. In this connection it is said that one day Akbar hit upon the idea of building a fortress at the Ṭillā and garrisoning troops there. To this end he sent a unit of his army there and they began building a fort. On several occasions the Mughal soldiery also mistreated the yogis there. One day, upset by the conduct of the troops, the yogis went to Zindā Pīr and lodged a complaint, and he replied that he would figure out some way to send them packing. Having heard the yogis' tales of woe, Zindā Pīr caused all the wells and tanks and other water sources to dry up. Faced with the sudden lack of drinking water, the Mughal forces were in a quandary. Eventually this information made its way up the chain of command to the Mughal emperor. Finally, when Akbar came to know of the reason behind this water scarcity, he immediately ordered his troops to depart. But for some time afterward the drinking water problems continued at the Ṭillā. In the end, the yogis gathered together and once again went to the head of the Ṭillā and informed him of their hardships. At this, Zindā Pīr ordered that "daliyā" be made and distributed at a "laṅgar" [a communal feast]. It is said that after the distribution of the "daliyā" a torrential rainfall occurred and all the wells and tanks were filled with water. From then on, every year on the fifteenth day of Āṣāḍh "daliyā" is distributed at the Ṭillā. People maintain that on this day the monsoon winds and rain begin in the Panjab region.

Akbar's visit to the Bālnāth Ṭillā

(From Antonio Monserrate, *The Commentary of Father Monserrate, SJ, on his Journey to the Court of Akbar*, trans. John S. Hoyland and S. N. Bannerjee [London: Oxford University Press, 1922], pp. 113–16.)

This Balnat Thile, that is crag of Balnat, is very high and steep. Ascent is difficult, and cannot be accomplished on horse-back. On the crest itself is a level space; on this are built several small dwellings, in which it is said that a certain

Balnat used to live, with his sister. He was the founder of a sect of which the following are the customs. For the space of two years before novices are admitted to full membership and allowed to wear the peculiar dress of the sect, they have to act as servants to others who live in that place, helping the cook, cutting the wood, bringing it to the kitchen, pasturing the flocks and herds, fetching water (a very arduous task, especially in summer), and acting as table-servants to the full members, of whom about three hundred are always to be found living here. If the novices perform these duties diligently and carefully for two whole years, they are then invested with the garments of the sect. But first they must promise to keep themselves for ever pure and chaste, and to do nothing contrary to the dignity and rules of their order. The garments mentioned above are a cloak, a turban and a long dress coming down to the feet (similar to that which was vulgarly called by the ancients the "toga harmiclausa," and which some in our time call the "scapulare"). These are all dyed with a species of red chalk, so that they look as though painted red. Those who have been invested with these garments may go where they will and live by begging. If they do anything unworthy, they are dismissed from the sect. They have one leader, who, once he has been raised to that dignity, may never leave the hill. He has also with him a number of old men to help him by their advice and authority. When the leader dies, these old men elect his successor. The mark of this leader's rank is a fillet; round this are loosely wrapped bands of silk, which hang down and move to and fro. There are three or four of these bands. It is absurd enough that they should adopt this sign for their high priests. By this alone he whose heart has been enlightened by the last gleam of the true faith, can clearly recognize the vanity of their superstition. For although they are not enslaved to the superstitious beliefs either of the Musalmans or of the Hindus, they have others of their own not less full of absurdity and ignorance. For they honor a certain Balnat as though he were a prophet and servant of God. He lived as a hermit on this mountain with his sister three hundred years ago, or so they say. Since then he has been no more seen: but he is still an object of universal reverence, since it is said that he still lives and shows himself in various places and under various forms, like Prometheus, and hangs strips of cloth on the tops of trees or in high and precipitous places, which are signs of his having been there. They say that he taught the right way of worshipping God, namely that at dawn all should turn towards the east, and greet the rising sun with the concerted sounds of flutes and conches. They do the same in the evening, facing westwards. When they eat, they give thanks, as it were, to God. Balnat laid upon his followers no restriction with regard to food or human society. Their mode of living, when at home, is exceedingly frugal: for they eat only cooked lentils and ghi [clarified butter].

There are two orders amongst them, one of married people and the other of celibates. The former wear a shorter dress. The latter only differ from the former in their view of chastity and in their duty of teaching. They give oracles ostensibly from Balnat, and are devoted to divination, so that they may more properly be called magicians than religious teachers. Our Priests considered Balnat himself to be a devil, since he deceived the ancestors of these people by false miracles, and still shows himself to them from time to time. For the Evil One has beguiled these foolish Hindus into calling and worshipping himself by many names which end in "nat" [nāth]: such as Manquinat, Septenat, Jagarnat, etc. In honour of Balnat travelers hang strips of cloth on trees along the road-side.

At the time that Zelaldinus [Akbar] visited this place the high priest was an old man who was said to be 200 years of age. In reality he can hardly have been 80. For this type of man is accustomed to claim that he is of very great age, in order to impress the common people, as though virtue and sanctity could be measured by the number of years a man has lived. When they heard of the King's approaching visit, a huge number of the members of that sect gathered at this place, many of whom in order to show off their sanctity, betook themselves stark naked to certain caves which either nature or the art of man has made there. Many people did reverence to these naked ascetics and proclaimed their sanctity abroad. They are however extremely greedy of money. All their trickery and pretended sanctity is aimed at the acquisition of gain. The King, who has a leaning towards superstition in all its forms, was conducted by the Balnataei to the place where Balnat is said to have lived. Thereupon he did reverence to the place and to the prophet with bare feet and loosened hair.

While the King was dallying with Balnat, the army was halted for four days on the plain below. Thence it marched, in two days, to Ruytasium, and encamped on the bank of the stream which almost surrounds that fortress.

Akbar and Śakarnāth

(From Bali, *Ṭillā Gorakṣanāth*, pp. 13–14.)

There is also a cave at Ṭillā Gorakh Nāth that is very famous. In this cave Śakarnāth used to sit and do *tapasya* [austerities]. Previously he had some other name, but one day he revealed the "sugar rain" [miracle], [so from then on] he was called by the name Śakarnāth ["Lord of Sugar"]. In this connection it was said that he was a first class siddha and he would carry water to serve the monastery. This was roughly around the time when Emperor Akbar ruled India. In those days Siddha Śakarnāth would fetch water daily from the Ganga and bring it for his guru's bath, and it was said that he had an intimate relationship with Akbar as well. One day Akbar went with his army to the Ṭillā and met with the Pīr. There the emperor assigned some estates in the name of the Ṭillā. But in the midst of this some of Akbar's soldiers got into an argument. Śakarnāth was an extremely peace-loving sādhu and was disturbed by all the commotion caused by the soldiers; he ordered the army to leave the place immediately. One of them asked him to demonstrate some powers. At this Śakarnāth filled the skies with clouds with his own yoga-śakti. While they were watching, it began to rain, and after a little while it began to appear that snow was falling. But in fact it wasn't a snowstorm or blizzard, rather it was sugar [*śakkar*]. It was absolutely sweet sugar, [in fact] all four directions were jammed with heaps of sugar. Seeing the sugar falling, Akbar's troops were shocked [pulled their ears] and many people began filling their clothes and pots and pans with it and took it to their houses. Seeing all this Siddha Śakarnāth turned all the sugar into dirt. Everyone was amazed at this miraculous power (*siddhi*) and they all returned to their homes singing his praises. From this time on, this cave has been known as Śakarnāth's Cave. Even till today there are piles of dirt near this cave that look like sugar had fallen there.

Śakarnāth, the Demon, and Jhāfar Village

(From Bali, *Ṭillā Gorakṣanāth*, pp. 16–17.)

Śakarnāth-ji was considered a great siddha yogi there. Later some ancient sādhus told the author that visions of him would appear to them in the tank at the Ṭillā. Sometimes the ancient yogis would see him in their dreams. Baba Barakhānāth-ji of Delhi, who is one of the oldest yogis, told the author that he would sometimes have a vision of both Zindā Pīr and Śakarnāth at the Ṭillā. Śakarnāth-ji went to a place called Jhāfar when it was time to die [lit., when he was ready to abandon his body]. At that place lived a demon who every day would kill and eat one person. Before this he used to terrorize the surrounding villages. And he used to kill lots of people. So in time the people of that region decided that they would send a person to the demon every day, along with other things to eat. The demon agreed. And he put a stop to his attacks on that region. Later, when Śakarnāth-ji went to that village, [it so happened that] a member of the family in whose house he was staying was about to be handed over to the demon that very evening. When Śakarnāth learned of this, he decided that he himself would go to the demon that very night. He ignored the warnings [of the people] and at the appointed time he set off in the direction of the demon's lair. When the demon came in the night he saw that Śakarnāth was eating the accompanying food intended for him [the demon]. They both commenced fighting over it. When the demon raised his hand to smite Śakarnāth, he suddenly became lifeless. The next day when the villagers came there they saw Yogī Śakarnāth fast asleep and the demon's dead body [as a pillow] beneath his head. Śakarnāth lived there a long time. Toward the end of his time he took a Saiyad Musalman [a high-class Muslim] as his own disciple and placed him on his throne [*gaddī*]. With respect to this it is said that all the people in the village in which he lived were Saiyad Musalmans.

At the very last, he asked three times, "Do any Hindus live here?" Each time, a Saiyad Musalman responded, "Yes, I live here." Then Śakarnāth cut a hole in his ear, made him his disciple, and entrusted him with the care of the site. From then on Saiyad Muslim fakirs ran the seat at Jhāfar village. In their lineage lists they also refer [to him as] "Pīr Jhāfar." In the end, Śakarnāth said to that Saiyad that "the Pīrī [office of the Pīr] will be yours, and Fakīrī [the fakirs] will belong to the Ṭillā." The yogis of this *gaddī* are called Jhāpar Yogīs and they regard the Ṭillā as their principal place. At the time of Partition, Pīr Lāl Nāth was the monastic head of the site. Some people believed that Pīr Jhāfar was not a Saiyad Musalman but in fact a Hindu, and worked as a maker of pots and pans [*bartan*]. But because he lived in a village of Saiyads, people also referred to him as a Saiyad. The Jhāfar Yogīs were indistinguishable from the [other] yogis gathered at the Ṭillā, so one of the Pīrs at some point decreed that they should use some other utensil for their begging bowl. From that time onward they began to hang their begging bowls upside down. This is the main way to recognize Jhāfar Yogīs.

Patronage, Servitude, and Devotion at the Ṭillā

(From Bali, *Ṭillā Gorakṣanāth*, pp. 29, 34–35.)

There is a practice among the pīrs of the Ṭillā that after being made the head of the monastery the abbot for the remainder of his life may not descend from the Ṭillā. Of course, yogis think travel and pilgrimage is good, and indeed many yogis of the Ṭillā continually visit India's lovely regions and go on pilgrimage. However, whosoever becomes the chief of the Ṭillā must remain there his entire life and even after he dies his *samādhi* [burial tumulus] is built at the Ṭillā . . .

At the tail end of the eighteenth century the head of the Ṭillā was Pīr Icchyā Nāth. In connection with him it is well known that he was related to Maharajah Ranjit Singh [who ruled over the Punjab from 1799 to 1839]. Ranjit Singh's father was also a servant-devotee of the Ṭillā. It is said that due to a boon by "Ṭillādhīsh" [Ṭillā chief] Ichhyā Nāth, [his] precious son was born to him. Some documents from the time of Ranjit Singh and his father have been shown to the author [K. K. Bali] according to which they assigned land in the name of the Ṭillā to support the Ṭillā monastery. It is also said that Maharajah Ranjit Singh presented the Pīr of the Ṭillā with a *hookah*. The base of the *hookah* was made of silver and its *chilam* [the bowl that holds the tobacco] of gold. Up until Partition this *hookah* was still at the Ṭillā in Pakistan, but the yogis did not bring it with them to India.

In the first half of the nineteenth century Gauhar Nāth was the heir-apparent at the Ṭillā. In connection with Gauhar Nāth it has already been related that he was born into the Jammu and Kashmir royal house but that later he became a yogi. Even after becoming a yogi he kept his sword and bow and arrows etc. by his side. He took great pleasure in hunting. During his time there was another great siddha yogi at the Ṭillā whose name was Siddha Śām Nāth. He is famous for having served as a water carrier at the Ṭillā until the age of twelve. The office buildings of the Ṭillā were quite a distance from the well, and the constant and heavy demand for water made the job of carrying the water very difficult. It is said that Siddha Śām Nāth's forehead developed terrible sores in which insects began to fester, but that despite the pain he never once uttered a complaint and remained constantly devoted to the work of serving the Ṭillā. But one day this fact became known to Pīr Gauhar Nāth. He was very upset by this and conveyed an order to Siddha Śām Nāth to cease immediately carrying water and get some medicine for his sores. But Siddha Śām Nāth would not accept the Ṭillā's food without doing service. As a result, he was given responsibility for looking after the cows of the Ṭillā. From then on he spent all his time herding cows. But one day, as luck would have it, one of the cows fell off a cliff at the Ṭillā. Seeing a cow of the monastery tumbling down, Yogī Śām Nāth immediately leapt up and began to race down the mountain. Meanwhile, Lakṣman-deva [Rām's younger brother], pleased at his [Śām Nāth's] concern for the welfare of the cow, bestowed all kinds of powers [siddhis] on him, and in addition restored the cow of the Ṭillā Bhavan [offices] to life.

Akbar's Interviews with the Jogīs

(From Abdu-l Q̱ādir Badāūnī, *Muntak̲h̲abu't Tawārīḳh*, vol. 2, trans. George S. A. Ranking (Calcutta: Asiatic Society of Bengal, 1898–1925), pp. 334–36.)

In the same year [1583] His Majesty built outside the town [Agra or Lahore] two places for feeding poor Hindus and Musalmans, one of them being called Khairpurah, and the other Dharmpurah. Some of Abu'l Faẓl's people were put in charge of them. They spent His Majesty's money in feeding the poor. As an immense number of Jogīs also flocked to this establishment, a third place was built, which got the name of Jogipurah.

His Majesty also called on some of the Jogīs, and gave them at night private interviews, enquiring into abstract truths; their articles of faith; their occupation; the influence of pensiveness: their several practices and usages; the power of being absent from the body; or into alchemy, physiognomy, and the power of omnipresence of the soul.

His Majesty even learned alchemy, and showed in public some of the gold made by him. On a fixed night, which came once a year, a great meeting was held of Jogīs from all parts. This night they called Sivrat [Śivarātri]. The Emperor ate and drank with the principal Jogīs, who promised him that he should live three or four times as long as ordinary men. His Majesty fully believed it, and connecting their promises with other inferences he had drawn, it became impressed on his mind as indelibly as though it were engraved on a rock. Fawning court doctors, wisely enough, found proofs of the longevity of the Emperor, and said that the cycle of the moon, during which the lives of men are short, was drawing to its close, and that the cycle of Saturn was at hand, with which a new cycle of ages, and consequently the original longevity of mankind, would again commence. Thus they said, it was mentioned in some holy books that men used to live up to the age of one thousand years; and in Thibet there was even now a class of Lamahs, or devotees, and recluses, and hermits of Cathay, who live two hundred years, and more. For this reason His Majesty, in imitation of the usages of these Lamahs, limited the time he spent in the Haram, curtailed his food and drink, but especially abstained from meat. He also shaved the hair of the crown of his head, and let the hair at the sides grow, because he believed that the soul of perfect beings, at the time of death, passes out by the crown (which is the tenth opening of the human body) with a noise resembling thunder, which the dying man may look upon as a proof of his happiness and salvation from sin, and as a sign that his soul by metempsychosis will pass into the body of some grand and mighty king. His Majesty gave his religious system the name of Tauhīd-i-Ilāhī:

You want to have this world at your wish,
And also the right Religion:
These two are not compatible,
Heaven is not your slave.

And a number of disciples, who thought themselves something particular, he called Chelah [disciple], in accordance with the technical term of the Jogīs. . . .

Śām Nāth Restores a Boy to Life

(From Bali, *Ṭillā Gorakṣanāth*, pp. 35–36.)

Some time later [after *Śām Nāth* was granted powers by Lakṣman, the brother of Rām], a woman came to the Ṭillā and prayed that Pīr Gauhar Nāth grant her a child. By the grace of Pīr-jī, a son was soon born into her household. When the boy got bigger, his mother and father remembered their vow. So they took the child and headed to the Ṭillā. But on the road the child fell ill and by the time they arrived at the Ṭillā he was dead. However his parents [lit., "guardians"] took the dead child to the Ṭillā Pīr and explained the circumstances. They begged the Pīr-jī to restore the boy to life, but Pīr Gauhar Nāth felt that it was improper to contradict the laws of nature. When that woman was taking the dead child back [home], she met Yogī Śām Nāth on the road . . . When he became apprised of the circumstances, he restored that boy to life with his own yoga-śakti. When the Ṭillā chief got wind of this incident, he was furious. He asked Siddha Śām Nāth why he had revealed these powers in spite of [the decision of] his own guru. From then on there was a dispute between these two, and Siddha Śām Nāth was expelled from the monastery and went to live by the banks of the Jhelum below.

Yogis Congregate at Lahore, 1596

(From Jerome Xavier, letter to Fr. Francisco Cabral S. J., Provincial, 8 September 1596, in *Documenta Indica*, XVII (1595–1597), vol. 133 of the *Monumenta Historical Societatis Iesu*, ed. Joseph Wicki (Rome: Jesuit Historical Research Institute, 1988), pp. 550–53 (paragraphs 26–32). Translated by William R. Pinch and Javier Castro-Ibaseta. (Note: Italicized text indicates Latin in the original.)

Before I leave this side of the river I will tell something you would like to know. In the month of March [and] the end of February, I saw a swarm of jogīs crowded onto the open space on the opposite bank of the river; all of them gathered in two or three days and they camped in that area of God in groups of ten or twenty, and they said that every year they gather together at this same time, because the King [Akbar] visits them and gives them alms. He converses with them and, knowing the abilities of all, he chooses those who are most able in sorcery or the most wild in appearance, or according to some other ability, and orders that they be given food and a place to live.

Lots of people go to see these jogīs, and we likewise visited nearly all of them. There will have been about five thousand of them, and with many of them we spoke about God and his works. They listened attentively to all this; they were surprised at all this fruitless labor [on our part], but they remained deceived in their knowledge of God and the true law . . . Some told us that they would be pleased to listen to us so that they could learn and take the right path, but there was no time or place for more, and after the second or third day they all dispersed and I neither heard nor saw them again.

Most of them worship Baba Adam, that is, father Adam, believing that there is no other god and that he made all of them, and in front of his seat and place they have done a portrait that they venerate. *To the pure, all things are pure* [from Titus 1.15], so I will [now] say what I saw that astonished me most of all, that is, that the part of Adam that they had represented and that they venerated as god, joining their hands before their faces in front of such a spectacle and bowing before such a figure, as if they were venerating and adoring God, were the reproductive organs of both sexes, made of clay, with so many leaves around. This figure had [attracted] many groups and crowds of these animals; they had this figure at their door or entrance [to their tents?]. How will such people guard their chastity when they worship as god the instrument of its opposite [i.e., lust]? And some spoke about their worship with so little shame that sometimes we left them in mid-sentence and went to give others the same [Christian] doctrine.

Most of these jogīs said that Adam is their god that they worship and the earth from which he was formed; others say that all men are god, and that all men are a man-god with various figures, and that men do not die but sleep. And we saw an old man so certain and so sure of this doctrine that we were amazed . . . He did not acknowledge his old age, nor admit past time, nor change, nor youth, and he said everything was the same, nor did he give any credit to [believe in] the evidence of his aging, nor to those of his friends, acquaintances, and companions who had died: he was completely covered in red [vermelhão, "vermillion"] and incapable of mere reason, so that it seems more sure to [the meaning of the remainder of the sentence is altogether unclear].

Of these jogīs, some used their ordinary clothes made of improperly patched rags, others [were] more unclothed, others naked, and thus they showed themselves to the sight of people of *both sexes*, as though they were dressed in the best silks and brocades in the world . . . so powerful is the custom when there is corruption, and so dull the needle of understanding where there is sin. Only one garment covered them all, and it was the ashes with which they washed and decorated their faces. We met some that were adorning themselves with these golden colors with as much care and attention as more diligent [or ordinary people] would use to adorn themselves [with makeup]. They said that they covered themselves with these ashes because everything is earth and made of earth, and so they put this over their head like their god. All these jogīs have the King's guards [to defend them], so that no one can harm them.

When we were coming back, we saw the secretary of the King go to them; he went to count them and give them alms, and to be informed of the most rare of their exhibitions, so that when the King came to visit them he [the secretary] would know and could thus inform him [the King] about everything and present him with those that were the most remarkable. The following day, in the morning, the King went, embarking from our entrance. He visited them all, and they were waiting for him, each of them seated in his place or in his squalor. And taking a seat at a certain place, he was presented with the most remarkable [among them], with whom he spoke. He brought some horns ["cornetas"] to give them that look like things for snorting, because the jogīs use them a lot, and he gave the bugles to the jogīs . . . although not all of them, as we saw him coming back with some extras.

These jogīs believe that when they blow these horns they expel with their breath all the sins they have committed, and [also] the devil, and thus they blow them in the morning and during the Ave-Marias, especially when the King appears at the window as I mentioned. And it seems that for this or some other reason, the King sometimes himself blows his own horn . . . which, to tell the truth, is more proper for those who guard the pigs in the villages, to call and herd them, than for the pleasure of the King, not to mention for expelling sins or scaring away demons. Into these and other errors fall those who do not follow the light of Jesus Christ.

—16—

Yogic Language in Village Performance: Hymns of the Householder Nāths

Ann Grodzins Gold and Daniel Gold

This chapter presents the texts of eleven bhajans—choral devotional songs or "hymns"—translated from transcribed oral performances. All were recorded at all-night ritualized singing sessions known as *jāgaraṇs* in rural Rajasthan. The core performers belong to locally formed singing groups called bhajan maṇḍalī or bhajan parties—as the English word is quite commonly used. Most but never all of the members of the several bhajan parties we recorded belonged to the birth-group or caste community called Nāth. All the lead singers are Nāths and most of the authors of these songs, whose names appear in the final "signature" verse, are identified as Nāths. The Nāths' bhajans are similar to many sung throughout North India, but the yogic language sometimes used in them has added significances for the householder Nāths. In this introduction we describe the Nāths of Rajasthan, locate them within broader traditions, and sketch the performance context for our recordings. We then examine the substance of the hymns themselves, paying particular attention to the Nāths' use of a somewhat obscure yogic language.

Persons known as Nāths or jogīs—a vernacular pronunciation of yogi—live in Rajasthan as well as many other regions of North India and neighboring Nepal. In rural Rajasthan, members of the Nāth *jāti* (community or "caste") marry, raise children, and own land just as other householders do, but they claim particular affinities, both spiritual and genealogical, with world-renouncers. The term Nāth may also refer to an ascetic sect whose members would prescriptively be celibate and without possessions. Nāth householders trace their ancestral lineage to fallen yogis: world-renouncers who were drawn back into the illusory snares of marriage, procreation, and inheritance.

Our subjects here for the most part are those Nāths who are born into their identity and spend their entire lives within village society. Now and then, however, a born Nāth will give up worldly life, returning to compelling ascetic roots. A few members of the bhajan parties we recorded were such persons, who may still keep company with householder Nāths and possess special status among them.

Nāth means "master" and the Nāths are understood to be masters of religious knowledge and yogic powers. Jogī castes have a somewhat dubious reputation in other parts of India where they may be itinerant minstrels and beggars. In central Rajasthan where these hymns were recorded, Nāth is generally used as a surname by all members of the community, and considered to be the most respectful term of reference. However, Nāths will comfortably refer to themselves as "jogīs."

In the vicinity of Ghatiyali, the Rajasthan village where we have based our ethnographic work, householder Nāths are well integrated into local society. Nāths own land and livestock, and participate in many other occupations, from shopkeeping and snack-vending to local politics and public administration. Respected religious experts, Nāths perform a number of roles explicitly connected with their yogic identities. They serve as worship priests (*pujārī*s) in many regional Śiva temples and shrines, and as repositories of healing and protective knowledge, possessing spells that provide succor for various afflictions. The latter are often called *gāyatrī*s (after the name of a well-known Sanskrit mantra)—a term that is also occasionally applied to the verses of bhajans sung by the Nāths (see bhajan #1, verse 4).

A very few Nāths—either by familial tradition, personal inclination, or most often a combination of both—learn to play a stringed instrument called a sārangī and to sing and perform religious epics. Chief among these are the tales of two renouncer kings—Gopī Chand and his uncle Bhartṛhari (called Bharthari in Rajasthani). The sole narrative bhajan included here (#4) describes a famous episode in the latter king's tale.

Nāth death rites are arguably the most distinctive element of householder Nāths' identity, setting them apart from other Hindu villagers. Nāths bury their dead near their homes, rather than cremating them outside the village as is the custom for most Hindus. In practicing burial, Nāths make a significant ritual claim to their ongoing renouncer identity: Hindu world renouncers, who are symbolically cremated at initiation, are traditionally buried after their physical deaths because cremation can only happen once. Householder Nāths, moreover, refer to their family members' graves as "*samādhi*s"—the same term used to refer to the revered resting places of holy persons, whose bodies are often thought to continue to serve as repositories of their ascetic power.

Nāth gurus officiate at death rituals for members of an esoteric sect. Although this sect is strongly associated with Nāths, persons from other communities may choose initiation and participate in the funeral rituals also. The night preceding burial, Nāths and other initiates gather to worship the goddess Hiṅg Lāj Mā in a private ceremony accompanied by all-night bhajan performance. This ritual replaces the normative culminating Hindu death ritual known as *sapiṇḍikaraṇa* that other castes perform on the morning of the twelfth day following a death—a ritual whose purpose is to unite the spirit of a recently deceased person with three generations of ancestors. Nāths, by contrast, explicitly state that Hiṅg Lāj Mā's ritual worship will liberate the soul forever. The majority of texts included here were recorded at such funeral *jāgaraṇ*s.

Nāth tradition seems to have emerged in the tenth or eleventh century as a particular ascetic style that gave attention to the esoteric powers accessible through yogic practices focused on the body. Looming large in early Nāth legends is the shadowy but imposing figure of Gorakh Nāth (Skt. Gorakṣa Nātha), whom we know through stories laden with magical exploits of mythic proportions. Many cultural historians believe, however, that a living and highly influential yogi named Gorakh existed not later than 1200 CE and that he came originally from Eastern Bengal. While Nāth Yogī lineages are contested, a prevalent version says that Gorakh Nāth is a disciple of Macchendra (Skt. Matsyendra) Nāth, who obtained his knowledge directly from the great god Śiva.

As Nāth teachings spread within popular Hinduism, both their content and mode of transmission changed. From secret instructions transmitted from guru to disciple, Nāth ideas passed into publicly performed folklore. In the process, Nāth teachings were transformed, veiled, perhaps watered down, perhaps fragmented—as we see in some texts presented here. Yet references to yogic practices emerge lyrically and vividly in these bhajans and sometimes do suggest a living tradition of continued esoteric yogic practice among some householder Nāths.

Vigils, called *jāgaraṇ*s, are among the most commonplace devotional events in the region of Rajasthan where these hymns were recorded, and in many other parts of North India as well. In Rajasthan, *jāgaraṇ*s are occasionally undertaken for no special reason, out of pure pleasure—as it is conventional to say. More often they are specifically motivated. Many *jāgaraṇ*s prescriptively precede life cycle rituals: children's first haircuts, weddings, and, of course funerals. To sponsor a *jāgaraṇ* entails large expenditures of resources, time, and energy, all in a self-sacrificial mode intended to serve and please both the community and the divine.

The sponsor of a *jāgaraṇ* will first ensure the availability of his bhajan party of choice. Such groups are not composed of professional performers, but rather of persons with "day jobs"—mostly as farmers and herders, although some we have encountered are metalsmiths, potters, and carpenters. Most often the group will sing well-known bhajans passed down over generations, incorporating the authorial stamps (*chāp*s or signatures) of renowned figures greatly revered in Hindu North India, including Gorakh Nāth and Kabīr. Traditional bhajans, orally transmitted, seem to undergo little change over time. Ann Gold re-recorded the "Cool Seed" bhajan (#7) in 2003 from two different persons and found it word-for-word the same as the version transcribed in 1980. However, the bhajan corpus is both flexible and permeable, incorporating numerous more recent and local compositions—some by living singers. Each party's repertoire is somewhat different.

Seven of the eleven texts included here were recorded at three different funeral *jāgaraṇ*s in 1980 in the context of Hiṅg Lāj Mā worship. Neither translator has witnessed this ritual, as it is closed to all but initiates. Ann Gold's close collaboration with two members of the Nāth community allowed her to send a cassette recorder to these events, at each of which the roster of participants partially overlapped. She later took notes on the transcribed texts from two men who had participated in the ritual—although they did not reveal all its secrets.

These bhajans performed in conjunction with death rites are considered particularly deep and serious, and are understood to contain edifying spiritual instruction—*śikṣā*, or education for the soul. However, only one bhajan of which we are aware is restricted to Hiṅg Lāj Mā worship. Other bhajans performed at funerals, such as those translated here, may well be encountered on other occasions. One bhajan included in our selection was recorded at a *jāgaraṇ* preceding a firstborn son's first haircut ritual. The boy's life was dedicated to—and received with gratitude as a gift from—Jaipālji, a local hero deity whose hillside shrine overlooks the Nāth neighborhood in Ghatiyali. Ann Gold attended this all-night song session as well as many other nonfunereal *jāgaraṇ*s. Three other bhajans, performed by different sets of lead singers, were recorded by Daniel Gold at a *jāgaraṇ* he sponsored to express gratitude near the end of a fruitful research period in 1993. Daniel Gold invited Nāths he had met from many surrounding villages, and no single bhajan party controlled the program at this memorable foreigners' *jāgaraṇ*.

In Ghatiyali, the type of hymns sung in the Nāth bhajan parties are called *nirguṇ* bhajans, songs that speak of a Formless Lord (in Hindi, *nir-* means "without" and *guṇ* means "quality"). The tradition of *nirguṇ* bhajans also encompasses the songs of the North Indian Sants, "poet-saints," who have a broader social base than the Nāths and who are often more devotional in their tone, but with whom Nāths clearly interacted. The esoteric vocabulary that both use seems to have originated with the Nāths, while the popular Nāth singers use poetic figures found everywhere among the more numerous Sants. Nāths and Sants mention one another in their verse—sometimes respectfully, sometimes less so. Thus, bhajan #9 seems to be presented as a teaching by the great Sant Kabīr to the great Nāth Gorakh, while bhajan #11 ends with a challenge from Gorakh to Kabīr and bhajan #3 presents Kabīr as only ambivalently accomplished. In that song, Kabīr is respected as a sincere seeker notwithstanding his low caste, but one who hasn't really found an effective path: the less than positive reference to Rāmānand ("Bliss of Rām") in the song is undoubtedly a reference to Swami Rāmānand, traditionally taken as Kabīr's guru. Sants and Nāths thus recognize one another, but may engage in rivalries too.

In Ghatiyali, as in North India generally, *nirguṇ* bhajans—which encompass hymns by Sant poets as well as our Nāth singers—are normally contrasted to their *saguṇ* counterpart, hymns to the Lord with form (*sa-* means "with"). These hymns generally describe the exploits of an embodied Hindu divinity such as Rām or Kṛṣṇa and often dwell on the image of the deity in loving detail. In *nirguṇ* verse the visual images are more abstract, and often seem to be derived from yogic experience: flames, lights, and colors (see bhajans #8 and #10). Instead of visualized divinities, the experience of sound comes to the fore. Sound is frequently referenced as an utterable divine name (*nām*, as in bhajan #5, refrain). This is often a common Vaiṣṇava name (such as Hari, in the refrain to #6), regularly used by our nominally Śaiva Nāths as well as by Sants; for both Nāths and Sants, however, a name such as Hari normally refers to a formless being, one also aptly called Alakh, "the Unseeable One," as invoked at the end of the same bhajan (#6). For the yogically adept, repeating the divine name can lead to inward experiences of primal vibration (*śabda*: see bhajan #8), which sometimes seems to come from on high (#8, opening verse) and sometimes seems to emerge from yogic practice (#8, v. 1). With no envisioned mythic deity, the guru gains added importance as an object of faith. While in Sant songs the elevation of the guru can lead to a mysteriously sweet guru devotion, in the Nāth bhajans the importance of the guru appears sooner as a reverential acknowledgment of lineage. For mysteries, the householder Nāths are more likely to highlight their inherited secrets of the subtle body.

The Nāth songs thus present the *nirguṇ* tradition in a decidedly yogic aspect, with elements common to the broader *nirguṇ* tradition often given a recognizable Nāth yogic turn. These include: (1) frequent imprecations to abandon the illusory truths of the world and follow the path of the true guru, here sometimes alluding to figures of Nāth legend; (2) images of what happens to the disciples as they travel that path, sometimes elaborately figured, which here is more often one of yogic transformation than of sweet devotion; and (3) references to yogic physiology through which practitioners ideally experience the body as a microcosm of the universe, about which Nāths particularly like to sing. These three elements are frequent throughout the Nāth bhajans we present, which we have ordered according to the prominence a particular bhajan gives to one or another of them.

1. *Wake up and follow the true guru's path.* The first four bhajans are, in different ways, largely exhortations to follow the path of the guru. The meaning of guru in *nirguṇ* verse is ambiguous, sometimes referring clearly to a living person, sometimes apparently to a transcendent divinity, and sometimes, possibly, to both at once. Alongside the term guru, we find the term *satguru*, "the true guru." Although it is tempting to see the two terms as distinguishing between the guru's human and divine aspects, in general poetic practice they seem interchangeable—their usage perhaps determined in part by metrics. Nāths usually cite a human guru in the last verse of a song, where the singer traditionally gives his name. Sometimes this citation is simple, but it can also be more elaborate. In bhajan #2, for example, the singer's guru is, unusually, his wife, the "great Jogī Nāth Gulāb" and her husband, the singer Bhavānī Nāth, tells us that he "drank what she gave him to drink." Some singers, like Bhavānī Nāth, can make a song their own and end it with their own names. Other bhajans are represented as giving a teaching from a legendary Nāth, such as Gorakh in bhajan #3, who "takes shelter" in his guru Macchindar. That song, with its ambivalence toward Kabīr, is an interesting example of the way in which householder Nāths can take heroes and verses from the standard Sant repertoire and frame them from their own sectarian perspective: verse 3 of that bhajan, using the figure of the millstones, is a very familiar saying attributed (as here) to Kabīr, who, we are told elsewhere in the song, nevertheless doesn't know the true way. Yet at the same time as the Nāths alter hymns in the standard *nirguṇ* repertoire, they also add to it. Bhajan #4 is anomalous in a *jāgaraṇ* and in our collection, offering a brief selection from the Nāth narrative tradition sung in the context of hymns. Describing the pathos of King Bharthari as he abandons his wife and kingdom to follow his guru Gorakh, it advocates renunciation while also reflecting the householder Nāth's ambivalence toward it.

2. *Images of Spiritual Practice.* Bhajans 5–7 focus on images that suggest some dynamics of spiritual practice. Some of these are stock metaphors that can be fairly easily understood: the guru as a smith who must painfully forge his disciple into shape (#5, v. 4); spiritual virtues as weapons and shields (#6, v. 2). But the images can also be somewhat riddling and liable to different inter-

pretations: are the "five thieves" (of #6, v. 3) the five senses? Or are they the five "faults" (*doṣa*s) frequently enumerated by popular preachers: lust, anger, envy, attachment, and egoism? And just what are the twenty-five that also need to be "killed"? Of the three bhajans, the last, "Cool Seed," is the most integrated whole, developing a single poetic metaphor that resonates on three levels: farming, sexual reproduction, and spiritual practice. All these songs also make occasional allusions to the yoga of the subtle body, often using the Nāths' esoteric language. Those scattered allusions, in the contexts of these songs, serve largely to present tantalizing visions that hint at potential inward experience.

3. *The World Within the Body*. For many listeners, the esoteric allusions in bhajans 8–11 will have much the same effect as their scattered appearances in the previous set of songs, but for those practiced in yoga, the more sustained usage of them here may also describe paths through the subtle body that they have at least in part experienced. And because the body is taken as a microcosm of the universe, the travels described in these songs sometimes appear as metaphysical experiences in worlds beyond. Thus, in bhajan #11 v. 2, the fourteen worlds over which the deathless Rāval Yogi is spread (Rāval is an important Nāth sublineage) could refer to the seven yogic plexuses of the body and their nether counterparts (sometimes diagrammed in the legs), but they also seem macrocosmically imagined as the seven heavens and hells found in Hindu lore. Much of the language used to describe the subtle physiology in these bhajans is common to other yogic traditions: the central spinal channel as Mount Meru, the pole of the universe; *triveṇī*, "the three veins," the point between the eyes where three major yogic channels meet; the lotuses at the navel and the base of the spine. Other terms are often used conventionally in the later Hindi *nirguṇ* corpus (and can be read coherently here) to refer to a sequence of places in the head: above the *triveṇī* is the tenth door, which leads to the void (*sunna*) in the central forehead, at the top of which is *sohaṅ* (a commonly used mantra that means "I am that"); in this usage the yellow Niranjan ("the Spotless One": #10, v. 3) is situated below the *triveṇi* at the beginning of the entire sequence. Other expressions seem mysterious and may be intentionally mystifying: the "fingers" mentioned in #8, vv. 3 and 4, probably echo a more widespread yogic usage referring to small divisions near the top of the head, with a finger's breadth serving as a unit of measure. But what it means when it says that some "fingers" are served and others are burst remains a puzzle about which most can only speculate. Reasons for such obscure references in the bhajans, however, are not too hard to find: although yogic language in the Nāths' songs may indeed record inner experience and point to religious mysteries, its sometimes mystifying nature and its frequent interjec-

tion in songs of diverse types may also help reinforce the image of the householder Nāths as bearers of esoteric secrets, enhancing their yogic identity in their community and among themselves.

Whatever the intent of the esoteric references in the Nāths' bhajans, the latter are performed at *jāgaraṇ*s with verve and gusto. They almost always end with cheers—often to Mother Hiṅg Lāj or Gorakh Nāth—which are also sometimes inserted into songs, alongside frequent interjections of "hey," "yes, brother," and "sādhu"—a general term for someone dedicated to religious practice. When bhajans are performed, the singers regularly repeat entire verses, as well as lines within verses—most of which we have deleted, although we sometimes hint at this practice with a half line. The performance of the bhajans, moreover, leaves considerable room for verbal improvisation and wordplay. Sometimes singers introduce a song with a line or two that doesn't quite qualify as a regular verse, which we have noted as "opening." Singers may also vary refrains after different verses. In bhajan #2, the wordplay seemed interesting, with Bhavānī Nāth interchanging words of positive value with similar sounds (*satī sūdā sīdhā*) to describe the path to be followed—and so we have given his various versions. In bhajan #7, only one refrain repeats; the others each poetically vary in ways that echo the preceding verse, and we have therefore chosen to include refrains there as well.

The songs also have puns, some of which are common in the language of the *nirguṇ* tradition. In particular, *bānī* (or *bān*), a term that can mean both word (or sound) and arrow, is frequently used in the *nirguṇ* corpus to produce a double entendre. The term was used in the last line of bhajan #11, which was repeated in performance and which we have also repeated, while translating the different senses of *bān*. Other wordplay is more specific to an individual song: in bhajan #6, for example, the word for moment in the last stanza (*rati*) can in Rajasthani also mean an action—particularly a ritual action—which gives a double meaning to the song's last line.

Finally, we should remember that the bhajans really are meant to be sung, composed with rhythm and some rhyme. Although rhymes were beyond us, we at least tried to suggest the musical nature of this verse by giving our translations some rhythm. To do this we, like our singers, allowed ourselves license with the final a's in Hindi names, which are often pronounced in poetry but not in common speech. They come and go as meter demands.

All the bhajans translated here were recorded at all-night singing sessions in Ajmer district, Rajasthan in 1980 and 1993. The translations are based on transcriptions made by literate members of the Nāth community (Nāthu Natisar Nāth in 1980 and Shambhu Natisar Nāth in 1993) shortly after the performances—in both cases with the assistance of one of the lead singers (Ūgmā Nāthji Natisar Nāth).

Suggestions for Further Reading

For the broader context of North Indian religions in which Nāth and Sant traditions mingle, Charlotte Vaudeville's *Kabīr* (London: Oxford University Press, 1974) remains a comprehensive resource. David White's *The Alchemical Body: Siddha Traditions in Medieval India* (Chicago: University of Chicago Press, 1998) examines Nāth textual sources within the larger history of Indian religions. For a consideration of the Nāths as an esoteric tradition comparable to others worldwide (and for a translation from Hindi of an important Nāth text, the *Gorakh Bānī*), see Gordan Djurdjevic, "Masters of Magical Powers: The Nāth Siddhas in the Light of Esoteric Notions" (Ph.D. thesis, University of British Columbia, Department of Asian Studies, 2005). Ethnomusicologist Edward O. Henry presents Jogī minstrels and their bhajans in his *Chant the Names of God: Music and Culture in Bhojpuri-speaking India* (San Diego: San Diego State University Press, 1988). For more on the performative traditions of Rajasthan's householder Nāths, see Ann Grodzins Gold's *A Carnival of Parting: The Tales of King Bharthari and King Gopi Chand* (Berkeley: University of California Press, 1992). Daniel Gold explores Nāth rituals and values in his "Experiences of Ear-Cutting: The Significances of a Ritual of Bodily Alteration for Householder Yogis," *Journal of Ritual Studies* 10 (1996), pp. 91–112; and "Nāth Yogis as Established Alternatives: Householders and Ascetics Today," *Journal of Asian and African Studies* 34 (1999), pp. 68–88.

Wake Up and Follow the True Guru's Path

1. FUTILELY WANDERS

Futilely wanders, he futilely wanders
through eighty-four hundred thousand births:
yes, he futilely wanders. (refrain)
He doesn't know what's right
so prideful at his root,
so prideful.
That person without knowledge goes to dissolution—
yes, he goes to dissolution. (1)

Listen to the guru's warning—
he shows the path, yes shows the path.
Without the guru, just deep darkness:
the path is never found. (2)
He's become barely conscious
inside a dream,
looking out on four sides,
in confusion. (3)
Composed by Guru Srāvan Nāth,
these Gāyatrīs were then recorded.
Har Nāth recites them now. (4)

2. GRAB THE ROPE!

Yes grab the tree and climb, my soul,
let's take the beneficial path—
hey, take the beneficial path. (opening)
Yes grab the rope of Rāma's name,
grab tight the rope of songs to God!
The gracious guru's there:
absorb your mind in his.
Let's take the path that's true, my friend,
let's take the path that's true. (1)
Go where the swan goes, yes, my soul—
don't go where the heron goes.
Be like a swan and swallow pearls,
friend, go swallow pearls.
Don't be like the heron
with his mind absorbed in fish.
Let's take the path that's straight, my friend
let's take the path that's straight. (2)
Speak in the cuckoo's voice, my soul—
don't speak like a crow.
The cuckoo roams the gardens, hey,
the crow, though, roams in filth, o mind.
Let's take the path that's straight, my friend,
let's take the path that's straight. (3)
When saints come, serve them, wash their feet,
yes, rinse their feet and take that nectar—
Brother, rinse their holy feet.

Yes, O mind, let's splash in Rām!
Let's take the path that's true, my friend,
let's take the path that's true. (4)
I've met great Jogī Nāth Gulāb
and drunk what she gave me to drink.
Nāth Bhavānī's just a servant
to her holy feet. He's understood
the essence and not strayed, O mind.
Let's take the path that's straight. (5)

3. THAT ANCIENT HOME

I'll tell Kabīr about that home, about that well-worn home,
yes, I'll tell Kabīr about that ancient home. (refrain)
Gorakh staked banners in all the four ages
yes, Gorakh staked banners in all the four ages,
but never, sādhu brother, did he reach Rāmānand.
Why are you wasting your time then, my brother Kabīr? (1)
Kabīr lives with the butchers.
in an alley off the village square.
Hey, sādhu brother,
your actions go with you, not caste:
who is the father and who is the son? (2)
He saw the moving mill and wept.
Hey, sādhu brother, Kabīr wept.
Yes, between two grindstones
none remains uncrushed. (3)
Now Rām's by caste a ruler, sādhu brother,
and Kṛṣṇa's a cowherd,
but running to rest in yoga,
Kabīr strove many millions of times in vain. (4)
Taking shelter in Machhindar, Gorakh spoke:
I've meditated like a silent sage, O sādhu brother,
but never did I meet Rāmānand.
Why are you wasting your time, then, Kabīr? (5)

4. BHAJAN OF KING BHARTHARI'S DEPARTURE

For the Master's sake became a yogi-fakir,
for the Master's sake became a yogi-fakir. (Refrain)

The king went into the palace, on his begging rounds, on his begging rounds.
"Drop in alms, O Piṅgalā Mother, don't delay;
put in some alms, O Piṅgalā Mother, don't delay.
This strength King Bharthari earned, your Bharthari earned this strength." (1)
"My blouse never dampened, O Husband, my blouse,
by your wish I never nursed a baby boy in my lap."(2)
Yes, standing in the palace the queen tore her hair, crying,
"Why has the king torn apart our hands once joined in love?" (3)
Yes, the queen took a platter of pearls, her heart throbbing with misery, throbbing with misery:
"Let your Gorakh Nāth die, who made you leave your kingdom!" (4)
"O Queen, don't fault the guru, Piṅgalā Mother, O my Piṅgalā,
fortune inscribed this fate for me,
and it won't be removed by removing the guru.
I received Gorakh Nāth, and Macchindra." (5)

Images of Spiritual Practice

5. NOT WET, NOT DRY

Take the name of Hari every second—
keep it on your tongue, Oh yes!
Not wet, not dry: the name of
Hari every second. (refrain)
In the subtle body there are seven seas so full,
seven seas so full.
Oh yes, brother, sit right here and bathe.
If you see a fault within the subtle body,
sit down on the shore and get it out. (1)
All the steps that lead you to the sea
will count, according to the guru's wisdom:
oh yes, they all will count.
Whoever plunges deep into the guru's wisdom
will find there diamonds naturally. (2)
The likeness of truth can deceive, O yes
so learn discrimination
from the Sants.

The likeness of truth can deceive. (3)
The Sant will grab the tongs
and put you on the iron slab
and with the hammer give a mighty blow.
Droplets of hope, those pearls of the mind,
will jell together in the oyster. (4)
The knowledge that the guru gives—stamp it on your head;
the knowledge that the guru gives—stamp it on your body:
keep joined to his steadfastness. (5)
You take a bite, and hunger flees—
if thirsty, take a drink;
at an upside down house in the sky, says Lakshman,
that's where to have your feast. (6)

6. THE DIAMOND-TRUTH

Always, always praise to Hari,
realize the diamond-truth.
Keep this understanding, yes,
as strongly as you can.
My grace-giver's playing
in all the eight lotuses:
a different report is a lie. (refrain)
Make *satsang* your fist,
make patience your shield,
make *satsang* your weapon, yes.
Beat back rage and binding time—
it's then I'll know your princely valor. (1)
In the body dwell five thieves,
five thieves dwell in the body.
Just grab them by their pigtails, yes,
by their pigtails, yes!
Kill all five! Kill twenty-five!
It's then I'll know your princely valor (2)
Fine rain falls: drip drop drip drop:
these hundreds of souls here, just what will they do?
Fine rain falls: plip plop plip plop:
in Triveṇī's color palace
they swallow exceptional pearls, O soul
they swallow exceptional pearls. (3)

Hey, make sure your clock's on time:
don't advance its hands a moment.
Hey, make sure your clock's on time
Taking shelter with Macchindar, Gorakh said:
keep repeating Alakh and all moments will be true. (4)

7. COOL SEED

At Triveṇī the rivers are full to the brim. (opening)
Now make your cool drops rain, my brother.
Drink the cup of love that holds
the special name, my soul. (opening refrain)
Yoke, my soul, both mantra-oxen—
aum and *saum*—to karma as the plough.
Its iron sides are knowledge, soul,
but make the plough blade love. (verse 1)
Now make your cool field ready, soul,
and drink, my brother, drink—
with hope fixed in that special name
you need to sow as seed. (refrain 1)
Faith comes when the seed has sprouted.
All comes, soul, from your Lord. (verse 2)
Now have your cool seed sown, my soul—
brother, drink love's cup:
The seed that holds the special name,
in which your hope is fixed. (refrain 2)
Firmly stake, my soul, a platform in the fields
from which you'll aim your slingshot—knowledge—
and let fly round stones.
Now shoo away your evil thought-crows, brother,
those peacocks of doubt—shoo away! (verse 3)
Now have your cool seed sown, my soul—
brother, drink love's cup:
The seed that holds the special name,
in which your hope is fixed. (refrain 3)
Rising up in water at the hearth of a renouncer,
a flame, my soul, keeps burning without end.
Load up the wooden cart, my soul, and bring it home:
all comes, soul, from your Lord. (verse 4)
Now, brother, have your cool seed sown.

Have your cool crop brought home. (refrain 4)
The sādhu Bhuvānī Nāth, my soul,
takes shelter in fate and says:
The heart's deceptions are removed
for those touched by the Lord.
Now as your Lord keeps you, brother,
So should you remain. (verse 5)

The World within the Body

8. INTO WHICH VALLEY?

To which land are you headed, soul?
From which land did the sound emerge?
In which land will you wander? (opening)
The king inside the mind—into which valley will he go
when he penetrates the screen of confusion?
He's taken through the valley by the true guru:
the king inside the mind—into which valley will he go? (refrain)
My breath came from the eastern land
and will go wandering in the west—
my breath came from the eastern land.
From the navel's lotus comes the sound:
It rings out and goes wandering. (1)
Yes consciousness flames high and low—
keep the wick mild like the moon,
yes consciousness flames high and low.
Love of the name is the oil that fills the wick—
keep it burning day and night. (2)
Twelve fingers served, sixteen fingers burst,
if you've got them in a cluster, in its midst you'll see the Lord
in the cluster, see the Lord.
Yes, above, the Lord sits, splendid:
It's He who is our Lord. (3)
Twelve fingers served, sixteen fingers burst,
the sādhu's cloth, red-orange, gives color to the body,
the color of Triveṇī's vale. (4)
Yes, Gorakh spoke,
as Macchindar has spoken:

We're oil-pressers by caste!
Extract the oil, and take the oil,
then pass out the dregs to the world.

9. NO KARMA EXISTS WITHOUT MIND

No karma exists without mind:
no earth, no sky, no void.
Before you, Gorakh, who was there?
No karma exists without mind. (refrain)
In the beautiful grove of the Unseeable One
you sit and drink the immortal drop.
That drop made everything spread out.
The Unseeable One became two, O Gorakh! (1)
Yes, mother and father met and came together:
they did the worship-act of karma.
First father was alone and then
a son was born, another person. (2)
No seven seas existed in the body,
no eight mountains, no nine rivers
nor eighteen million plants as hairs:
where then was the body's shame? (3)
No Brahma existed
no Vishnu existed
Lord Shankar wasn't there—
and no temple either, says Kabīr. (4)

10. COME SUBTLY

First close up the base lotus
then turn the wind inside and up. (opening)
With no true guru you've got no knowledge:
which voids will you enter?
Make yourself small, my groom, my prince
come subtly my groom, prince Hari. (refrain)
First look at the five essentials—
five lights that glisten.
Concentrate attention, see the
inner moon and sky, and lose yourself. (1)
Yes, piercing the sphere of the stars,
approach the fort at *soham̐'s* peak.

In the fort at *sohaṅ's* peak, the Lord resides:
there find his holy presence. (2)
Yes, colors and colors—gaze at
black Kṛṣṇa and yellow Niranjan, brother.
Gorakh says, hey, listen Kabīr:
If you're a singer, come! (3)

11. THE RĀVAL YOGI

A Rāval Yogi's there: he's older
than all the four ages—take a look!
Hardly any sādhu can discern him:
it's only the brave Sant who sees.
The one who owns the truth
becomes the Lord's. (refrain)
In the subtle home you see
Triveṇī; then the tenth door opens.
In the void an arrow glistens,
ahead, oh yes, beyond the self! (1)
Where is his seat, hey, where is his cushion?
Where then is his place?
Here is his seat, yes, and here is his cushion.
Right here is his place.
No death for that Rāval Yogi,
spread across the fourteen worlds. (2)
There's twenty-one steps up to Meru's peak:
climb and take a look!
There's millions of Śivas to contemplate there—
the light of a diamond (3)
No lips there, no throat—not a trace of a tongue.
And a finger-breadth's distance above the light:
the base of liberation. (4)
Yes, keep on with your work, renouncer,
carrying your arrow.
Yes, keep on with your work,
holding to the sound.
Roam in bliss, hey, roam in bliss
So says Bihāri Lāl. (5)

Yoga in the Colonial and Post-Colonial Periods

—17—

The Yoga System of the Josmanīs

Sthaneshwar Timalsina

Hinduism is built upon a conglomeration of regional traditions or sects. The Josmanīs, a distinct sect of yoga in Nepal, share multiple nuances common to other regional bhakti traditions and the writings of poet-saints devoted to an attributeless god (*nirguṇ* Sants). The most salient feature of the Josmanī system is its rejection of orthodoxy. Although many of the sect's teachers were from the brahmin caste, people from all castes and creeds were not only initiated, but were also given the authority to teach and continue the lineage. Following a similar trend found among the *nirguṇ* Sants, Josmanīs also stressed the formless nature of god and often rejected image worship. Their influence in society and their tendency to popularize yoga brought yoga from select practitioners to wider strata of householders and common laypersons. While yoga practice and religious authority in Hindu society are mainly vested in the monastic orders, Josmanīs allowed people to choose between marriage and monasticism, and gave the same rank and order to both householders and monks in their practice of yoga. Josmanīs were aware of the Christian missionaries and British colonialism, and some of their social activism appears to have been directed against proselytization. Unlike traditional hermits practicing yoga in isolation, Josmanīs played an active role in their society and worked against corruption and for social transformation.

As with many other religious movements in India, there are many lacunae in the history of the Josmanīs. Historians suggest that the sect was founded by Jyotimuni Dās in the eighteenth century. The most influential Sant of this tradition is Śaśidhara, a disciple of Jyotimuni born in 1747 in Resunga, in western Nepal. Although many of his writings are in Sanskrit, the text translated in this chapter, *The Garb of Dispassion* (*Vairāgyāṃvara*), is written in an archaic form of the Nepalese language. Before becoming active in Nepal, Śaśidhara had gained popularity in the Garhwal region of India both as a Sant and as the first poet of Garhwali language. Two different narratives recount the story of Śaśidhara's marital life, one of which suggests that he married at the age of forty. Śaśidhara founded one order in Garhwal while a celibate, and another in Nepal, after he had become a householder.

Epitomized by the Nāth Siddhas, practitioners of yoga, ascetic hermits for the most part were actively engaged in blessing kings, offering ministerial counsel, and sometimes acting as power brokers. Śaśidhara, besides being a yogin and prolific author, also appears to have been keen on political activities from the time of his yoga practice in Garhwal. He was successful in influencing the king of Garhwal, Pratap Shah, and he also counseled Pṛthvī Nārāyaṇ Śāh, the architect of modern Nepal, and some of his ministers. The fact that Raṇa Bahadur, the grandson of Pṛthvī, took initiation from Śaśidhara to become an ascetic under the name Nirvāṇānanda, suggests the depth of Josmanī penetration within the Nepalese royal court.

It may not be the case that Śaśidhara and other Josmanīs actively sought political influence. Rather, it is possible that the political leaders of the time recognized the need for a religious movement to promote their sociopolitical agenda. Pṛthvī Nārāyaṇ Śāh was a perceptive king who was aware of British colonialism and saw the strength of Hindu unity as a vehicle for keeping Nepali national and religious identities alive. In order for this to be possible, a religious leadership shared by the different castes was necessary. Four of the individuals who promoted the Josmanī sect and also worked in the royal court came from different castes. Śaśidhara was successful not only in popularizing yoga, but also in establishing a tradition with multiple disciples hailing from different castes and creeds within Nepali society. With their focus on yoga and devotion rather than ritualism, acceptance of all castes and creeds in their lineage, and countering of different forms of social corruption, the Josmanīs' openness helped to transform Hindu society. A later Sant, Jñānadil, was possibly the most prominent among them in both his writings and his social activism.

Basic Principles

Josmanī soteriology is grounded in such pan-Indian assumptions as: liberation is the final goal of life; this liberation can be achieved through the immediate experience of the self when the mind resides in its true nature in absorption (*samādhi*); and this experience is possible through the practice of yoga. These shared features do not, however, render them identical to other Indic traditions. Different traditions define liberation in a variety of ways, and their descriptions of *samādhi* and the practice of yoga also vary.

By the time of the Josmanīs, many esoteric systems in India had reached their zenith. The rationalist systems championed by Buddha and Mahāvīra had waxed and waned, and devotion was more widely practiced than philosophy. Traditional boundaries had been dismantled and rebuilt, and cultural tension and fusion had become widespread. In the ongoing reformulation of the religious path and the goal, the Josmanīs, while a relatively small sect, nevertheless reflected general trends in the religiosity of the time. Even a cursory reading of their literature reveals a fusion of Bhakti, Sāṃkhya, Advaita, Yoga, Tantra, and numerous other systems. However, this should not lead one to imagine that the Josmanīs figured among the elite literati of their time. In fact, most of the Josmanīs emerged from the lower strata of Nepalese society. They shared the wisdom they learned, often in the process of hearing the teachings of their masters, the distilled knowledge of the various systems that had saturated India for over two millennia.

Although theirs was a yoga tradition, the Josmanīs seem to have been especially influenced by Advaita Vedānta. Relying on the Upanishadic literature, Advaitins hold that *brahman* is the sole reality, that the individual self is identical to *brahman*, and that the world is illusory and the product of ignorance. *Brahman* is described in terms of being (*sat*), awareness (*cid*), and bliss (*ānanda*). We can see traces of these Advaita concepts throughout the Josmanī literature. While the Yoga system of Patañjali borrowed multiple categories from the earlier dualistic Sāṃkhya system yet paid no heed to *māyā*, Nāth yoga relied on the concept of *māyā* to describe the world. Although the application of *samādhi* found in Josmanī writings aligns with the Patañjalian understanding, their treatment of *māyā* is identical to its use in Śaṅkara's Advaita philosophy.

Although the Josmanīs may have randomly borrowed from all strands of esoteric practices from within the Hindu system, the *Vairāgyāṃvara* (VA) reveals a disproportional influence of Advaita. Their lifestyle, however, differs from that of the monks of the Advaita orders, more closely resembling those of the Nāth Yogīs and other Sants from across India. The Advaita categories introduced in VA are appropriated in their yogic context. For example, the realization of the identity of the *brahman* and the self as taught in the phrase "thou art that" (*Chāndogyopaniṣad* 6.8.7) is not interpreted in Advaita texts in terms of the union (*yoga*) of *jīva* and *brahman*, as is the case in the Josmanī literature. Other examples, including that of waves and the ocean in order to describe the identity of the individual self and the absolute, are clearly borrowed from Advaita. The Josmanī cosmogony nevertheless differs from that of Advaita. While accepting *brahman* as the primordial principle, they identify the manifestation of the world in the sequence of *māya*, volition (*icchā*), cognition (*jñāna*), and action (*kriyā*). This description resonates with Tantric categories that are largely borrowed from early Śaiva Siddhānta literature. Their doctrinal inclusiveness makes it very difficult to provide a systematic analysis of categories.

Widespread in medieval India and commonly found among Siddhas, Nāth Yogīs, and Sants are the Josmanī practices of *nāda*, the belief in the serpentine force (*kuṇḍalinī* or Kuṇḍalī), and the visualization of various *cakras* that constitute the subtle physiology. These practices are central to Tantric literature, but absent from the yoga system of Patañjali. *Nāda* appears in Śaiva literature as the emanation of *māyā* and a cosmic force in itself that brings the material world into being. This *nāda* is situated in the body and gives rise to Kuṇḍalī. On this cosmological ground, inner or external sound becomes instrumental in the process of yogic awakening. Josmanīs use musical instruments such as the one-string *ektār* to keep the mind focused on *nāda* as the inner sound they believe manifests in nine different forms. The playing of a flute, often occurring in Josmanī songs, comes as a metaphor for the inner sound that manifests and upon which a yogin is supposed to rest his mind.

The yoga practice of Josmanīs, identified as "action" (*kriyā*), consists mainly of various breathing exercises. The VA gives lengthy detail of the minute measurements of time involved in the processes of inhaling, holding the breath, and exhaling. Time in this depiction is not merely external, as found in the movement of the planets, but also can be felt in each and every breath. This is why the Josmanīs identify "time" as one of the synonyms of the *brahman*. Knowing the proper measurement of time becomes essential to knowing proper breathing, as a yogin is supposed to take 21,600 breaths in one day. This attention to breathing distinguishes Josmanī yoga from the Advaita and Patañjalian traditions. Such counting is, however, commonly found in Tantric and *haṭha yoga* literature.

The Josmanī practice of *prāṇa* relies on the precise measurement of the flow of breath, with a focus on the duration for which the breath is held or allowed to flow as inhalation or exhalation. Śāśidhara's identification of the *brahman* with time is noteworthy in that it deviates from the Advaita identification of time as illusion. Both his focus on minute measurements of time in the process of breathing and his elevation of time from illusion to the supreme reality support the concept of liberation that is granted through bodily means and not by mere contemplation, as is the case in Advaita. The measurement of time in the Josmanī system relies on Indian astronomy, in which a day of twenty-four hours is divided into sixty *ghaṭīs*, with each *ghaṭī* bcing segmented into sixty *palā*s. The measurement is used to attune one's breathing so as to match the ideal number of 21,600 breaths in a day.

It could be argued that although the methods of liberation may vary among the Yoga, Tantra, and Advaita systems, their goal of liberation is identical. Particularly in the case of Josmanīs, this concept is virtually indistinguishable from that of Advaita, as they explicitly identify liberation as identity with the *brahman*, described in terms of the freedom of individual self (*jīva*) from *māyā*. This comparison, however, can be misleading. While accepting some Advaita categories, Josmanīs adhere to the corporeal nuances of yoga found in Nāth and Tantric traditions. Borrowing from Nāth literature, they describe the highest realization in terms of the identity of the individual body (*piṇḍa*) with the cosmos (*brahmāṇḍa*). Here, realization is not merely disembodied and transcendental consciousness. Parallel to the Śaiva systems, they describe a bodily purity that is integral to mental purification. The karmic residues that first imprint the mind ultimately result in conditioning the body and limiting its natural powers. Attainment of the *siddhi*s results from the removal of bodily defilements through practice that involves both body and mind, and issues in the body's freedom from karmic residues.

The VA describes in detail the (often unpleasant) physical symptoms that accompany the rise of Kuṇḍalī. Josmanīs compare this rise to the enflaming of the body: just as flames reduce beings to ashes, this inner yogic fire is believed to incinerate karmic residue. The pranic flow in the inner channels is believed to touch different physical centers and this contact triggers a variety of experiences. The VA details the process of inner sacrifice (*antaryāga*) in which a libation is made to the inner fire of Kuṇḍalī. Equating all external objects including the individual self with sacrificial objects, and the higher self with the center upon which offerings are made, this sacrifice is reminiscent of a Tantric ritual that internalizes the Vedic fire ritual within the body.

Some of the yogic practices found in *haṭha yoga* texts betray a Tantric influence. Five of the key practices found in the *haṭha yoga* literature are also discussed in the VA: "roaming in the void" (*khecarī*), "roaming on the ground" (*bhūcarī*), "roaming in the dry sphere" (*cācarī*), "roaming beyond the senses" (*agocarī*), and "beyond the mind" (*unmanī*). Before bringing these earlier texts into our discussion, it is essential to understand these practices in their own terms and context. The VA defines the practice of *khecarī* as touching the tonsils with the tip of the tongue. The *bhūcarī* practice is defined as focusing the eyes of the mind upon the tip of the nose. Similarly, *cācarī* indicates the practice of remaining focused with the eyes closed. The practice called *agocarī* involves focusing the mind on the ears. The ultimate and optimal practice of *unmanī* is defined as seeing *brahman* with the eyes of the mind.

In the preceding section, I have highlighted the many borrowings of the Josmanī from the Advaita tradition, a key concept being *māyā*. Śaśidhara defines *māyā* as momentary consciousness and *brahman* as the absolute. This definition, while deviating from the classical interpretation, provides a new premise upon which to explain the nature of the world. The objective of yoga thus becomes a matter of freeing the mind from momentary consciousness and thereby entering into unbound awareness, the innate nature of the self. The objective of the VA is to instruct individuals in how to free the self from *māyā* or the awareness of time and to experience an identity with *brahman*. In this sense, the yoga practiced by Josmanīs differs from *haṭha* or Patañjalian Yoga, and is closer to Advaita Vedānta. In summary, the Josmanī yoga practice, as found in the VA, is a synthesis of multiple and often contrasting esoteric philosophical traditions. Its broad appropriation of terminology from these sources can sometimes be confusing, as the terms borrowed are not always used in their original sense. Although its synthetizing tendency may fall short of the subtlety of classical philosophy in all its hairsplitting detail, the Josmanī system nevertheless had a meaningful impact on the Nepalese society of its time.

The following translation of selections from the *Vairāgyāṃvara* of Śaśidhara is based on the edition found in *Josmanī santa paramparā ra sāhitya*, edited by Janaklal Sharma (Kathmandu: Royal Nepal Academy, 1963), pp. 195–209.

Suggestions for Further Reading

Apart from Sthaneshwar Timalsina, "Songs of Transformation: Vernacular Josmanī Literature and the Yoga of Cosmic Awareness," *International Journal of Hindu Studies* 14:2–3 (2010):201–28, there are virtually no English-language studies devoted specifically to the Josmanī tradition. However, substantive studies on Kabīr and the *nirguṇ* tradition, the Nāth and Siddha tradition, and the Sahajīyā literature have shed light on similar religious movements in medieval India. The pioneering work of David Gordon White, *The Alchemical Body: Siddha Traditions in Medieval India* (Chicago: University of Chicago Press, 1996) on the Siddha tradition; and Edward C. Dimock, Jr., *The Place of the Hidden Moon: Erotic Mysticism in the Vaiṣṇava-sahajiyā Cult of Bengal* (Chicago: University of Chicago Press, 1966; reprint Phoenix Press, 1989), are helpful in further understanding these traditions. For the Sant tradition, Karine Schomer and W. H. McLeod, eds., *The Sants: Studies in a Devotional Tradition of India* (Delhi: Motilal Banarsidass, 1987) is helpful. Works by Glen Heyes on the Sahajiyā tradition, particularly "The Vaiṣṇava Sahajiyā Traditions of Medieval Bengal," in Donald S. Lopez, Jr., ed., *Religions of India in Practice* (Princeton, NJ: Princeton University Press, 1995), pp. 333–51; and "The

Necklace of Immortality: A Seventeenth-Century Vaiṣṇava Sahajiyā Text," in David Gordon White, ed., *Tantra in Practice* (Princeton, NJ: Princeton University Press 2000), pp. 308–25, are helpful in understanding a theologically parallel tradition from Bengal.

The Garb of Dispassion

First Teaching

[. . .] First, one should know the condition of the body, mind, and the essential self, and [thus] analyze: [Here is] the cause of the mind. The mind is that which is endowed with the sixteen properties of passion, anger, greed, delusion, drunkenness, envy, mind, intellect, thought (*citta*), ego-sense, [the three qualities of] *sattva*, *rajas*, and *tamas*, and fear, grief, and joy. *Māyā* is the specific intellect that registers [notions] such as body, pain and pleasure, action, and activities [in the mind]. The individual self is one who is bound by *māyā* and does not have self-discrimination and remains in control of *māyā*, thinking that "I will be ruined if I abandon *māyā*." When defilements of the individual self are removed, whatever [remains] is the essential nature of the self. The nature of the self is beyond the syllable (*akṣara*), beyond qualities, beyond the word principle; it is in eternal peace, and is the primordial cause. A devotee is one who has devotion with knowledge of the nature (*gati*) of the self and abides in this nature, being endowed with knowledge and dispassion, compassion and forgiveness, peace, good conduct, and faith. One should serve Lord Kṛṣṇa, the very self, by abiding in the essential nature by means of the yoga of devotion and with the quality arising from that, having abandoned the nature of the body and mind.

I [now] elaborate upon the discrimination of serving the non-dual being [alone]. If one is free from thinking, that is the nature of the self; thinking is the nature of mind. The nature of the self is free from determinations; determination is the nature of mind. [Effortless breathing] free from counting is the nature of the self; counting is the nature of mind. Freedom from difference and freedom from the end is the nature of the self; the one that differentiates, that brings [something to an end] and [itself] comes to an end—the one that distinguishes between actions and their limitations [and is endowed with] passion, aversion, and so forth—has the nature of the mind. The nature of the self is that which is beyond movement, free from division, immediate, non-dual, immeasurable, free from thought, free from counting etc., free from delusion—and [this is] the non-dual cause. One should serve the self with the yoga of devotion following this discrimination, [aware of] the nature of the actions of mind. One should constantly practice the yoga of devotion.

Following this, I focus upon actions concerning the body, such as [what] food [is appropriate] for a sage in the state of practice. One should sit fixed in a comfortable position and should practice controlling the breath etc., at morning, midday, dusk, and midnight, having studied and understood the actions of *prāṇa* as it is written in the *Garb of Dispassion*. After that, one should repeat *nāda* every day by finding the proper moment and sitting in a quiet place: repeat a three-letter mantra, *a-ha-m*, loudly and continuously, 5-10-15-20-25-30-35-40 [times], as much as one can. [*Nāda*] arises with the sound of a great bell and ends in the same manner. One should make *nāda* with a continuous sound, and when practicing *nāda*, one should listen only to the sound of *nāda*. The mind should not move to any other object. After this practice, one should constantly meditate every day upon the essential nature of the self that is in eternal peace. The mind is stilled with the power of dispassion.

When blocked, the fire of *brahman* illuminates. With its heat, fingers and toes start throbbing. It feels like the entire body is being cooked. Sometimes, Kuṇḍalī rises and comes up to the neck. Sometimes, it causes headache. Sometimes it [makes one] giddy. Sometimes it makes [one] feel faint. Sometimes smoke of different colors mixed with white and gray comes out of the mouth and nose. Sometimes [one] feels sweetness in the mouth. [One] feels acute bliss. Sometimes, it feels like a burning in the belly. Sometimes, one feels the dryness [of dehydration] in the mouth. Sometimes one's stomach growls. Sometimes one sees fearsome dreams. One feels some pain in the body. These symptoms remain for two to four *palās*, 8 to 10 *ghaṭīs* [or even as long as] five to seven days. A headache can last all day and night. However, these impediments that arise automatically will subside on their own. One should not worry. If [the practice of] yoga has caused [these physical symptoms], one will not have other diseases. One should remain peaceful. The fire rises in order to demonstrate the faults of sense organs. When these faults are subdued, the symptoms will not repeat. One will feel bliss.

If these symptoms arise in the body, [one should do as follows]: if one feels hot, one should drink cold buffalo-milk. One should drink buffalo-milk that is still warm [after milking] if one feels giddy. If one feels cold, one should drink cow-milk warmed with dry ginger and *ajowan*. If one is suffering from *vāta* (an over-accumulation of wind), one should eat a warm porridge of *mung* beans with black salt, dry ginger, nutmeg, and ghee. If the digestive fire is dead, one should warm up cold rice mixed with ghee and eat it mixed with rock salt. One should not drink water but rather drink cold milk if the bile is increased. One who is [engaged] in practice should eat rice, milk, ghee, *mung* dāl, bread made from old wheat, dry ginger among the spices, molasses among the sweets, and rock salt among the salts. Furthermore, one should contemplate these things. Whatever keeps [one] healthy, [one] should eat that. There is no discrimination in food. Whatever does [you] good, eat that. If [one's health] is good, one feels joy. One can practice if the body is in [a state of] bliss. This is what food is for.

Furthermore, if one eats [excessive] salt, one will have asthma. If one eats [excessively] sour [food, the belly] will swell. If one eats sweets, the bodily fluids will curdle. If one eats [raw] greens, one will have a bellyache. If one consumes [excessive] oil, one will have pain throughout the body. Coughing will increase if one drinks buttermilk. *Vāta* will increase if one eats yogurt. If one eats raw [food], the bile will increase. If one eats bitter and spicy [foods], one's bodily fluids will curdle. If one eats [food that is] too hot, one's power of lunar digits [within the body] will decrease. If one eats [food that is] too cold, the digestive fire will die, and *vāta* will increase. If it is too hot, one will feel uneasy and the mind will be restless. With regard to fire, [the practitioner should not] see the flame of a lamp. One should stay away from fire. If it is too cold, one will feel lazy and sleepy. Therefore, one who knows should take care of oneself.

For the sake of maintaining the practice of yoga, one should think of things that are good for the body and eat mild, warm food. Not all [people] have the same body. With this insight [in mind], one should think of one's body and eat the things that are good for one[self]. This body is impermanent. One should be dispassionate toward [worldly] objects and keep practicing as long as the mind does not dissolve in the abode of Hari. One should not talk too much. One should not walk too much. One should keep one's body pure and at peace in these ways, and being endowed with love and the yoga of devotion one should practice a self that is eternally at peace. All [one's] defilements will be removed through the glory of [this] non-dual practice. One's primordial form will be illuminated. Furthermore, the bliss that is free from all fears will be natural. The more the non-dual self is practiced, the more [one's] heightened bliss will be revealed. The more [one's] heightened bliss is revealed, the more the mind will dissolve in the self. The more the mind is dissolved, the more one will hear various sounds, such as [that of] a flute. Among all the sounds, one very blissful sound will be heard. On certain occasions, something like lightning will appear around the eyebrows. One should hear that [blissful] sound and be immersed in the practice of sound. Due to the good conduct [observed] in previous lives, some will realize these symptoms quickly. Not everyone will have the same symptoms of yoga due to the kindling of the Brahma fire. There is no rule with regard to the sequence [of the symptoms].

Furthermore, one should be free of anxiety (*cintā*) and practice mindlessness. If one can abide [in this state] for one *ghaṭī*, an instant of *siddhi* can arise. One should not have fear, anxiety, and greed, [but rather] abide in the non-dual absorption of [pure] being. All perfections will be attained. One will be united with the lotus feet of Kṛṣṇa [who is] free from distinctions. One will be of the nature of innate bliss. One should also explore the literature of other yogas, methods, [and paths to] knowledge, dispassion, devotion, or the grace of truth, and so forth. This is revealed in the *Garb of Dispassion*. One should explore that and understand and [one] should serve the lotus feet of Hari. One should read the scriptures. There are many methods explained [and] all are for the pacification of mind. When the mind is pacified [and] one has understood everything, everything has been achieved. If one abides peacefully in the self alone, without thinking anything, that is the yoga of the self. One does not need to do anything [. . .]

There is no other mantra equal to the *ajapā*, which describes the non-duality of the individual self and *brahman*. There is no other [form of] counting that affords [such a] great result with [so] little effort. There never has been [any] other wisdom or literature [that could] grant the non-dual experience equal to [that of the] *ajapā*, nor will there ever be. [. . .] One should contemplate the self in this way. The supreme self is at the center; in the surrounding four corners, there is the girdle of the individual self; surrounding this is the girdle of awareness. At the center of this sacrificial altar [whose] four corners are decorated with gates of bliss, [there] is the fire enflaming the vulva of the power goddess Yoganidrā. On top of that is the triangular sacrificial altar of the crescent moon [that is] endowed with sound (*nāda*) and drop (*bindu*); and when this is known, one should [offer into the fire] the clarified butter of virtue and vice, with the ladle of mind illuminated with the wisdom of reality of the nature of emptiness [lit. the sky]. With the air [of *prāṇa*] and the ladle of [the central channel] *suṣumnā*, I make the oblation of the clarified butter of virtue and vice in a fire of the sort that burns without any fuel. In such an inner fire [is to be found the power] that dispels the darkness of illusion and illuminates wisdom. At the center of such a fire, there is a shining space and I offer as an oblation upon this altar the elements starting with earth, water, fire, air, and sky—all of these according to the [ritual] act—at the [level of the] *svādhiṣṭhāna* [*cakra*].

[. . .] *Brahman* is one, non-dual, and pure consciousness. That which is other than *brahman* is *māyā*. The *māyā* of *brahman* is comparable to a tree and its shadow. A tree and its shadow are not separate. There cannot be a shadow in the absence of a tree. Such is their relation. *Brahman* is pure consciousness. *Māyā* is momentary consciousness. *Brahman* is above *māyā* and there is nothing above *brahman*. The supreme *brahman* is described as free from distinctions. Three powers keep arising from the *brahman* with the desire to become many. These three powers are volition, cognition, and action. With these three powers arise three further powers of doubt, non-cognition, and contrary cognition. *Brahman* has five names: *brahman*, individual self, time, action, and the essential nature. It is called *brahman* because it is free from distinctions. It is [called] the individual self due to not knowing oneself. It is time due to not knowing itself and seeing time. It acts, dwelling in multiple bodies. It is called the essential nature because it experiences various symptoms such as irritationality and loathing, the bitter and the spicy, honor and insult. *Māyā* is also called by five names: illusion, sky, void, power, and the procreative force (*prakṛti*). It is called *māyā* due to its association with *brahman*, sky due to the oneness of the body and the cosmos, void due to seeing the insentient, power since it knows the entire world, and *prakṛti* since it moves forth. Creation is due to the union of these two.

The sky element evolves from the divided *brahman*, air from the sky, fire from air, water from fire, earth from water—and all the bodies and the universes [that exist] have evolved from earth. *Māyā* is their cause and it is unconscious. Due to this cause [affecting] the *brahman*, it is called the individual self. Therefore the *brahman* is pure consciousness and *māyā* is the unconscious (*jaḍ*) consciousness. The body is the momentary consciousness. This is why *brahman* and *māyā* are always intimate. They are not separate. The colors of the five elements are [as follows]: earth is yellow, water is white, fire is red, air is blue, and the sky is of mixed colors.

The names of twenty-five *prakṛti*s [associated with] five elements [are as follows]: The body is the limb of earth; the mind is the limb of water. Ego is the limb of fire [and] intellect is the limb of air. The sense organs are the limbs of the sky. Furthermore, sound is the limb of sky. Touch is the limb of air. Form is the limb of fire. Taste is the limb of water. Smell is the limb of earth. These are the five subtle portions (*tanmātrās*). [Ear is the limb of sky.] Skin is the limb of air. The eye is the limb of fire. Tongue is the limb of water. Nose is the limb of earth. These are called the five sense-organs. The organ of speech is the limb of sky. Hands are the limbs of air. Feet are the limbs of fire. The reproductive organ is the limb of water. Anus is the limb of earth. These are called five motor-organs. These twenty-five elements are [collectively] called *māyā*. The one principle [above these] is called *brahman*. There are four states: waking, dreaming, deep sleep, and the transcendent. [Consciousness] conditioned by actions is the waking [state; when] conditioned by illusion [it] is the dream [state]; to not know any of [these] illusory systems is [the state of] deep sleep; and the determination that this individual self is the very *brahman* is identified as the transcendent [state]. Thus, it is stated in the entire Vedantic corpus that *brahman* and the individual self are identical [. . .]

There are five [yogic] practices as well: *khecarī*, *bhūcarī*, *cācarī*, *agocarī*, and *unmanī*. *Khecarī* is the practice of placing the tongue upward [touching the tonsils]. Focusing the eyes of the mind upon the middle of the nose is the practice called *bhūcarī*. Staying focused with closed eyes is the practice called *cācarī*. The practice called *agocarī* [involves] keeping the mind focused in the ears. The practice of *unmanī* is seeing the *brahman* with the mind. In all of the yogas, *unmanī* is considered the highest. Therefore one should abide in its practice and stay determined that "I shall [offer my] life [as] sacrifice" while [engaged] in this practice.

[. . .] The true guru himself is the complete *brahman*. He appears in bodily form and so forth and his true characteristics are mentioned above. With great compassion for those who are embodied, when Śiva assumes the form of the *jīva* in the human body, seeing grace in the body, [he] grants them experience and awakens [individuals] so that they maintain his actions. The *jīva* is the very self, a part of the self, full of grace. Whatever action the *jīva* supports, he accomplishes that. Therefore, one does not find the nature of the guru and the true guru is not recognized for so long as one does not abandon all actions, thinking with proper insight [lit. agreement] that all is false. Even in the words written [by someone endowed] with dispassion [who has refrained] from all actions, the [reader's] mind becomes the agent [in construing meaning] and even the best *nirguṇ* words are understood following [the reader's] actions and the true intention [of the teaching] is not grasped. Once the mind has been conquered, one attains discriminatory wisdom and the truthful words of the true guru will be revealed as they were intended by the guru who spoke [them]. Having abandoned the state of the self and merged with the waves of mind, when the individual self enjoys the sweetness of objects; [it] forgets [its true nature]. Time absorbs all that flows. For instance, some of the water drops coming from the ocean are absorbed by air, some by earth, and some by the sun. If water remains in water, it merges with the ocean and is the very ocean. The true guru is like the ocean. You should know that the individual self is like the drop [. . .]

This is the first teaching in *The Garb of Dispassion* [presented] in [everyday] language.

The Second Teaching

[. . .] If practices such as controlling the breath are maintained [for a duration of one] *palā* up to one *muhūrta*, the body will become pure, peaceful, and free from disease. Physical faults such as slumber, laziness, or disease gradually diminish. This practice is [now] described. In this very body, by virtue of the strength of the self, [breath] enters into the body for a measure of time, starting with one *nimiṣa* [i.e., a blink of the eye]: accordingly, faults such as slumber or laziness and afflictions such as cough or pain dissolve, and pleasure arises. Therefore, the wise ones control faults with the same [instruments as those] by which they arise, and dwell in peace.

One breath is [comprised of] one inhalation and exhalation. One *palā* is six breaths. One *ghaṭī* is sixty *palās*. One *muhūrta* is two *ghaṭīs*. The practice of the breath is [effective for] up until one *muhūrta*. One should breathe in slowly with the left nostril, plug both channels and hold [the breath for] as long as possible, and breathe out slowly with the right nostril. If the flow of breath that occurs in one *palā* is controlled, sleep and laziness will disappear for half a *ghaṭī*. If the flow of breath that occurs in two *palās* is controlled, slumber and laziness will vanish for one *ghaṭī*. If controlled for four *palās*, slumber and laziness will [be] remove[d] for two *ghaṭīs*. If the breath is controlled for eight *palās*, slumber and laziness will [be] remove[d] for four *ghaṭīs*. If the breath is controlled for twelve *palās*, slumber and laziness will recede for six *ghaṭīs*. If the breath is controlled for twenty *palās*, slumber and sluggishness will disappear for ten *ghaṭīs*. If *prāṇa* is controlled for forty *palās*, slumber and sluggishness will [be] remove[d] for twenty *ghaṭīs*. If the flow of *prāṇa* that occurs in one *ghaṭī* is controlled, slumber and sluggishness will cease for thirty *ghaṭīs*. If the flow of *prāṇa* that occurs in one *muhūrta* is stopped, slumber and sluggishness will be removed for a day and night. This is *prāṇa*. One should continue the practice in this way and the body will be pure.

[. . .] One should encourage the mind with love to listen to *nāda* and remain immersed [in it]. One aspires to self-nature through the grace of the self [i.e., of the nature of] consciousness, and [the mind] becomes tranquil on its own. If the mind becomes pure and peaceful due to dispassion and discrimination, keep inquiring into the self. The self-nature will be obtained, and other actions and *haṭha* [yoga practices] will not be required. If the mind is not fixed [because it is] empowered by earlier mental conditioning (*vāsanā*s, literally, "perfumes"), practice *nāda*. After that, if the body is burdnened with sluggishness, slumber, and afflictions such as cough, one should perform the aforementioned practices of controlling *prāṇa* and so forth, and when [these obstacles] are removed, one should abandon all these actions, become free from actions, and engage in search of the self. For so long as the mental conditionings are not removed, one should repeat the practice in the same sequence as mentioned above, [so that the mind] will be stilled.

This is the second teaching in *The Garb of Dispassion* [presented] in [colloquial] language.

Third Teaching

[. . .] The supreme *brahman*, full [in itself], free from division, [and eternally] complete, is the abode of power, quality, intellect, and *māyā*. From an abode endowed with *māyā*, the world comprised of five elements expands on its own and after that, quality and cognition arise according to the [limitations of the] body. [One] sees the other due to this very quality and cognition, and due to *māyā*, one merges into *māyā*, and then the same condition arises once more. [It] has forgotten [the self] again and again and so it lacks the insight to distinguish its primordial indestructible state. It is in a way similar to a fruit that has fallen to the ground, being separated from the tree. [It] becomes a plant on its own through association with the agents of water, heat, time, and so on. Time, the cause, does not disassociate [from it] and [it] again becomes the same [embodied being]. If the fruit does not touch the ground, it will [be] free from the condition of becoming a tree and the fruit will turn into a *jīva* and go to another form. In the same way, the *jīva* has a seed in the form of the mind and the ground [has a seed] in the form of *māyā*, and time [has] contact in the form of *karma*—and [so from the seed that has fallen on the ground] a plant arises, [in this case,] the body with its five elements, on its own. It cannot discriminate itself. Again and again, it follows the cause that is *māyā* and is not [ever] freed from the eighty-four [cycles of birth]. Whatever action one performs, one obtains the same condition. A wise man abandons the net of passion and delusion [and remains on] the ground devoid of *māyā*, [with] the seed of mindlessness, and the association of knowledge and dispassion. [Just] as a seed turns into a plant on its own soon after falling on the ground, in the same way when one becomes free from the desire to enjoy objects and [is] free from *māyā* and actions, this very individual self becomes associated with the cause [that leads to] becoming the luminous self, the complete *brahman*. By means of the yoga of the self, it autonomously becomes the luminous self, the *brahman*.

This is the third teaching in *The Garb of Dispassion* [presented] in [conversational] language.

Fourth Teaching

Now the analysis of the individual self and the supreme self is explained. The *jīva* is one's very self. What binds it is the fact that it has not realized the insight [that comes with the] full knowledge that "I am the self, consciousness in itself," and so it has to be awakened with the sentence [*tat tvam asi*] given by the guru. One should have conviction in the words of the true guru. [It is] like this: The water in a pond does not have discrimination [arising from] the knowledge that "I am clean." If [a blockage] is opened, it flows out; if plugged, it gets mucky. Due to its own deeds, it becomes covered with muck and this continues due to its [own] action. In the same way, the individual self does not gain the insight that "I am the self" and so is covered with the ten sense-organs and actions such as seeing, eating, walking, [or] speaking. The *jīva* is the one guiding [these] various actions. The one connected to it is in *māyā* and this is the entire world. When isolated from all of these, this very *jīva* is [none other than] the effulgent *brahman*. And the *jīva* is awakened by the guru in his teachings on the truth with sentences like "thou art that," that you are the [supreme] self alone. With the discrimination of knowledge, one removes the stain [of *māyā*], one abandons *māyā* that gives rise to defilement, and one awakens through the practice of the meditation on fearlessness. One obtains one's [true] nature. If one does not obtain the discrimination of the knowledge [imparted by] guru, the *jīva* is bound and will never be freed from suffering. Therefore, a wise [man] should abandon the ego-sense [found] in the body and engage in the discrimination of knowledge and dispassion. The mind remains restless for so long as the mental conditionings have not been destroyed. Maintain practice as described in the second instruction. What is experienced in the highest and fixed absorption is innate to the self [that is identical to] bliss. This is the self.

This is the fourth teaching in *The Garb of Dispassion*, [presented] in [colloquial] language.

Fifth Teaching

Now the practice of the actions that cause establishment in yoga is explained. When the sentence ["*tat tvam asi*" expressed by] guru is realized, knowledge and dispassion become established. Once armed with its conviction [in this] knowledge and dispassion, if the mind remains in that [absolute] essence, that is the practice of the self. All the qualities and appearances of the self in the past will dissolve one after the other, due to this conviction and practice of dispassion.

Now the practice of discrimination that causes the dissolution [of the mind] is explained. The mind holds onto the second [cause], if the first cause is dissolved. The mind remains in the third if the second cause is dissolved. The mind remains in the fourth if the third cause is dissolved . . . The mind remains in the tenth [cause] if the ninth is dissolved. This is the essence of the practice that comprises discrimination and dispassion, [a practice] that [allows] the mind to remain in the tenth [cause] and dissolve sequentially.

Now the practice of the self is explained. In the first exercise, the intellect becomes fixed, freed from error and comprised of the nature of wisdom and discrimination. In the second exercise, one has an intellect that does not distinguish [the difference] between anything, that is in equipoise and free from activity. In the third exercise, one obtains an intellect that is free of desire and thoughts of enjoyment. In the fourth exercise, the intellect becomes enlightened and free of anger. In the fifth exercise, the intellect becomes free of greed and freed from cause and effect. In the sixth exercise, the intellect becomes equal to the self, and freed from the ego-sense. In the seventh exercise, the intellect becomes freed from the qualities (*guṇa*s) and realizes a nature that is without attributes (*nirguṇ*). In the eighth exercise, the strength of the intellect becomes the state of the self, freed from the intellection of qualities and desires. In the ninth exercise, devoid of knowledge, the intellect becomes luminous with the essential form of the self. In the tenth exercise, devoid of dispassion and devoid of intellect, one becomes the complete Nārāyaṇa, the supreme *brahman*, the non-dual Self, having the nature of Being, and one dissolves in union with the yoga of bliss [. . .]

This is the fifth teaching in the *Garb of Dispassion* presented in [folk] language.

—18—

Songs to the Highest God (Īśvara) of Sāṃkhya-Yoga

Knut A. Jacobsen

A form of meditation focusing on Īśvara is part of Sāṃkhya-Yoga (or Pātañjala Yoga), the school of Yoga that is based on the *Yoga Sūtra* with Vyāsa's commentary (*bhāṣya*) and the philosophy known as Sāṃkhya. Īśvara, God, is defined in Sāṃkhya-Yoga as a particular self (*puruṣa-viśeṣa*) and not as a separate principle (*tattva*) beyond the twenty-five principles that, according to Sāṃkhya and Sāṃkhya-Yoga, constitute reality. In Sāṃkhya and Sāṃkhya-Yoga the *puruṣa* principle is the twenty-fifth and final principle. In many of the theistic philosophies of Hinduism, the supreme God is postulated as a separate principle beyond the *puruṣa* principle, and these philosophies usually also postulate additional principles between the *puruṣa* and the supreme God. Mādhavācārya's fourteenth-century *Sarvadarśanasaṃgraha* ("Compendium of All Philosophies") claimed that of the two Sāṃkhya systems, Sāṃkhya and Sāṃkhya-Yoga or Pātañjala Yoga, the first was non-theistic ("Sāṃkhya without Īśvara," *nirīśvarasāṃkhya*) and the second was theistic ("Sāṃkhya with Īśvara," *seśvarasāṃkhya*), and that according to Pātañjala Yoga, Īśvara was a twenty-sixth principle. That Īśvara should be a separate twenty-sixth principle (*tattva*) goes against the evidence from the classical Sāṃkhya-Yoga texts. In Sāṃkhya-Yoga, Īśvara is one among many *puruṣas*, but he is a particular and unique *puruṣa* in that he has never been bound to matter; and he is not a separate or a twenty-sixth principle (*tattva*). This Īśvara is always autonomous and free, and plays no active part in either creation or liberation of the universe and its creatures. The Īśvara of the *Yoga Sūtra* is neither a creator god nor a savior god, but a model of eternal liberation. Meditation on this Īśvara is one of the methods for attaining the goal of Sāṃkhya-Yoga. Īśvara's most important function, therefore, is to make possible the use in Sāṃkhya-Yoga of the sentiment of devotion for the attainment of liberation.

The Sāṃkhya system of religious thought as it is presented in the *Sāṃkhya-*

kārikās, the foundation text of the Sāṃkhya system of religious thought, has often been interpreted by scholars as "atheistic," but this assessment is based on a misunderstanding. In this case, "atheistic" simply means the denial of a particular type of god, the god of theism, rather than the plurality of gods found in India's polytheistic context. In Sāṃkhya the gods are not denied; but gods, like all living beings, are products of the association of the principle of consciousness (*puruṣa*) and the material principle (*prakṛti*). Gods have a *puruṣa* component and a *prakṛti* component, and the principle of consciousness (*puruṣa*) and the material principle (*prakṛti*) are the sole ultimate principles in this system. These two ultimate principles are impersonal. The fifty-fourth verse of the *Sāṃkhyakārikās* refers to the hierarchy of beings with the god Brahmā at the top and leaves of grass at the bottom. The gods Brahmā and so forth have a *puruṣa* component and a *prakṛti* component and therefore are not ultimate principles. In *Yoga Sūtra* 3.26, a hierarchy of beings in a number of realms superior to the human realm is also presented. The understanding of the plurality of gods such as it is found in Sāṃkhya and Sāṃkhya-Yoga is therefore far more complicated than the simplistic concepts of theistic and atheistic. Īśvara is also a quite unusual god. The Īśvara of Sāṃkhya-Yoga is similar to the other gods in the sense of having a *puruṣa* component and a *prakṛti* component, but this god is nevertheless very different from the others. Īśvara is content-less consciousness and its *prakṛti* component is perfect *sattva* in which the other two constituents (*guṇas*) of *prakṛti*—i.e., *rajas* and *tamas*—are present but not operative. *Prakṛti* consists of or is identical to the three *guṇas*—*sattva*, *rajas*, and *tamas*—and all material things and sentient beings are mixtures of the three *guṇa*s. In the unmanifest state of *prakṛti* the *guṇa*s are in equilibrium, but manifestation follows from the presence of the *puruṣa* principle, which disturbs the equilibrium. When *prakṛti* is manifest one of the *guṇa*s dominates, but, in contrast to the case of Īśvara, the other two are still operative (Jacobsen 1999). As Gerald James Larson has argued (in Larson and Bhattacharya 2008), Īśvara therefore cannot be either a thing or an entity, nor can it be personal in an intelligible way. Īśvara is the exemplar of permanent liberation but is also always present in the cycles of creation.

The hymns translated here to Īśvara, the highest god of Sāṃkhya-Yoga, were composed by Hariharananda Aranya (1869–1947) and are sung in the Kāpila Maṭha ("Kapila's Lodge," named after Kapila, the founder of the Sāṃkhya system of religious thought [see Jacobsen 2008]), the monastery founded by him in the north-central Indian state of Jharkhand. Hariharananda Aranya was one of the most important religious thinkers of early twentieth-century Bengal. He was from a wealthy family in Kolkata (Calcutta), but after a few years of college study of Sanskrit he became a Sāṃkhya-Yoga renouncer and for many years lived the life of a renunciant yogin in the Barabar Hills of Bihar, the Himalayas, and Bengal, before finally settling in Madhupur in Jharkhand, where he founded the Kāpila Maṭha. Aranya lived a solitary life in caves, a lifestyle he continued in the Kāpila Maṭha. There he lived enclosed in an artificial cave whose sole entrance was blocked for more than twenty years, from May 14, 1926 until his death in 1947. Aranya followed and renewed the Sāṃkhya-Yoga tradition. He believed that Yoga was one of the traditions of Sāṃkhya and that the function of Yoga was to realize the twenty-five principles of Sāṃkhya. His reputation is based on his ascetic lifestyle, his personal charisma, and the large number of books on Sāṃkhya and Yoga that he authored in Sanskrit and Bengali. Hariharananda Aranya forbade his disciples from writing his biography. Therefore less is known about him and his influence than would otherwise have been the case. However, his religious thoughts are accessible through his books. He wrote a number of philosophical works, among them a Sanskrit and a Bengali commentary on the *Yoga Sūtra* and Vyāsa's *Yogabhāṣya* commentary. His Sanskrit commentary, the *Bhāsvatī*, is recognized as one of the classical Sanskrit commentaries on the *Yoga Sūtra*.

According to Aranya, Yoga is mental concentration, *samādhi*, an interpretation that follows that of Vyāsa's commentary on the first verse of the *Yoga Sūtra*. Following the teachings of *Yoga Sūtra* 1.2, he defines Yoga as the "suppression of the fluctuations of the mind" (*yogaścittavṛttinirodhaḥ*) (Aranya 1961 [1983]): 7). For him, suppression of the mind means "keeping the mind fixed on any particular desired object." As he explains, "acquiring by practice the power of holding the mind undisturbed in the contemplation of any particular object . . . is called Yoga" (ibid., 7). The goal of yoga is liberation, and "liberation cannot be attained unless one passes through the process of concentration" (8). In this mental concentration, the Sāṃkhyan *tattva*s are to be realized, that is, to be known in immediate experience. Yoga is mental concentration leading to *samādhi* and the realization of the *tattva*s of Sāṃkhya. This is the cause of liberation, *mokṣa* or *kaivalyam*.

For Hariharananda Aranya, Yoga is one of the schools of Sāṃkhya philosophy. Yoga philosophy is found in particular in the *Yogabhāṣya*, the earliest commentary on the *Yoga Sūtra*. Like the *Yoga Sūtra*, it dates from between 350 and 450 CE. The *Yogabhāṣya* is a Sāṃkhya text, but the Sāṃkhya philosophy it presents differs on a few important points from that of the *Sāṃkhyakārikā*s of Īśvarakṛṣṇa, the foundational text of the other important school of Sāṃkhya philosophy. A salient difference between the two schools is that in Sāṃkhya-Yoga the yogin is encouraged to make use of the sentiment of devotion to Īśvara for the attainment of liberation.

Hariharananda Aranya composed several hymns in Sanskrit that explore the sentiment of devotion in Sāṃkhya-Yoga. The hymns of the yoga of devotion to Īśvara are based on descriptions found in *Yoga Sūtra* 1.23–1.29. Aranya argues that devotion to Īśvara (*īśvarapraṇidhāna*) means feeling the existence of God in the innermost core of the heart and resting content with this (ibid., 56). It is inside the heart that devotion to Īśvara is practiced (see "Devotion to the Supreme Lord" verses 3–4; "The Great Lord of Yoga" verse 10). In his *Yoga Philosophy of Patañjali*, Aranya explains that the heart is the inner part of the chest where one feels pleasure if there is love and happiness, and sadness if there is unhappiness and fear. Locating the heart is attained by identifying the locus of these feelings, and not by analyzing human anatomy. The heart is the center of I-ness, while the brain is the center of mental fluctuations. Aranya argues that when the mental fluctuations stop for a time, the yogin is able to feel that the sense of ego drops down to the heart. By meditating on the region of the heart, the yogin will then realize the subtle I-sense. This subtle I-sense can be pursued upward into the brain, where the most subtle center of I-sense is located. Then, Aranya argues, the heart and the brain become one. Aranya recommends that in the initial stages of practice the yogin should perform *īśvarapraṇidhāna* to God with a form. Aranya recommends imagining a luminous figure of God inside the heart. The luminous figure in the heart should be imagined as calm and peaceful, similar to the liberated person. When one's own mind becomes calm and able to rest in the feeling of godliness, then one should imagine a transparent white limitless luminous sky within the heart. Next, knowing that God pervades that space, the devotee should know that his whole self is in God who is present in his heart. Finally, the mind should be merged with the mind of Īśvara residing in the void-like space within his heart. When this is practiced, it leads to the realization of the self. Commenting on *Yoga Sūtra* 1.28–29, Aranya finally argues that devotion to Īśvara is a means to liberation, because to understand a thing is to become similar to that thing.

Several properties of Īśvara are described in the hymns translated here. Īśvara is devoid of ignorance, the sense of ego, attachment, detachment, and desires. He is not an effect of anything, nor is he the one who creates and maintains suffering and worldly pleasure. God is totally devoid of defects and is full of great noble qualities. Among the noble qualities are that he is ever concentrated, ever peaceful, that he knows his own Self and is established in himself. He realizes himself within himself and his mind is controlled. He is the beginningless reality, the omnipresent essence of the world, and the great Lord of Yoga, the highest and the greatest of all. God is beyond delusion and is compassion personified. He is the sole shelter of gods and humans, who removes disease in the form of birth and effaces the experience of things different from the Self. Īśvara is the shelter of yogins to whom he grants peace of mind. But perhaps most importantly, God is not a savior because, unless the dissolution of the mind is effected by oneself, it can never be permanent. The purpose of this characterization of Īśvara is to assist the yogin in the practice of *īśvarapraṇidhāna*. The hymns are part of the practice of Yoga, explaining what is meant by *īśvarapraṇidhāna* and, as such, means to *īśvarapraṇidhāna*. They illustrate a particular devotional sentiment integral to Sāṃkhya-Yoga.

The *Īśvarapraṇidhānastotram*, *Mahāyogeśvarastotram*, and *Maheśvaranamaskāraḥ*, the first hymns translated here, are instruments in the practice of devotion to Īśvara. Devotion to the Īśvara of Sāṃkhya-Yoga is a method for controlling the mind and is one of the means for realizing *samādhi*. *Samādhiṣaṭkam*, the final hymn translated here, is a description of the person who practices *samādhi*.

The hymns are translated from *Kāpilāśramīya-Stotrasāṃgrahaḥ* (Sarnath: Kapil Samkhyayogasrama, 1997).

Suggestions for Further Reading

Aranya had a large literary production. His books have been published in Bengali and Sanskrit (printed in Bengali script) by the Kāpila Maṭha in Jharkhand. The Sāṃkhyayogāśrama in Varanasi has published many of his books in Hindi, while the Kāpila Maṭha in Jharkhand has published English translations of a number of his works. An English translation of the *Bhāsvatī* was published in 2000 by the University of Calcutta and a Sanskrit volume of classical *Yoga Sūtra* commentaries (*Sāṃkhya Yogadarśana* [Varanasi: Chaukhambha Sanskrit Sansthan, 1989]) includes the *Bhāsvatī* together with the *Tattvavaiśāradī*, *Pātañjala Rahasya*, and *Yogavārtika* commentaries. His Bengali commentary—which was translated into English in 1961 (University of Calcutta Press) under the title *Yoga Philosophy of Patañjali*—was republished in the United States in 1983 by the State University of New York Press. Detailed summaries of several of his philosophical works on Yoga are found in *Yoga: India's Philosophy of Meditation*, edited by Gerald James Larson and Ram Shankar Bhattacharya (Delhi: Motilal Banarsidass, 2008), 367–96. An overview of the Kāpila Maṭha and the cave tradition is found in Knut A. Jacobsen, "In Kapila's Cave: A Sāṃkhya-Yoga Renaissance in Bengal," in *Theory and Practice of Yoga: Essays in Honour of Gerald James Larson*, edited by Knut A. Jacobsen (Leiden: Brill, 2005), pp. 333–49. A translation of one of Aranya's hymns (which is not included here) from the *Stotrasaṃgrahaḥ* is found in

Knut A. Jacobsen, *Kapila: Founder of Sāṃkhya and Avatāra of Viṣṇu* (New Delhi: Munshiram Manoharlal, 2008), pp. 204–8. The material principle, the *guṇa*s and divinities are analyzed in Knut A. Jacobsen, *Prakṛti in Sāṃkhya-Yoga* (New York: Peter Lang, 1999).

Devotion to the Supreme Lord (*Īśvarapraṇidhānastotram*)

Homage to that God
who is devoid of ignorance,
in whom the sense of ego is totally absent,
totally free from desire and aversion,
fearless.
homage to Him
again and again. (1)

Homage to that God
who is ever concentrated,
ever peaceful,
devoid of attachment,
indifferent,
[who] properly knows his own Self,
self established. (2)

My body and sense organs exist in You
while You are seated in my inner Self.
Please shine in the space in my heart
free from all confusion. (3)

OṂ,
my complete being is established in You,
and You are established in my heart.
Please keep me remembering You,
please pacify my mind. (4)

May I remember that God
who is peaceful and pure consciousness,
the pure Self established
only in You. (5)

The Great Lord of Yoga (*Mahāyogeśvara-stotram*)

I give my homage to that beginningless God
who is not an effect of anything,
whose mind is controlled,
realizing himself within himself,
free from various kinds of worldly things since he is the beginningless reality.
You are that very God. (1)

Suffering is clearly poison,
but worldly pleasure
is just poison put into honey, O omnipotent one.

You are full of compassion,
and therefore not the one
who creates and maintains
suffering and worldly pleasure. (2)

O Lord, You are thus the greatest of all.
Being tortured by worldly pleasures
and suffering born
of the ripening of the beginningless series of acts,
I wish that
I may attain
perfect peace by meditating on you. (3)

I think of you as the father,
but a father is a human being.
Thinking of you as a mother is likewise wrong,
because a mother is also a human being.
No simile can illustrate the sense of highest devotion
that is suitable to the Great Lord. (4)

O Lord who art not performing any acts!
People with deluded minds
superimpose on you
the act of granting wishes.

They do not know the glory of Your divine powers
which lead to attaining
the desired fruit
simply by the act of meditating on You. (5)

The unmanifest
activated by highest consciousness
is enough for creating and destroying the universe.
Therefore, O God,
although You are capable
of creating and resolving the universe,
You are established in yourself,
restricting the mind. (6)

Your will
is the only means to all things,
just a moment is enough
for accomplishing acts,
therefore thinking
that You take up various means
to perform various acts
is just an imagination
caused by ignorance. (7)

What should I expect of You?
Should I ask for liberation from You?
No!
This is to be accomplished
only by oneself.
O Lord, why do You not cause my mind to be dissolved?
Because if the dissolution of the mind
is not done by myself,
it will not be permanent. (8)

You have been sung and praised
as being consciousness only.
You are listened to and respected
in the sacred scripture
as being self-established.

You are the source of the highest good
    and have controlled even your godly marks. (9)

I desire to meet You directly.
But alas,
    the limitations placed on my sense organs
    obstruct me,
O Lord,
having realized You,
    as entered into my heart,
the fire of suffering of bereavement of separation,
    O Dear One,
    is pacified. (10)
O Lord,
when will I be able to develop
    the highest love for You
    which means even giving up
    the inclination of my mind
    to sing Your names
    because that involves speech? (11)

When shall I
    having dedicated myself to You,
    be over-flooded by nectar
    in the form of remembering you constantly
    while giving up small drops of tears
    born of bliss
and be established in You forever? (12)

When shall I attain
    by means of meditation
    the highest seat called *mokṣa*
    where You have been shining
    for unlimited time? (13)

The greatest mantra
    OṂ
    is the expression of You,
    O Lord of greatest Yoga!

With the syllable O Īśvara should be remembered
and with the syllable M meditated upon. (14)

Homage to the Supreme God (*Maheśvaranamaskāraḥ*)

I offer my homage to You
who are the highest among the gods (*īśvara*s)
and therefore the supreme God (Īśvara),
to You who are highest divinity (*deva*) among the divinities (*deva*s),
the Greatest Lord of all the Lords,
the ever illuminating
and praiseworthy Lord of the universe. (1)

My homage to You,
whose presence is peaceful and dispels fear,
O Auspicious One,
who causes auspiciousness. (2)
You are both greatness and divinity
and therefore forever the Great Lord,
my homage to You the Great Lord
who are totally free from attachment and aversion. (3)

My homage to you
who are the Greatest God,
whose great knowledge has caused the manifestation of the world
and what is beyond the world,
and whose mercy and meditation are great. (4)

My homage to the omnipresent Viṣṇu
whose great amazing powers pervade the universe
and whose very nature
is the Great Self. (5)

Homage to You again and again,
who are completely free from great delusion.
totally devoid of defects
and who are full of great noble qualities. (6)

Homage to that God
who removes the experience of things different from the Self,

to the highest omnipresent Lord,
to the God who is the only shelter of gods and humans,
homage to Him
  who is the Lord of the universe,
to the omnipresent Lord
  who is superior to all other gods,
homage to that Lord of all beings
  who removes the suffering of his devotees,
homage to that God
  who is the shelter of yogins,
  and grants peace of mind
and to the Lord
  who grants auspiciousness. (7)

Homage to my single Lord,
  the highest,
  beyond delusion,
  compassion personified,
  the essence of the world,
  who removes disease in the form of birth,
  always located in the lotus
  in the form of my heart. (8)

O Lord,
You are the forehead,
  and the ornament on my head,
You are the light of my eyes
  and the light of immortality,
You are the sandal paste on the outside of my body
  and the elixir of life within it,
You are the garland over my chest
  and the life within it as well. (9)

Six Verses on Concentration (*Samādhiṣaṭkam*)

Such a person
who has not experienced the happy feeling
  caused by control of the sense organs,
cannot attain *samādhi*,
whether in the day or by night. (1)

Such a person
who has not given up hope
  of worldly success
  properly and completely,
cannot attain *samādhi*,
whether in the day or by night. (2)

A person
all the physical activities of whom
generate lasting and happy remembrance
  of concentration on one single thing,
is very close to *samādhi*. (3)

The main means to *samādhi*
  are the eradication of all confusion,
  stilling the speech organ,
  and always viewing one's own mind
  as an object. (4)

Such a person
is first and foremost entitled to *samādhi*
who does not see anything,
does not hear anything,
does not commit any lapses,
and is devoid of attachment
  for worldly objects. (5)

Such a person
is the real practitioner of *samādhi*
who is always engaged
  in not experiencing
  any worldly objects
  with his sense organs,
is totally free
  from the desire
  to know
  those things that do not really exist. (6)

—19—

Yoga Makaranda of T. Krishnamacharya

Introductory Essay and Further Reading by Mark Singleton

Translation by M. Narasimhan and M. A. Jayashree, edited by Mark Singleton

Tirumalai Krishnamacharya (1888–1989) is one of the most significant figures in the creation of a global, English language–based yoga in the twentieth century. This is largely thanks to the propagation and development of his teachings by influential disciples such as B.K.S. Iyengar (b. 1918), K. Pattabhi Jois (1915–2009), Indra Devi (1900–2002), and his son T.K.V. Desikachar. In recent years, Krishnamacharya has attracted the reverence of thousands of yoga practitioners worldwide, and is considered by many to be the grandfather of yoga in the modern era.

Born in Muchukundapuram, Karnataka State, Tirumalai Krishnamacharya was the eldest child of a distinguished Vaiṣṇava brahmin family. His great-grandfather had been head of the Śrī Parakālamaṭha in Mysore, which was, according to T.K.V. Desikachar, the "first great center of Vaishnavite learning in South India" (1998: 34). From a young age his father began to initiate him into this culture, and to instruct him in the bases of yoga. He divided his early studies between Benares and Mysore, and mastered several of the orthodox *darśana*s. In 1915, eager to learn more about the practice of yoga, he set out to find one Rammohan Brahmacari who was, according to Krishnamacharya's preceptor in Benares, the only person capable of teaching him the full meaning of Patañjali's *Yoga Sūtra* (Desikachar 2005: 54). After seven years under his tutelage at Lake Mansarovar in Tibet, Krishnamacharya had absorbed "all of the philosophy and mental science of Yoga; its use in diagnosing and treating the ill; and the practice and perfection of *asana* and *pranayama*" (Desikachar 1998: 43). At the end of his apprenticeship, his guru instructed him to go back to India, start a family, and teach yoga. In accordance with these instructions he returned to Mysore in 1925, married a young girl called Namagiriamma, and for the next five years toured the region promoting the message of yoga (Chapelle 1989: 30).

In 1931, he was invited by the Maharaja to teach at the Sanskrit College (*paṭhaśālā*) in Mysore, and two years later was given a wing of the Jaganmohan Palace in which to teach yoga. It was during this time that two of his most influential students, B.K.S. Iyengar and Pattabhi Jois, studied under him. Patronage, however, came to an end soon after Independence and the *yogaśālā* closed forever. In 1952, Krishnamacharya was invited to Chennai by a leading jurist, and took over the evening yoga classes at the Vivekananda College there (Chapelle 1989: 31). He remained in Chennai until his death in 1989. In 1976, his son, T.K.V. Desikachar, established the Krishnamacharya Yoga Mandiram in his honor, and it remains the principal organ for the dissemination of Desikachar's vision of his father's teaching.

The *Yoga Makaranda* of 1934 (hereafter YM), written shortly after he began teaching yoga at the Jaganmohan Palace, represents an early phase of Krishnamacharya's career. His stated intention in the book is to "answer all the possible questions that might arise" on the topic of yoga (1), but in practice the YM is largely concerned with the practical performance of *āsanas* (postures) and has far less to say about other aspects such as *prāṇāyāma* (breathing exercises) or meditation. T.K.V. Desikachar asserts that this is because the book was conceived as the first in a series of works on yoga—none of which were ever written or published due to the death in 1940 of the project's sponsor, the Maharaja of Mysore, Krishnaraja Wodiyar IV (Desikachar 1993: 5). While this is probably true, it is also the case that Krishnamacharya's teaching during this period focused very heavily (and, for many students—such as B.K.S. Iyengar—exclusively) on the practice of *āsana*, and the book reflects this tendency. Indeed, Krishnamacharya's *Yogāsanagalu*, from around 1941, is, as the name suggests, another instruction manual of *āsana* practice. These posture-based forms are also the aspect of his teaching that has contributed most to the popularization of yoga in the West, mainly via Iyengar Yoga and the Ashtanga Vinyasa Yoga of Pattabhi Jois, as well as through Western spinoffs such as Power Yoga, and the various forms of "Flow," "Hatha," and "Vinyasa" Yoga that abound in America today.

YM was written in only seven days and nights (Desikachar 1993: 4), a fact that surely contributes to its incomplete, uneven character. In spite of its editorial and expository shortcomings, however, the text is a vital document for understanding the evolution of Krishnamacharya's teaching and its influence on modern, transnational yoga. It begins with an introductory discussion of yoga and why one should practice it. This is followed by a delineation of the eight limbs (*aṣṭāṅga*) of Patañjali's "Classical Yoga," namely: (1) the ethical principles (*yama*); (2) the personal rules (*niyama*); (3) posture (*āsana*); (4) yogic breathing (*prāṇāyāma*); (5) withdrawal of the senses (*pratyāhāra*); (6) single-pointed focus (*dhāraṇā*); (7) meditation (*dhyāna*); and (8) meditative absorption (*samādhi*). Included in the *prāṇāyāma* discussion is a description of the ten principal *cakras* (the ritually constructed, corporeal "wheels" or energy centers of *haṭha yoga* and Tantra). The subsequent section deals with criteria for eligibility, arguing that people of all castes, genders, and ages may freely practice yoga. Krishnamacharya then returns in more detail to the first four of the eight limbs of Pātañjala Yoga, with a particular emphasis on the third limb, *āsana*. Following this is advice on the construction of a suitable abode for yoga practice (*yogābhyāsa mandira*), what foods to eat, and what kinds of activities to avoid or embrace in one's life. There are then three fairly lengthy chapters on, respectively, the subtle channels of the body (*nāḍī*), the six purificatory practices of *haṭha yoga* (*ṣaṭkriyā*), and the internal bodily "winds" (*vāyu*).

A chapter with brief instructions on how to perform hathayogic *mudrās* and *bandhas* (bodily "seals" and "locks") is followed by an extended treatment of the practical technique of *āsana*, and the linking sequences (*vinyāsa*) that join them. Thirty-eight *āsanas* are presented, illustrated with photos of Krishnamacharya and his early students. In total, a little less than half the entire work is given over to *āsanas*. Krishnamacharya often recommends maintaining the postures for a long time (anywhere from three to thirty minutes), sometimes holding the breath in or out during that period according to the student's constitution and the demands of the *āsana* itself. This is clearly very different from the method taught by Krishnamacharya's early student Pattabhi Jois, currently popular in the West as Ashtanga Vinyasa Yoga, in which each posture is held for only five to eight breaths. Details regarding the health benefits of each posture reflect a modern emphasis on *yogāsana* as a kind of curative gymnastics, in line with the historical "medicalization" of yoga that really took hold in India during the 1920s with Swami Kuvalayananda and Shri Yogendra. Often, the presentation of *āsanas* in the *Yoga Makaranda* is not particularly cohesive, insofar as simple and advanced postures follow one another without apparent concern for graded sequencing. This may be one reason for the Krishnamacharya Yoga Mandiram's reluctance to publish a widely available translation of *Yoga Makaranda*, especially in light of their emphasis on proper *āsana* sequencing as the basis for successful teaching. It also suggests once again the pilot status of this text within Krishnamacharya's overall pedagogy.

Much of the first portion of the book is taken directly from classical texts on yoga, in particular Patañjali's *Yoga Sūtra* and late medieval *haṭha yoga* texts such as the *Haṭhapradīpikā* and the *Gheraṇḍa Saṃhitā*. Krishnamacharya maintained a life-long commitment to teaching yoga on the basis of the *Yoga Sūtra*, and the YM reflects this tendency. In this regard, Krishnamacharya is an important figure in the establishment of Patañjali as the source authority for yoga in the modern, global era. The attention given to the procedures of *haṭha yoga* in the YM is a little more difficult to explain. Krishnamacharya had an ambivalent and often openly hostile attitude toward *haṭha* practice, as is more than clear from the following excerpt from *Yogāsanagalu*:

> It is distasteful that some people propagate through books that *nauli*, *neti*, *basti*, *vajrolī*, *dhauti*, and *khecarī* and other *kriyās* (Cleansing Acts) are part of Yoga . . . But the main source for yoga, Patañjali Darśana, does not include them. Nor do they appear in the Upaniṣads or other works on Yoga . . . It is gravely disappointing that they defile the name of Yoga (Jacobsen and Sundaram 2006: 17–18).

It may seem strange, therefore, that Krishnamacharya devotes so much space in the YM to the description of fundamental hathayogic practices, such as *kriyā*, *mudrā*, *bandha*, and *āsana*. Desikachar asserts that the purpose of the book was merely to lay out the different techniques of yoga, "whether relevant or not," and to this end Krishnamacharya included descriptions of certain *kriyās* which he himself did not recommend (1993: 5). While this goes some way toward explaining this apparent discrepancy in the YM, it does not satisfactorily account for the fact that the treatment of *āsana* is obviously practical and instructional in intent. Before we investigate this problem further, we should note that Krishnamacharya's antipathy toward *haṭha yoga*—notwithstanding a certain degree of borrowing from it—is characteristic of the way Indians (and, increasingly, foreigners) were presenting practical yoga during this period. For instance, when Krishnamacharya refers in the extracts below to the "strange types of practice, of which the only function is to enthrall the audience" (34), he is echoing a typical criticism within the modern Indian yoga renaissance against panhandling street "yogis" who perform contortions in return for cash.

What, then, of Krishnamacharya's emphasis in YM on the practice of *āsana*? It is obvious that there is no such emphasis in Krishnamacharya's source text, the *Yoga Sūtra* of Patañjali, nor in the Upaniṣads and Vedas. Where Patañjali does mention *āsana* (II.46–48) it is almost certainly with reference to the seated positions of meditation, and not to the kinds of postures described in the second half of YM. Even in the *Dhyānabindu Upaniṣad*, cited by Krishnamacharya as evidence of a vast, vanished, tradition of *āsana* (39), only four seated postures are actually mentioned (*siddha*, *bhadra*, *siṃha*, and *padma*: DU 42–43). In Krishnamacharya's account, those Vedas which delineated the enormous range of *āsanas* at the origins of the YM's postural forms have been obscured by the "enemies of the eternal religion [*sanātana dharma*]," and are therefore not available to us (39). Krishnamacharya also refers here to an extant tradition of eighty-four postures, but even this claim is difficult to substantiate. As Gudrun Bühnemann has argued, an ancient tradition of eighty-four postures, such as that referred to by Krishnamacharya, is not accessible to us, nor is there any evidence that it ever existed (2007a, 2007b).

According to Krishnamacharya, his guru Ram Mohan Brahmacari personally practiced seven thousand *āsanas*, and Krishnamacharya learned approximately seven hundred of these from him (40). By his own estimation, therefore, Krishnamacharya is familiar with over eight times more *āsanas* than any of his contemporaries (the best of whom know about eighty-four), making him a major authority within this vastly diminished tradition. The deference to *śāstra* and *guru* in the YM's account of *āsana*, as well as in other sections of the book, is a habitual mode of exposition for an orthodox *paṇḍita* like Krishnamacharya, and functions to play down the author's personal innovations within the teachings he expounds. Indeed, there is little doubt that Krishnamacharya's presentation of *āsana* represents a new synthesis of tradition and modernity, adapted to the current social, political, and cultural conditions of early twentieth-century India. For example, the evolution of his *āsana* teaching during the Mysore phase certainly owes a debt to pervasive forms of international physical culture, as well as to the biomedical yoga experiments of Swami Kuvalayananda, whose Bombay institute Krishnamacharya had visited in 1933. Moreover, the dynamic forms of "jumping" yoga which emerged from the Jaganmohan Palace *yogaśālā*, and which form the basis of today's popular Ashtanga Vinyasa Yoga, were formulated as a physical practice suited to the children in Krishnamacharya's charge, and drew heavily on the standard forms of pedagogic gymnastics of the time—forms which were already being popularized across India, as yoga, by the likes of Kuvalayananda.

In sum, Krishnamacharya's teaching during the period of the YM's composition was, at least in practical terms, based on a foregrounding of *āsana* as the primary expression of the yoga *sādhana*. Until the early years of the twentieth century, *āsana* had almost always played a provisional, preparatory, and relatively minor role in Indian yoga traditions. Due to a range of cultural and historical factors, popular yoga was, by the 1920s, becoming increasingly identified with the performance of postures. For Krishnamacharya, the sparse references to *āsana* in orthodox texts—especially the *Yoga Sūtra*—provided sufficient grounds for radical enlargement upon the scope of the concept, and the development of an unprecedented approach to postural yoga practice. (Conversely, the absence of discussion of the six purificatory actions in Patañjali, as well as their association with the perceived inferior *haṭha yoga*, were enough to keep them out of Krishnamacharya's yogic portfolio.) While the marked emphasis on *āsana* practice in the YM is by no means representative of Krishnamacharya's entire teaching career, it is this aspect that has had the greatest influence on the creation of a global, posture-based culture of yoga practice.

The translation presents selections from the 1935 Kannada language edition of *Yoga Makaranda*, published by the Bangalore Press, with a preface by V. Subrahmanya Iyer, the de facto "Reader in Philosophy" to the Maharaja of Mysore. According to Sjoman (1996), there exists an earlier edition with a different preface in the Mysore Palace archives. Square-bracketed numbers in the translation refer to page numbers from the 1935 edition.

Suggestions for Further Reading

The Krishnamacharya Yoga Mandiram (KYM) published a celebratory issue of its magazine on the occasion of Krishnamacharya's one hundredth birthday (*Viniyoga* 24, December 1989). The issue contains several important articles, including an interview with Krishnamacharya about his early life by one "Hastam," which includes some intriguing details about the period before and after the composition of the YM ("Le Jeune Homme et le Rajah," 14–20). Chapelle's article in the same issue gives a useful overview of Krishnamacharya's career ("La Traversée d'un siècle," 27–32). Krishnamacharya has been the subject of two full-length biographies, one by his disciple Mala Srivatsan (*Sri Krishnamacharya, the Purnacarya* [Chennai: KYM, 1997]), and the other by his grandson, Kausthub Desikachar (*The Yoga of the Yogi: The Legacy of T. Krishnamacharya* [Chennai: KYM, 2005]). T. K. V. Desikachar's *Health, Healing and Beyond* combines biographical stories with lessons on yoga's healing power (New York: Aperture, 1998). Kausthub Desikachar's recent "family album," *Masters in Focus* (Chennai: Krishnamacharya Healing and Yoga Foundation, 2009), is conceived as a photographic tribute to the major figures of twentieth-century yoga, with Krishnamacharya at the center.

Between 1993 and 1995, the KYM published selections from the YM (translated by K. Vijayalakshmi and A. V. Balasubramaniam) in its magazine *Darśanam*. T.K.V. Desikachar's introduction to the project (*Darśanam* 1993 [2:3], pp. 3–5) and his on-going editorial comments (such as *Darśanam* 1995 [3:5], p. 4) are intriguing insofar as they suggest a certain ambivalence regarding the desirability of republishing his father's early work. In March 2011, the Krishnamacharya Yoga Mandiram did publish a complete translation of the YM by T.K.V. Desikachar. In the same month, Nandini and Lakshmi Ranganathan made available (for free download) their own translation of the text at http://redcrowyogashala.com/pdf/YogaMakaranda.pdf. Another book from the Mysore period, the *āsana* primer *Yogāsanagalu*, delineates the dynamic series of postures that would eventually form the basis of the internationally popular Ashtanga Vinyasa Yoga. First appearing in 1941, the book's second edition was published at the University of Mysore in 1973. A 2006 translation of the 1973 edition, by Autumn Jacobsen and R. V. S. Sundaram, remains unpublished. Some other translated works of Krishnamacharya are available through the KYM's website, www.kym.org.

Norman Sjoman's *The Yoga Tradition of the Mysore Palace* (New Delhi: Abhinav Publications, 1996) is a study of Krishnamacharya's *āsana* teaching during his time at the Jaganmohan Palace. Sjoman suggests that the postural forms developed by Krishnamacharya stem from an extant royal tradition of gymnastics in Mysore, as represented by the nineteenth-century texts, *Śrītattvanidhi* and *Vyāyāmadīpikā*. Chapter 9 of Mark Singleton's *Yoga Body, The Origins of Modern Posture Practice* (New York: Oxford University Press, 2010) contextualizes Krishnamacharya's teaching during the Mysore period within the broader history of the early twentieth-century *āsana* revival, and links his postural forms to the predominant styles of gymnastics in India at the time. Elliott Goldberg's as-yet unpublished *Radiant Bodies: The Formation of Modern Hatha Yoga*, contains new suggestions about the possible influence of contemporary South Indian bodybuilder K. V. Iyer on the evolution of Krishnamacharya's *āsana* teaching. Articles by Klas Nevrin ("Modern Yoga and Śrī Vaishnavism," 14:1, pp. 65–93) and Eddie Sterne ("The Yoga of Krishnamacharya," 14:1, pp. 95–106) in the Fall 2005 issue of *The Journal of Vaishnava Studies* consider Krishnamacharya's teachings in relation to his allegiance to the Śrī Vaiṣṇava tradition. Gudrun Bühnemann's 2007 book, *Eighty-Four Āsanas in Yoga: A Survey of Traditions* (New Delhi: D.K. Printworld, 2007), and her article in the 2007 special yoga issue of *Asian Medicine, Tradition and Modernity* (2007, 3:1, pp. 156–76) are invaluable studies of the place of *āsana* within Indian yoga traditions, ancient and modern.

For a general background on the development of yoga in the modern period, the two most important books to date are Elizabeth De Michelis's *A History of Modern Yoga, Patañjali and Western Esotericism* (London: Continuum, 2004) and Joseph Alter's *Yoga in Modern India: The Body between Science and Philosophy* (Princeton, NJ: Princeton University Press, 2004). The collection *Yoga in the Modern World, Contemporary Perspectives*, edited by Mark Singleton and Jean Byrne (London: Routledge, 2008), may also be useful as a resource for the study of popular yoga in the twentieth and early twenty-first centuries. De Michelis's survey of "Modern Yoga Studies" in this collection provides a particularly convenient departure point for those new to the field. See also Suzanne Newcombe's 2009 article, "The Development of Modern Yoga: A Survey of the Field" (*Religion Compass* 3, pp. 1–17). The website www

.modernyogaresearch.org, managed by Mark Singleton and Suzanne Newcombe, is a developing online community for the academic study of yoga in the modern age.

Yoga Makaranda

[1] Why should I practice yoga? What will I get out of it? How much time is needed, and what benefit will I get from setting aside time for practice? People frequently ask questions such as these. Many come and meet me personally at the Sanskrit College [*pāṭhaśālā*] to inquire about these and many other matters. Therefore, by means of this book, I hope to answer all possible questions that might arise.

I have something extremely important to say right at the outset. There seems to have been of late an increase in the numbers of commercially minded people. Such a tendency is highly detrimental to one's evolution. Merchants who wander in the marketplace like to get what they want without delay, and are ready to pay any amount to obtain what they desire. This sort of expectation is known as the "commercial mentality." **[2]** Introducing such commercial-mindedness into this ancient dharmic society of ours, and into the path leading to evolution and elevation, is frankly detrimental not only to society but to the individual as well. We should never insist on, nor even hope for, immediate results in return for an hour or two repeating mantras or engaging in worship (*pūjā*), yoga practice, or dawn and evening prayers etc. If we do, we are like the coolie who considers that it is not worth doing a couple of hours work if he does not receive his wages. Ever since monetary considerations of this kind have caught hold of our minds, we have become victims of the venal mindset and are growing meaner by the day.

Discipline in yoga (*yogābhāsya*) is not like the activities that one sees in the bazaar. Nowadays in every aspect of life, including the domain of *dharmic* action, people are losing interest simply because there is no quick monetary return. Because of this tendency our minds are becoming distanced from elevated thinking and higher aspirations, and we are mired in doubt and crisis at each and every moment. This is the primary and paramount point that our dear readers should know.

[8] By applying oneself, at least for some time, to the study of education or agriculture, one can gain knowledge of these subjects. In the same way, if one practices yoga, the desired benefits of health, strength, happiness, and stability of the mind (based on the quality of goodness (*sattvaguṇa*) will be gained after a few days without much difficulty. Imagine a mango tree full of fruit, and that somebody has given you permission to pick the mangoes and eat them. If you just stay where you are and don't go anywhere near the tree—let alone climb it, stretch forth your hand, pluck the fruit, and put it in your mouth—how will you ever enjoy the taste of the mango? It is clear that the greatest pleasure comes in eating the mango and not in climbing the tree, plucking the fruit, etc. To put it plainly, there can be no result without effort. And this is true even in yoga. **[9]** It should also be borne in mind that you cannot reap the full benefits if you do not practice with total faith and confidence. You know very well that gaining the fruits of action depends solely on following a proper plan. Until you practice with total devotion, pursuing a single objective, practicing at a designated place at a designated time, you will not get the full benefit. He who wants to climb the hill at Tirupati must proceed step-by-step, and gradually reach the higher mountain planes. At the end of his ascent he enjoys the blissful vision of the Lord. In the same way, if you follow in sequence the ethical principles (*yama*), the personal restraints (*niyama*), posture (*āsana*), yogic breathing (*prāṇāyāma*), withdrawal of the senses (*pratyāhāra*), single-pointed focus (*dhāraṇā*), meditation (*dhyāna*) and meditative absorption (*samādhi*) which are the steps of [Patañjali's] yoga teaching, in the end you will gain infinite bliss . . .

[11] The practice of postures regulates blood flow in the body. The efficiency of the nerves and muscles increases. The internal organs function properly. Everyone knows the relationship between proper blood flow, the neural centers, the different organs, the body, and health. This should provide an answer to those who ask, "What is the benefit of practicing postures?" What more do you want? This is the money you earn for this work, and it can be invested for future profit . . .

[19] In essence there will be no loss if one practices yoga following the injunctions of the teachings (*śāstra*). Depending on the sincerity, strength, and diligence of the practice, the results will naturally follow. If you practice daily, following all the rules of personal restraint (*niyama*s) for two to three hours, then within one year you will obtain appropriate benefits. Bodily and mental strength will increase, which will in turn bring happiness. There is no branch of traditional knowledge other than yoga that can bring such immediate results. However, if one practices yoga along with indiscriminate eating, drinking, traveling, entertainment, etc., one will not get all the benefits. One may get a little relief and nothing else. If a physician prescribes the correct medicine and a proper diet, but the patient does not follow his advice and indulges in improper food (resulting in the increase of disease), whose responsibility is that? Is it that of physician, the medicine, or the sick person? **[20]** In the same way, if the practitioner of yoga does not follow the injunctions of the masters as given in the yoga teachings, the suffering that he will face is not due to some fault in the science of yoga (*yogavidyā*). Every one of us knows that even in worldly activities like agriculture, commerce, and administration, one will get into difficulties if one does not follow the law of the land. There is no doubt that all benefits will accrue to those who practice yoga according to the rules . . . Each person should make a firm resolve to practice those things by which one can understand the true nature of creation and the soul. It is a waste of time to know other things, which are transient. It is only the Yoga Teachings (*yogaśāstra*) that will teach you and allow you to experience the form, function, and quality of creation and the soul. Therefore you should understand the secrets of yoga and practice it.

[22] You might ask, "It may be true for Indians, but what about foreigners who are healthy and long-lived, without any practice of yoga? Are they not intelligent? Are they not happy?" You are right, but you should realize that God has created an appropriate system of educational activity according to the geographical conditions of each country and the quality of air and vegetation. That is to say, the structure of knowledge has been created in accordance with the particular characteristics of the land, water, and air. That is why each society has its own unique features and traditions, and is different from others in terms of language, philosophy, culture, study, and pursuit of pleasure. This is well understood by our modern youths who go abroad so frequently. But it is not true that those people are not practicing physical exercises in conformity with our yoga system. We don't know what they were practicing in the past, but at present all of you should know for sure that they are practicing the same yoga discipline as us . . .

[24] Every individual is eligible for Yoga practice: the four main castes (*varṇas*) (namely those of the priest [brahmin], warrior [*kṣatriya*], merchant *vaiśya*] and low-caste persons [*śudra*]), as well as the sage (*jñānin*), women, men, youth, elders, very old people, the sick, the weak, boys and girls. None of these distinctions of age, condition, and hereditary position (*jāti*) will present an obstacle to the practice of yoga.

[25] The only secret is that it should be learned through a teacher who can convey even its inner core. Gheraṇḍācārya [the author of the hathayogic treatise entitled the *Gheraṇḍa Saṃhitā*] is of the opinion that the following types of person are not eligible for the practice of yoga: stubborn people, swindlers (*kapaṭī*), eaters of bad food, speakers of evil words, the lustful, pleasure seekers, dissemblers, cheats, jealous people, hateful people, abusers of the Vedas, and drinkers of alcohol. The reason for this is that even though yoga is a purifier, this knowledge will, in the hands of such unreliable people, bring suffering to society. The stories of the *Purāṇas* and our own experiences in the past are evidence of such misfortunes. Everybody knows that clean cow's milk is healthy, but that if one puts it in a pig- or dog-skin container it will lead to ill health. In the same way, in the hands of miscreants, this nectar of yoga (*yogāmṛta*) will bring trouble. A king once gave his sword to his evil son in order to conquer the enemy, but because of the son's misuse of that sword, the king lost his kingdom . . .

[33] If a man wants to live with a healthy body, not just for one hundred years but for as long as he desires, the cleansing of the internal wind known as *prāṇa* is the basic requisite. *Prāṇaśuddhi* means controlling the *prāṇa*. The most important means for such control is *prāṇāyāma*. Our ancients, following this method, lived as long as they wanted, and did service for the elevation of the world—and even now their name and fame remains with us. Nowadays we have given up this method for controlling the *prāṇa* and doubt the greatness of the ancients. Instead, people have taken up physical exercises, which are harmful to the *prāṇa*. Because of this, people are becoming old even before they reach the age of three, and are suffering unnecessarily. I will describe the *prāṇāyāma* method in the chapter on *prāṇāyāma*.

[34] In *haṭha* yoga, prominence is given to the technique of *āsana* practice. Also, too much emphasis is placed on some strange types of practice, of which the only function is to enthrall the audience. *Rāja yoga* explains the means of increasing the strength of the mind through meditation (*dhyāna*) and concentration (*dhāraṇā*). It also speaks of methods to keep the actions of the eleven senses centered in the third eye (*ājñācakra*), or in the thousand-petalled lotus (*sahasrāra*), thus keeping the mind turned inward and not outward. In this way, one can understand and realize the Soul (*ātman*), the Supreme Soul (*paramātman*), and the world. In this type of yoga *prāṇāyāma* practice is given in the beginning to cleanse the subtle channels (*nāḍī*s) . . .

[39] The Vedas tell us that there are as many postures of yoga as there are living beings: that is to say, 8.4 million. In ancient times human beings had a practical knowledge of all of them, but as time passed, many postures disappeared, due to changes of place, company, and lifestyle. The meaning of the Vedic scriptures which are the very foundation of these postures has been made obscure by the enemies of the eternal religion (*sanātana dharma*). Whatever Vedic scriptures are available today are only useful for debating, rather than for experiencing higher states of consciousness. What is more, some of those who have learned to chant the Vedas are using them as a means to gain renown and material wealth. Others are simply indifferent toward this sacred body of knowledge, **[40]** and still others complain that chanting the Vedas gives them a headache. It is very difficult to find anyone who is genuinely interested in this knowledge. The few interested people still remaining have to face many difficulties.

How are we to recognize such people? In our society, which exhibits a mixture of ignorance, indifference, and animosity toward the Vedas, who are those people that retain an interest? How many obstacles such people face! However, despite all these handicaps, some great people and pious kings in India are doing their best to bring [this knowledge] into the experience of the youths of their region, so that the next generation will have healthy, long lives and unbroken contentment. This in itself is a great relief.

According to the account of Śaṅkarācarya, in his day there were only 84,000 postures in practice, out of the total of 8.4 million. By the time of Rāmānuja, according to his biography, the number of postures was reduced to 64,000. By the time of Mādhavācarya and Nigamānta Mahādeśika it was down to 24,000. I myself have heard from the lips of Jagadguru Narasimha Bharati that he knew and practiced sixteen hundred postures. With my own eyes I have seen Guru Maharaj Shri Ram Mohan Brahmacari of Nepal practice seven thousand postures. From him, I have learned and practiced about seven hundred of them. **[41]** In works currently available on *yogāsana*, as well as among practitioners of today, we generally only find eighty-four postures in use. There may be some who know a few more . . .

[42] Where there is no mention of the position of the head in the *yogāsana* sequences, one should practice the chin lock (*jālandhara bandha*). In the same way, if the focus of the gaze is not specified, it should always be between the eyebrows. The hands should be kept as in the *siddhāsana* posture if no other position is specified. If there is no mention of how to grasp a part of the body with your hands, you should hold it with thumb, forefinger, and the middle finger. While practicing the postures, hands and legs should be alternated: that is to say, one should first do the pose on the right side and then on the left side. This principle should be put into practice whenever necessary. If not, the energy (*śakti*) will not spread itself uniformly through the body.

[43] *Vinyāsas* have been part and parcel of *yogāsana* and *prāṇāyāma* from time immemorial. In recent times and in many places, however, people leave out the *vinyāsas* but still claim to be doing *āsana* practice while they are merely sitting, stretching, or folding their legs and hands. It is not only in the yoga teachings that this is happening: even in Vedic chanting (*vedādhyayana*), mantra recitation (*mantropāsana*), and many other areas, people practice without consideration of the rules (*niyama*) and approach them like any other physical activity. If this goes on like this much longer, the Vedic literature will also disappear. Any activity done without practicing the rules will not bear fruit. Everybody knows this.

Some people, due to the company they keep, are interested in worldly gain and complain that there seems to be no benefit in practicing the eternal religion, ritual action (*karma*), and yoga. There are good reasons why they would make such statements, and we can find some instructive things hidden here. For example, **[44] s**uch people do not follow the proper steps (*vinyāsa*s) and other rules. Also, their teachers have not given them the secrets of receiving the proper experience, nor the correct information regarding the time and place, etc. of practice. Nor do they have correct knowledge of what kind of food and drink one must take. It is because of individuals like these that society is abandoning yoga, and that people are allowing their bodies to become abodes of disease and suffering. Instead of undertaking exercises that give proper strength to all parts of the body, they squander money on unsuitable games which are simply a waste of time. Others cover up their own defects and misguided ways by claiming that yoga practice leads to madness. Nevertheless, the youth of today are endeavoring to compile the fragmentary texts of yoga and, by undertaking the personal restraints to the best of their abilities are practicing the ancient system of yoga. I am sure God will reveal the secrets of yoga to such sincere seekers. After all, the modern age is the age of youth, and I firmly believe that the Lord of Yoga will give long life, health, and strength to these young seekers.

[45] In this book I will try to explain all the secrets that were taught to me by my Guru. *Āsana* and *prāṇāyāma* are of two types: "with mantra" and "without mantra." Only those who are authorized to receive the teachings of the Vedas are eligible for the practices of yoga with mantra. All human beings are eligible for the practice of yoga without mantra. Each *āsana* has between three and forty-eight *vinyāsas*. There is no *āsana* with fewer than three *vinyāsas*. While practicing *āsanas*, you should keep your inhalations and exhalations equal. Breathe only through the nostrils, and only perform *āsanas* along with their *vinyāsas*. Just as music will not bring mental absorption (*manolaya*) if sung without the appropriate tone (*śruti*) and rhythm (*laya*), so *āsana* practice without *vinyāsa* will not lead to good health, let alone long life.

While practicing yoga postures, the most effective breathing practices are of two types. One is called "the activity of expansion" (*brāhmaṇakriyā*) and the other "the activity of reduction" (*laṅghanakriyā*). Just as a physician prescribes medicines which are appropriate to the disease, so the *Yogaśāstra* prescribes practices suitable to the temperament and the body structure of the individual, leading to three benefits: long life, health, and happiness. Fat people should practice the activity of reduction and thin ones should practice the activity of expansion. People of moderate bodily proportions should practice both. **[46]** In the activity of expansion, one should take air in through the nostrils and hold the breath (holding the breath in like this is known as "internal retention" [*pūrakakumbhaka*]). In the activity of reduction, one should expel all the air from the body through the nostrils and hold the breath (holding the breath out like this is known as "external retention" [*recakakumbhaka*]).

[47] Some people say that yoga practice is meant only for men and not for women. Others say that it should be exclusively for those of the brahmin, *kṣatriya*, and *vaiśya* castes and not for others. For such people our answer is clear: you simply haven't studied the yoga texts properly. Others are trying to destroy control of the senses and family values in society by spreading the false notion that yoga practice leads to madness. We say these people are the enemies of the six systems of orthodox Hindu thought (*ṣaḍdarśana*). If one were to look at the *Bṛhadāraṇyaka Upaniṣad*, the *Yoga Yājñavalkya Saṃhitā*, and other *Upaniṣads* and compare them with the yoga texts, such derogatory statements could not be made.

The reader can see how many *vinyāsas* should be performed for each posture under each *āsana* description. Generally, in the *vinyāsas* where you have to raise your head, you should retain the breath internally (*pūrakakumbhaka*) and where the head has to be bent forward, you should perform external retention (*recakakumbhaka*). In the posture called *utpluthi*, overweight people should do external retention and thin ones internal retention.

If you take up yoga without following these rules, or by merely following pictures; if you complain on account of this that yoga has no effect, and start **[48]** abusing the yoga system and the eternal religion which is the foundation of practice; if you take up exercises which are not suitable to the air, water, and food of our country and thereby lose health, then you have only yourself to blame!

It is normal when one takes up physical exercise that some pain in the arms and legs will be experienced for some days. Don't think that this is exclusive to yoga discipline: such pains are common to all exercise. Physical exercises are of two types: whole body practices (*sarvāṅga sādhana*), and partial body practices (*āṅgabhāga sādhana*). Nowadays, thinking that it will make practice easier, some people have been importing expensive exercise-toys and are using them at inappropriate times. These types of practices increase the blood flow in one part of the body and reduce it in another, leading to weakness. This will certainly lead to strokes and will bring our body to an untimely death. **[49]** On top of this, we have seen that those who practice these extremely popular exercises shout loudly and breathe through their mouths. This is very dangerous. It reduces our lifespan. After all, we only live as long as the vital breath (*prāṇavāyu*) is sufficiently strong within our system. These types of practice are not suitable for the people of our country. It is advisable that such practitioners spend their money on improving their bodies rather than in purchasing equipment to do these kinds of exercise.

Exercises which give equal strength to all parts of the body, including the blood vessels and the joints, are of three types: the discipline of yoga, the science of wrestling (*mallavidyā*), and the science of archery (*dhanurvidyā*). We don't know why archery has been discarded in modern times. Even though we see wrestling practiced here and there, it is not performed in the proper order. What is more, it is geared toward winning competitions. This science of wrestling is only helpful in gaining physical strength and is not conducive to spiritual evolution. The great defect in this system is that it does not help to increase mental capacity or the equanimity of the body and mind, nor to effect other subtle changes. If a man wants to get the five benefits—namely health, long life, happiness, intelligence, and physical strength—he should practice yoga. Without these five, one will not be able to comprehend the essence of life itself. And in spite of our human birth, without such knowledge life is a waste.

[50] For some reason, in today's world we are buffeted by many strange ideas and thoughts. We must become extremely vigilant, and select what is good in these ideas and thoughts, and put it into practice. To this end, we need to be very agile, and in possession of these five strengths. The essence of these strengths is yoga. To achieve this there is no need to import costly apparatus. We have sufficient means at our disposal in our own country without spending all this money. By falling prey to the advertisements of those same foreigners who stole so much of our indigenous knowledge, we have indeed paid a high price. Now they claim that it is their own discovery! Perhaps in the future they will also sell back to us the science of yoga. The reason for this is that most of us have neither studied nor put into practice the texts of yoga. If we remain quiet, the foreigners will become our yoga gurus! It is nothing short of a tragedy that we have thrown away our golden cup and are drinking instead from this foul smelling leather flask brought from abroad. I sincerely hope that such ill fortune will not fall on future generations.

[51] For the exercises of yoga, the locally available tools are quite sufficient. Our hut alone will do—we need not spend any extra money. The only thing that Mother Yoga (*yogamāta*) begs from us is that we eat solely the pure food produced by Mother India. We are firm in our opinion that our youths, who are more than able to enlighten foreigners, are equally capable of resurrecting the indigenous, ancient knowledge systems. The importance of reviving this knowledge is well known, and is desired by all those scholars working in the field of education who know how to bring about transformation in an individual through yoga.

Yoga gives strength to the body, yoga gives us health, and only yoga can give us long life. Yoga enhances our intellect. Yoga makes us rich. Yoga makes us human beings. Yoga will bring back honor and respect to Mother India. Yoga tells us where our duty lies. It is yoga that unveils the purpose of our birth. Only yoga can answer the question, "Where is God?" Thus yoga and yoga alone will enhance our strength and evolution.

—20—

Theos Bernard and the Early Days of Tantric Yoga in America

Paul G. Hackett

Theos Casimir Hamati Bernard (1908–1947) was an early American pioneer in the field of Indo-Tibetan Tantric yoga. Following a successful and highly publicized trip to Tibet in 1937, Bernard established a yoga ashram in Manhattan's affluent Upper East Side in the late 1930s, advertising himself as a teacher of Indian and Buddhist philosophy and as a yoga instructor. To the general public, Bernard presented himself as a scholar of Indo-Tibetan religion, culture, and politics; to his students, however, Bernard presented himself as an accomplished yogi and religious adept. For many years, the only biographical sources on Bernard were his purportedly autobiographical works, *Heaven Lies Within Us* and *Penthouse of the Gods*, books written and published to support his claims. In these books and subsequent interviews, Bernard presented himself as an exemplar for anyone wishing to pursue personally transformative knowledge.

By his own account, Bernard was a second-generation American yogi, an intentionally conceived child of Tantric yogis, and the namesake of his parents' guru, Sylvais Hamati. Bernard's childhood was not that of an ordinary American boy, he claimed, but rather the life of a secret yogi in training. Following a college illness, Bernard claimed to have been visited by an old Indian yogi during his convalescence, and his life from the age of eighteen onward became solely a quest for the meaning of life. Bernard's years in Tucson, Arizona thus came to be described as a conscious spiritual mission in which his illness was framed as a spiritual trial by fire; in short, his ordeal and recovery were his "sacred rites." From that point on, as he claimed his teacher told him, he had become innately qualified for the yogic teachings. Claiming to have mastered all the preliminary practices and rituals of purification before ever leaving the fields of his adolescence, Bernard was a man on a quest for "mental and spiritual realization." He maintained that it was only in India and Tibet, however, that the fruits of his efforts truly ripened.

> It seemed so strange that I had come so far from the lonely deserts of Arizona to this devout land, from an environment so young to a culture so old. What had planted the seeds within me of this desire to come here? What had called me to this Land of Mystery? Why was I being accepted? It was clear, or so it seemed to me now, that all my effort to gain some understanding of the Laws of Life had not been in vain. The old saying that when the pupil was ready the teacher would appear flashed upon my mind, and I felt there was truth in it. I knew I was on the verge of being liberated, on the path to verify by experience what I had learned in theory . . . It was to be the start of a new life for me, of spiritual rebirth. The shackles of the personal consciousness would be forever removed. I would directly perceive the universal manifestation of the Divine Law. (Bernard 1939: 97–98)

Thrust into the public limelight in the wake of his much-publicized trip to Tibet, Bernard recounted his experiences in making his way to the Himalayan kingdom, where he claimed he was welcomed with open arms as a reincarnated Buddhist saint. Given secret teachings and highly esoteric "Tantric empowerments and transmissions" while in Tibet, he had returned to America, presenting himself as an emissary from the mystic East.

To the 1940s alternative religion and health communities of New York City, Bernard was thus part student and explorer, and part religious visionary and pioneer, with different aspects of his public persona receiving different emphases depending on whom he was talking with. Although highly personable, Bernard was described by many as a lackluster speaker, and his lectures often were not well attended. Consequently, unlike his predecessors and contemporaries, such as Swami Vivekananda, Paramahansa Yogananda, or others who would follow him—figures who founded institutions that survived them—Bernard left no lineage of students or practices in his wake. Instead, Bernard's legacy would prove to be a literary one, which would only flower in the years following his death. His Columbia University doctoral dissertation on *haṭha yoga* (*Haṭha Yoga: The Report of a Personal Experience*, 1943) would be translated into several languages, and his fictionalized account of his time in India (1939) would become required reading for many on the "hippie trail" to India and Nepal in the 1960s.

Throughout the decades that followed, as many new students began to have their own experiences in India and study directly with yoga teachers, the limitations of Bernard's books relegated him to obscurity. Over the course of the past ten years, however, numerous primary source materials have become available that shed light on Bernard's actual activities and the man behind the self-constructed mythology, revealing much of the content of his "autobiographies" to be fictitious or misrepresentative of the actual events in his life. When one examines the themes in Bernard's writings, interviews, and lectures today, one can see that so much of what he said and did may best be seen as a manifestation of broader cultural themes in mid-twentieth century America and part of the crafting of a distinctly American understanding of yoga—a yoga divorced from its religious dimensions and refashioned into an American lifestyle accessory. Introducing himself to the American public as "The White Lama"—a title he claimed to have received in Tibet—Bernard articulated precisely this approach to the practice of yoga.

> The general public is 99% wrong about what Yoga is. It is not a religion, although it is most distinctly a way of life. No one need sacrifice an iota of his religion to engage in Yoga . . . and that's why I try to adapt my instruction to Western civilization . . . The earnest student of Yoga soon learns the truth of the Biblical statement "To him who hath shall be given," and that is what I mean when I say that the deeper disciplines and joys will be disclosed as the student advances toward the light . . . Yoga is the key to happiness for many people who are maladjusted to life in the United States. (Robinson 1939: 14–15)

This message, of yoga's "non-denominationalism," was one that Bernard carefully constructed to reassure a nominally Christian populace that it would not be damned to hell for practicing yoga . . . or for paying him to attend his classes, at the very least. If anything, he explained, by doing so they would only deepen their own religiosity and gain insight into the sorts of religious practices that, unbeknownst to themselves, they were already engaged in. In his unpublished notes from a May 2, 1939 lecture entitled "General Analysis of Various Types of Yoga," Bernard explained that "Bhakti Yoga [is] the path of love and devotion" and that Christianity, "is a form of Bhakti Yoga."

> Everyone in the world is actually practicing one or another form of Yoga, but they lead lives of separateness, integrating nothing, and losing the value of their experiences. Yoga is designed to reach the creative flow, to conserve and then liberate it . . . The Tantras say that in this age of Kali Yuga, we are not vital enough to be aroused by any form of Yoga but Hatha Yoga. The Tantras teach that everything is energy, and Yoga is the means of releasing it. This experience cannot be described in words, but must be felt to be known.

The possibility of such experiences—personal, direct, and unmediated access to the divine—was an idea that American audiences steeped in a Protestant mythos could easily understand and embrace. Nonetheless, Bernard's "creative flow of life" was little more than a thinly disguised presentation of the Sāṃkhya notion of *prakṛti*, though he made great efforts to incorporate elements (or at least, terminology) from both Buddhism and Christianity into his lectures, participating in and perpetuating the populist notion of the equivalency of all religions, a commonplace approach that attempted to conflate and appropriate the elements of all religions under a common umbrella.

Bernard's lectures—as well as his father's correspondence with Indian informants—reveal a deep familiarity with much of the jargon of English-language neo-Vedānta philosophy that was enthusiastically promulgated in Indian intellectual circles as the foundation of both Yoga and Tantric Buddhism (the latter despite sufficient evidence to the contrary). Bernard, for example, makes repeated references to "name and form" (*nāma-rūpa*), the stock phrase used in Vedānta to refer to the illusory world (*māyā*) which ordinary beings inhabit. It is also, however, an idea that Bernard used reductionistically to dismiss the need to study different cultures. If different cultures are equally illusory—mere "name and form"—he argues, then one need never bother studying their claims in depth, but rather merely concentrate on developing one's own "innate spiritual knowledge" and by doing so come to "know" the truths of all cultures and religions. In this way, Bernard absolved himself of any responsibility for accuracy in his portrayals of Indian and Tibetan cultures. Far from being alone in doing so, Bernard and others who ascribed to this worldview were intellectually rooted in the pop eastern mysticism culture of the late nineteenth and early twentieth centuries, a culture that was heavily influenced by the works of Madame Blavatsky, the Theosophical Society, and Jiddu Krishnamurti: this last figure who had only recently (1929) repudiated all culturally bounded approaches to religious practice, including his own. This approach would have been familiar to Bernard's audience steeped in the counterculture of the day.

What is also evident from reading Bernard's writings is that many of his views, which can also be seen in present-day orientations toward yoga, are not recent innovations but rather simply typically American counterculture attitudes toward life and religious systems in general. In his *1939 Lectures* (a series of short talks that would precede actual *haṭha yoga* instruction), Bernard presented the ideas of egalitarianism in access to religious knowledge, the notion of "innate knowledge" as opposed to specific knowledge that must be derived from study and contemplation, the unity of all religions on a fundamental level underlying superficial cultural forms, and so forth, all wrapped up in a vaguely misleading conflation of traditions and terminologies.

The basic framework of Buddhist cosmology, which was the foundation for such discussions, presents six realms of possible rebirth within the "wheel of life" (*bhavacakra*, a pictographic description of cyclic existence, and Bernard's preferred term): gods, demi-gods, humans, animals, spirits/ghosts (*preta*s), and hell-beings. An individual born in any one of these realms would do so through the force of their karma—with the exception of only the most extraordinary beings, who could do so willfully. Thus, the individuals who functioned to their fullest in such a system were *bodhisattva*s—persons with a degree of spiritual realization who had also gained a certain level of control over the process of rebirth. A *bodhisattva*, strictly speaking, was an individual who had vowed to achieve the state of Buddhahood solely for the sake of benefiting and liberating all other sentient beings from cyclic existence. A yogi, on the other hand, was an individual who engaged in the spiritual discipline (*yoga*) of binding (from the Sanskrit root *yuj*) the mind. Bernard, like many of his contemporaries, employed these technical terms in much looser ways as, for example, Paramahansa Yogananda had done in identifying the Christian savior as "a bodhisattva." "Bodhisattva" and "yogi"—words that have gained increasing currency in modern parlance—for Bernard became generic terms divorced from their classical meanings and deployed at whim for the poetic inspiration and flattery of people, being applied to persons well outside their normal range of reference. Despite this cavalier attitude toward terminology, Bernard did attempt to remain true to the authentic teachings on *haṭha yoga*—or, at least, what he perceived them to be.

In its native context, along with bhakti ("devotional"), *dhyāna* ("meditational"), and karma ("action") yoga, *haṭha* ("exertion") yoga was considered but one among many equally valid forms of religious discipline ("yoga") that could be practiced by an individual. Singled out by Bernard and others as unique, however, *haṭha yoga* was presented as specifically appropriate for this day and age, the practices themselves having been spelled out by the fifteenth-century Indian author, Svātmarāma, in his text, the *Haṭhayogapradīikā*. In his work, Svātmarāma distinguished *haṭha yoga* from the earlier eight-part (*aṣṭāṅga*) system—which he referred to as *rāja* ("royal") yoga—as codified by the fourth-century author, Patañjali, the author or compiler of the *Yoga Sūtra*. As can be seen from the wealth of references in Bernard's books, the source for much of his understanding of yoga was the then recently translated *Haṭhayogapradīpikā*, along with another relatively late work, the circa seventeenth-century *Gheraṇḍa Saṃhitā*.

In addition to the postures (*āsanas*) of yoga practice, many preliminary purificatory exercises were also detailed in both the earlier yoga tradition and by Bernard in his books. In addition to the aforementioned texts, Bernard also drew upon the *Suśruta Saṃhitā*, a canonical work on Ayurvedic medicine, for his understanding of the purification techniques prerequisite to actual *haṭha yoga* practices. These techniques, it is claimed, were designed to both cleanse and render malleable the various organs of the body, and included both external and internal "washing," from cleansing the nasal passages with string (*neti*) and swallowing cloth to absorb excess acid in the stomach (*dhauti*), to rendering the abdominal muscles serviceable (*nauli*) and cleansing the rectum and anus (*basti*). All of these, however, were geared toward what Bernard considered the "key" yoga technique: *vajrolī mudrā.*

Harking back to the medieval Nāth Siddha traditions of Bengal and the founding figure of Gorakṣanātha, *vajrolī mudrā* was a practice that lay at the core of a sort of internalized sexual alchemy. Through the practice of *vajrolī mudrā* ("urethral suction") and precisely controlled "internal hydraulics" (to use White's term), the "power substances" of male and female sexual fluids are manipulated to induce a very specific state of mind for the practitioner, together with a host of secondary powers and benefits. This, at least, was Bernard's understanding of the practice based on his father's research.

The selections from the private papers of Theos Bernard presented here reflect all of these different components and paint a picture of the popular yoga world in circa 1940s New York. However, another selection from his research papers—a letter written by an Indian informant to Glen Bernard, Theos Bernard's father and research assistant—tells a different story, disclosing the then state-of-the-art knowledge of esoteric religious practices that ran counter to all of these popular notions, reinforcing the notion that the yoga *āsanas* were unequivocally religious practices and, moreover, merely the preliminary preparations to the primary practices—facts of which Bernard was well aware, and that he indeed attempted to secretly put into practice.

Suggestions for Further Reading

On Theos Bernard's life and writings, see Paul G. Hackett, *Barbarian Lands: Theos Bernard, Tibet, and the American Religious Life* (forthcoming); as well as Bernard's own writings: Theos Bernard, "Haṭha Yoga: The Report of a Personal Experience" (Ph.D. dissertation, Columbia University, 1943); and *Heaven Lies Within Us* (New York: Scribner's Sons, 1939). A 1939 interview with Bernard was published in Stewart Robinson, "The White Lama on Yoga," *Family Circle Magazine*, Aug. 25, 1939, pp. 14–21. A biography of Theos Bernard's uncle, Pierre Bernard (also known as Oom the Omnipotent), who pioneered his own brand of yoga teaching in New York a few decades before his nephew, is available in Robert Love, *The Great Oom* (New York: Viking, 2010). Stefanie Syman, *The Subtle Body: The Story of Yoga in America* (New York: Farrar, Straus and Giroux, 2010) contains a historical survey of yoga in America, from its inception in the nineteenth century down to the present. Elizabeth De Michelis, *A History of Modern Yoga* (New York: Continuum, 2004) provides an overview of several of the varieties of yoga found in contemporary settings, and examines the nineteenth- and twentieth-century presentations and reformulations of the "yoga" tradition that fed Euro-American cultural appetites for eastern mysticism. Joseph Alter, *Yoga and Modern India: The Body Between Science and Philosophy* (Princeton, NJ: Princeton University Press, 2004) offers an analysis of modernist Indian revisionings of yoga and its origins. For a discussion of the Nāth Siddhas and their practice of *haṭha yoga*, see David Gordon White, *The Alchemical Body* (Chicago: University of Chicago Press, 1996).

Selections from Lectures–1939, Theos Bernard Papers

MAY 4, 1939

As the light which is consciousness comes into the world, it brings little to the four kingdoms of nature. In the human kingdom, consciousness helps man find himself. Consciousness cannot be rationalized, it can only be perceived; it cannot be argued out, we can only live and learn it through our experiences. Yoga is the practical method of accomplishing this. Mind is the chief difficulty; we can achieve freedom more easily by proceeding naturally, instead of engaging in excessive mental activity. Mind is an instrument of consciousness, but most people lose themselves in the mind, forgetting it is only a vehicle. There is only one truth, one essence; when two mentalities disagree on fundamental truth, it is not because something is wrong with truth; something is wrong with the mind.

We must learn to look for the essence of things, and not stop at name and form. Happiness and suffering are transitory, existing only in the world of name and form; they cannot last. People, looking at a tree, observe only the name and form. The tree can be cut down, and, to the observer, is no more. The essence still remains, since another tree is evolved from the seed. When we learn to see the essence beyond external things, we banish illusion. All religions and philosophies teach this; if we cannot accept it, it is because we have not the capacity. The "spiritual tramp" who wanders from religion to philosophy is lost in name and form; he can not find the essence which was to be found in the very first religion he attempted. The essence can be discovered only by direct perception, and Yoga gives us the means.

The Yogi is not selfish when he retires from the world; the world of illusion (name and form) in which we live, tears down what the Yogi builds; thus, he seeks those who will stimulate and vitalize him. The developed soul manifests joyous vibrations, giving joy to those surrounding him; therein lies his own happiness.

MAY 8, 1939

The body has cravings so that it will keep healthy and living. We feel hungry, because, if we should not eat, we should sicken and die. All other physical indulgence[s] are just as simple. While we are seeking happiness, we cannot give happiness to others; it is only after we have found it that we can give it out. An old saying explains that because the King of the land had everything, he needed to give no attention to himself, and could be good to his people. So with the Yogi, who may be called a spiritual king; having happiness, he can devote himself to helping others.

The Bodhisattva (the perfected soul), having earned the right, [m]ay choose whether he will go on, or stay and help others. Since the Bodhisattva lives in universal consciousness, he doesn't wish to leave this plane until others have been helped. Christ is a soul who "arrived," came back to teach, and then went on. When the Bodhisattva comes back to this plane of consciousness, he comes again within the scope of its laws. There are laws in the realm of Bodhisattvas as well; as there are in every realm of consciousness. There is no great spiritual leader today; in the East, Gandhi comes closest; there is no one in the West; our consciousness does not seem to be directed that way.

There is nothing we can do about the wheel of life; we are chained to it; but instead of using it as a symbol, we can learn to use it in our every day life. The Tibetan philosophy divides it into six compartments, each compartment symbolizing a realm of consciousness:

Realm of Bodhisattvas—those who have "arrived"
Realm of Titans—not quite "arrived"
Realm of humankind
Realm of animals
Realm of hells—hot and cold
Realm of spirits.

Consciousness goes on after physical death, although not manifesting through a physical vehicle. In the realm of spirits, the consciousness must work off what has not yet been purified. [The Tibetans picture the greedy man in the realm of spirits as having an enormous stomach, and a neck so small that a pea can't get through.] We can develop if we live with understanding and free ourselves from our weaknesses.

There are many things about us of which we are not aware. If we could have a chart of our lives, we could analyze and really see ourselves. Certain incidents seem to happen to us all the time, forming a certain pattern; we should search deeply and try to understand why this is. Sometimes they may be due to uncontrolled energy, and by developing calmness, we could change the pattern.

Money and sex are the motivating forces in the life we lead today. Our emotional relationships begin so pleasantly and easily, but soon we find trivialities become irritating. That is being concerned unduly with name and form. One may like classical music, and one a brass band. Understanding that this is a clue to the emotional nature within, we can avoid being lost in name and form. It explains why we gravitate to people of the same emotional nature, although their external characteristics seem not at all to be what we think we like. When emotional relationships are unsatisfactory, the weakness is in ourselves; lack of understanding.

Let us not follow name and form; let us learn to get at the essence of things. Truth is not to be found in what people say. Let us learn to search for that which is behind the words. Know people with your consciousness; not with your mind.

MAY 9, 1939

How to be "smart"?

Nobody can give us the answer to that question. Suddenly at some future date, we will find the answer, never knowing how it happened, and never being able to tell anyone else about it. Each ego is a complete universe in itself, and the gap between two egos can be bridged only by symbols, i.e., name and form. Now we are acquiring knowledge of the Yogic philosophy of consciousness, and the problem is to apply it in order to avoid the long, arduous path of hard knocks. Yoga in its truest essence is to see life intuitively. First purify the instrument; the intelligence is so delicate and precise that we are always in danger of getting lost in it. Let us develop our feelings, and then our knowledge will be of use. When great scientists grow older, and are preparing themselves for old age and death, they usually grow philosophical and idealistic.

The Yogi knows that true knowledge is in the heart, not in the head. He knows that when a problem needs solution, the answer is in his consciousness, and by working at breathing and head stand, the consciousness will divulge the answer.

Reviewing and recalling our past experiences with understanding, getting them into our consciousness, we can begin to get realization, and in that way, lay out our future in a much better way.

Reveal Yoga only to a teacher or a fellow student. Revealing it to the outside world is manifesting pride. Learn to manifest Yoga by not doing what is expected of you; doing the expected is a manifestation of ego alone.

Therefore, if you want to be "smart," do nothing concrete. The smartness will manifest itself.

MAY 18, 1939

Why have religion?

All life is consciousness, and carrying that idea to its conclusion, nothing at all exists. Yoga calls the existence we know, Maya (illusion); consciousness alone lasts forever, and neither men, societies nor mechanical things last forever. The young boy should be taught that the most important thing for him is to find some way to enable the forces within him to manifest. Instead, he is taught that the profession or business he chooses is the most important thing in the world. But we see that professions change and forms change. A good profession of 50 years ago no longer exists, and new professions spring up today that were unheard of fifty years ago. We see that these forms are merely Maya and exist for society alone. Society functions to give man leisure time, but fails to teach him how to use his leisure to get acquainted with himself. People in action, using a full flow of consciousness, understand the unimportance of forms; they know there is something more to life, and they turn to religion to learn how to direct that flow of consciousness back to its original source. Consciousness makes the human being aware; he strives, not knowing why. If a child is abandoned all alone on a desert island, and can survive, in 20 or 30 years he will have religious feeling, though no-one has ever told him anything. Our life is a constant effort to establish contact with the ultimate source, and if we lose sight of that goal, we are frustrated and unhappy. The man who is in tune with himself (God) knows that nothing that happens to his body can matter. The church is Maya in one sense of the word, but for the understanding man, it is one pathway to consciousness. The most dynamic way to find knowledge of reality is through feeling, and the church can serve in that respect. The Yogi has no need for religion, because he knows how to contact reality; he prepares the body for the breath, and then works with the breath. Breathing exercises help us to get in contact with the rhythm of life; although in the beginning we retain awareness of ourselves, later, we lose ourselves in it, and find consciousness. We cannot tell anyone about it until we have "arrived," and even then we can't put it into words, because it is beyond the mind. We want to help others get the same understanding; most people can learn only through feeling, and they require something concrete, therefore devices have to be used to arouse it.

Explaining astral body: Mrs. Blavatsky had understanding, but knowing that it was impossible to give the masses philosophy, she gave them name and form. After the student has "arrived," lost in the light completely unaware of externals, he finds he can leave them behind. That is what is meant by astral body. After such an experience, you will never fear death, knowing what it is to leave the externals. Nor will you commit suicide, understanding that the problem must be solved, and killing the body does not annihilate the consciousness, and the problem still remains to be worked out. (In cases of incurable illness, only a full understanding could justify suicide.)

Religion is therefore merely a device to enable people to have feeling. Today it is almost impossible to find the meaning behind the forms. Let a new symbol come along, behind which we can find meaning and understanding, and there is our new religion.

Selection *from Letter written by Sukumar Chatterji to Glen Bernard, July 19, 1936* (from unpublished Theos Bernard Papers on the vajrolī-mudrā)

Regarding Bajroli—this is what I have—one school claims that it is not for women and only men, specially celibates should practice it. Another school known as Weerachari [Vīrācārī] Tantriks, claim that it is specifically meant for married persons who practice it with their wives, thereby interchanging each other's powers.

The blowing [of air into the bladder] is meant for the beginner and occasionally when proper function does not take place of suction owing to some watery or slimy liquids in the canal.

Just as water is sucked with or without Naoli [*nauli*] thru the rectum and a tube is used but when sufficient practice is done no tube [is] required but—if the water does not go in then finger is inserted to clean the passage. Same purpose is served by blowing in the bladder. Also there is an involuntary muscle which causes seminal discharge after Wajroli [*vajrolī*]; that muscle becomes voluntary and brain can control it.

There is no book which gives any detail but there are instructions imparted by word of mouth which I have carefully collected. The blowing of air in urethra as well as in the rectum is mentioned in one place to enable a person to control the air (Wayu [*vāyu*]) there with the breath. As shown, Wayu is situated below, it must be controlled by breath or Mudras or naoli & such.

It is to be practiced like all processes early in the morning and it takes from 3 to 6 months to complete it. The completion means the sucking of mercury. After which one can suck water, milk, honey, etc. without a tube and even when erection takes place. Another mention is made of introducing filtered oily medicines in the rectum and bladder for various purposes. Main function tho seems to be to be able to suck one's own and the wife's semen back into the urethra, both the semens being reabsorbed into the body from the pores. Also a mention is made to practice it just before discharge and how on doing it, so that no semen is discharged at all.

The followers of Gorakshanath practice it early in the morning and at midnight, as they sleep early in the evening and at noon and keep awake all night to forenoon.

—21—

Universalist and Missionary Jainism: Jain Yoga of the Terāpanthī Tradition

Olle Qvarnström and Jason Birch

From the early Christian era to the twelfth century, Jainism was a proselytizing religion with no universalistic claims. According to both its main sects, the Śvetāmbara ("White-Clad") and the Digambara ("Sky-Clad"), the Jain dharma or teaching could only be beneficially practiced by persons belonging to the Jain religion and living in different parts of India; and mendicants were not allowed to travel by any means of transportation other than their own bare feet. By the end of the twelfth century, mainly as a result of the expansion of Hindu theistic traditions and the increasing presence of Islam, proselytizing activities markedly declined.

As a result of various schisms centered around the issue of "true" ascetic practice, a number of Jain reform movements developed from the fifteenth century onward. Within the Śvetāmbara tradition, Ācārya Bhikṣu (1726–1803) founded the Terāpanthī, one of three non–image worshipping Śvetāmbara sectarian traditions. Ācārya Bhikṣu was, as noted by Paul Dundas, a reformist who adopted a "radical interpretation of Mahāvīra's doctrine," and in so doing, dismissed many traditional Jain religious practices as "buying merit." Ācārya Bhikṣu was also more interested in self-discipline, correct understanding, and maintaining the ascetic way of life. He thus emphasized the distinction between the ascetic and householder in an attempt to prevent ascetics from becoming "worldly." At the heart of his concern was a strict adherence to "nonviolence" (*ahiṃsā*) for the ultimate purpose of purifying the Self.

His successor, Acarya Tulsi (1914–1997), modernized the Śvetāmbara Terāpanthī sect and transformed it from an austere Indian monastic order into a global religion that expounds upon secular life, morals, education, social reform, and so on. To implement this, he established the *Jain Vishva Bharati Institute* at Ladnun, in the western Indian state of Rajasthan. The modernization of the Terāpanthī tradition was carried on and amplified by Acarya Mahaprajna (1920–), the tenth and current mendicant leader of the Śvetāmbara Terāpanthī sect. Acarya Mahaprajna interpreted Jainism in the light of contemporary society and modern scientific knowledge. He also contributed to the editing of the Terāpanthī version of the Śvetāmbara canonical scriptures as well as to the *aṇuvrat* (small-vow) movement initiated by Acarya Tulsi for the implementation of non-violence and morality in social life. In 1980, Acarya Mahaprajna established the *Science of Living* in order to promote non-violent living in schools and universities. His greatest legacy, however, is as the rediscoverer or reinventer of Jain meditation and yoga. In recognition of this, his predecessor, Acarya Tulsi, conferred on him the epithet *Jainayogapunaruddhāraka*, "the rebuilder of Jain Yoga."

As mentioned, mendicants of both main traditions, Śvetāmbara and Digambara, were not allowed to travel by mechanical transportation. In the post-canonical *Tattvārthasūtra* (AD 150–350), which was the first attempt to systematize Jain canonical teachings into a philosophical system (thus holding the same position in Śvetāmbara Jainism as that of the *Yoga Sūtra* in the Yoga tradition), travel on foot (*caryā*) is listed among the "endurances" (*parīṣaha*) that prevents deviation from the spiritual path and wears off accumulated karma (9.8). The prohibition against non-foot travel was, however, challenged during the twentieth century when Jain mendicant teachers or *ācārya*s either transgressed this rule or introduced new categories of novices who were permitted to use public transport as well as accept food that had been specially prepared for them. The most visible among those who broke mendicant rules and traveled to the west was Acarya Citrabhanu (1922–) of the Śvetāmbara image-worshipping (*mūrtipūjaka*) tradition, and Sushil Kumar (1926–1994) of the Sthānakavāsī sect. Citrabhanu established in 1971 the *Jain Meditation International Center* in New York, while Kumar founded the *Arhum Yoga System* in the United States in 1975. Acarya Tulsi, on the other hand, introduced a new type of male and female mendicant called *samaṇ* and *samaṇī*, respectively—an intermediate category between laypeople and monks and nuns—thereby opening the door for the emergence of a universalistic and missionary Jainism, especially in the United States. Jain doctrine and practice were not only made available outside of India by this new type of religious specialist, but more importantly, were interpreted and practiced in ways that deviated from orthodox Jainism and that shared certain elements with Buddhism, as interpreted by western scholars and Buddhist practitioners from the late nineteenth century onward. Peter Flügel has labeled this form of Jainism as "Jain modernism," in line with the German Indologist Heinz Bechert's term "Buddhist modernism." Based on field research among Gujarati Jains in Britain, Marcus Banks has called it "Jain neo-orthodoxy." A similar modernistic development was also evident among various religious thinkers in India during the latter half of the nineteenth century, notably in the person of Vivekananda, who claimed that Hinduism was a universal religion applicable to all cultures and periods. Since his time, this idea of a universal and missionary Hinduism has established itself in the West through new religious movements, various missionary activities, immigration, and a general influence of Indic currents of ideas.

The Terāpanthī sect has about 500,000 followers at present scattered across India and Nepal, the United Kingdom, and the United States. It is spreading rapidly worldwide by virtue of modern means of communication and the influence of the missionary activities of the *samaṇ*s and *samaṇī*s. In the following, we will examine an interesting development in Jain Modernism: the yoga system of the Śvetāmbara Terāpanthī sect, which was created by Acarya Mahaprajna in the second half of the twentieth century. We base our discussion on his books on *prekṣā* meditation as well as on interviews with Terāpanthī Samaṇīs and experienced lay practitioners in London.

The "Jain Yoga" of the Terāpanthī Tradition

The "Jain Yoga" of the Terāpanthī tradition is a combination of physical yoga techniques, such as postures (*āsana*s) and breathing exercises (*prāṇāyāma*), and a system of meditation (*prekṣādhyāna*). The Terāpanthī monk, Muni Kishan Lal, has explained their physical yoga in an instruction manual entitled "Yoga Postures and Health." *Prekṣā* meditation was created by the current Terāpanthī leader, Acarya Mahaprajna, who has written a series of books on the philosophical and scientific basis of his system of meditation, as well as its raison d'être, techniques, and benefits.

Over the centuries, the Jains have displayed a remarkable ability to integrate ideas from other traditions, and the Terāpanthīs are no exception, having combined a medley of practices from different Indian yoga traditions. Most of the postures and breathing exercises derive from traditional *haṭha yoga*, though the way they are performed and explained has been influenced by Western science and exercise systems. These are practiced in conjunction with *prekṣā* meditation, which is a combination of the traditional Jain practice of *kāyotsarga* (abandoning the body) and meditation techniques that appear to have been inspired by modern Buddhist Vipassanā, simple Tantric visualizations, and

Western relaxation therapy. On the whole, this system of yoga is much broader in its scope of practice and theory than most of the systems that are popular in the West today.

The Terāpanthīs avail themselves of a repertoire of more than fifty postures, the majority of which can be traced back to the *haṭha yoga* texts and unpublished manuscript sources listed in Gharote's *Encyclopedia of Traditional Āsanas.* By using this encyclopedia, one can trace twenty-nine of the forty floor poses in the Terāpanthīs' *āsana* manual to pre-twentieth-century sources, but only two of the ten standing poses. This confirms that the latter are late innovations. Indeed, the flowing sequences similar to the *sūryanamaskār* (named *aṣṭavandanāsana* by the Terāpanthīs) and coordinating movements with the breath appear to have been inspired by late developments in modern Indian yoga, which, as Mark Singleton has shown, was influenced by Western physical culture and exercise regimes. A few practices, such as *ardhaśankhaprakṣālana* (i.e., drinking salt water while performing gentle postures), are almost identical to those described in Swami Satyananda's *Āsana Prāṇāyāma Mudrā Bandha.*

It is important to note that the Terāpanthīs' Hindi instruction manual also quotes Sanskrit verses from such *haṭha* texts as the *Haṭhapradīpikā*, and paraphrases other verses, thus including many of the same instructions and discussions of the demonstrable benefits of the postures (for example, the greater steadiness, lightness, beauty, elegance of the body, etc.) as one finds in many *haṭha* texts. In fact, the link between traditional *haṭha yoga* and modern Indian yoga appears to be based on the inspiration modern Indian gurus have derived from the *haṭha* texts, and many gurus have published their own Hindi and English translations of them. Though it is uncertain whether early *haṭha yoga* ever developed more than the fifteen postures described in the *Haṭhapradīpikā* (ten of which date back to the twelfth- to thirteenth-century CE *Vasiṣṭhasaṃhitā*), the earliest texts, such as the *Vivekamārtaṇḍa* (eleventh to twelfth century CE), point to the possibility of innumerable *āsana*s; and several of the *āsana*s in the *Vasiṣṭhasaṃhitā* are advanced postures requiring an exceptional degree of spinal extension (*dhanurāsana*), spinal flexion (*paścimottānāsana*), twisting (*matysendrāsana*), strength, and balance (*mayūrāsana*). It is, of course, possible that these were considered the most important postures, and that other, intermediate *āsana*s were not mentioned. However, it is more likely that there was a proliferation of *āsana*s from the seventeenth century onward, with a list of eighty-four *āsana* names appearing in the *Haṭharatnāvalī*, and eighty-four described in the *Jogapradīpyakā*. Yet, further research is needed to determine the extent of this proliferation prior to the twentieth century, because there remains a substantial amount of unpublished manuscript material on *āsana* in Indian libraries that has not been properly examined. Specific examples include the eighteenth-century *Yogāsanamālā* (describing 108 āsanas with 90 illustrations); the *Āsanayoga or Kapāla-kuranṭaka-haṭhābhyāsapaddhati* (describing 112 *āsana*s and noted as "very old" in Kaivalyadhama's catalogue of yoga manuscripts); and the *Āsananāmāni* (mentioning 500 *āsana*s)—but one can also find, in various catalogues, manuscripts with titles such as *āsanalakṣaṇam*, *āsananirūpaṇa*, *āsanāni*, *āsanavidhi* and so forth, that may shed further light on the history of *āsana*.

The extent of the influence of the *haṭha yoga* tradition on the Terāpanthīs' yoga can be seen in their repertoire of *prāṇāyāma*, which is very similar to that of the *Haṭhapradīpikā* and eighteenth-century *Gheraṇḍa Saṃhitā*. They teach eight types of breath retention (*kumbhaka*), namely, opening the sun channel, i.e., the right nostril (*sūryabhedī*), alternative nostril breathing (both the *anulomaviloma* and *samavṛtti* variations), the cooling breath (*śītalī* or *śītakārī*), breathing with noise (*ujjāyī*), humming (*bhrāmarī*), bellows breath (*bhastrikā*), remaining without inhalation and exhalation (*kevalī*), and swooning (*mūrcchā*). Some other techniques have been included for beginners, such as lengthening the breath without retention (*dīrghaśvāsa*) and opening the moon channel, i.e., left nostril (*candrabhedī*). Apart from a few minor differences, such as redefining the swooning breath (*mūrcchā*) as fixing the gaze (*śāmbhavīmudrā*) during a breath retention, the Terāpanthīs' instructions on these techniques are in keeping with those of the *Haṭhapradīpikā*. The Samaṇīs (interviewed for this chapter) were familiar with all these breathing techniques, but said that they practiced only those varieties that most suited their needs, which, in their case, happened to be *sūryabhedī* (to counter the cold, damp weather of the UK) and *anulomaviloma* (for keeping the nervous system balanced amid their busy schedules).

If one attends a public yoga class at the Jain Vishva Bharati center in London, one might think that their yoga is exclusively devoted to practicing simple postures and alternate nostril breathing. However, these classes are designed to accommodate beginners, and it is clear from the interviews that the Samaṇīs incorporate more advanced techniques into their self-practice, including five of the traditional hathayogic *mudrā*s. These *mudrā*s were the most salient feature of traditional *haṭha yoga* and, unlike the *mudrā*s of earlier Tantric systems, they combine breath retention with posture (e.g., *mahāmudrā*, *mahāvedha*, etc.) while others lock or block a specific area of the body (e.g., *jālandharabandha* and *khecarīmudrā*), in order to force *kuṇḍalinī* to rise. The exclusion of these *mudrā*s from the Terāpanthīs' instruction manual on physical yoga stands in stark contrast to a traditional *haṭha* text such as the *Haṭhapradīpikā*, which devotes a separate chapter and nearly a quarter of its verses to them. In many systems of Modern Postural Yoga (as defined by Elizabeth De Michelis), most of these *mudrās* are no longer the focus of practice, but some of them (namely, the *bandhas*) are used while performing *āsana* and *prāṇāyāma*. This appears to be the case in the Terāpanthī Sect, because the Samaṇīs revealed that they apply both the root lock (*mūlabandha*) and throat lock (*jālandharabandha*) during breath retentions, and it is worth noting that they do not use the third lock (*uḍḍiyānabandha*) in *prāṇāyāma* (unlike the *Haṭhapradīpikā*, 2.45–46), but rather practice it separately as an *āsana* (i.e., *uḍḍiyānāsana*). The Samaṇīs report that only some advanced Terāpanthī Yogīs perform inversions (*viparītakaraṇī*) such as the head-stand (*śīrṣāsana*) and shoulder-stand (*sarvāṅgāsana*), whereas both monastic and lay Terāpanthīs practice a modified version of *khecarīmudrā*, where the tongue is turned back and upward, to press on the palate. Unlike the traditional *khecarīmudrā*, this version does not require that the frenum be cut because the tongue is not pushed into the nasopharyngeal cavity. The Samaṇīs claim that this modified version controls anger and inhibits discursive thinking before meditating.

In promoting the health benefits of *āsanas* and *prāṇāyāma*, the Terāpanthīs use a great deal of anatomical and scientific language. Most of the emphasis is on the physiological and psychological benefits of each technique. In fact, the instruction manual appears to be concerned with detailing the effects of each pose on the nervous system (i.e., the spine and internal organs) and the endocrine system (i.e., the glands). The physiological detail underlies the therapeutic possibilities of each technique. For example, a pose called *ardhamatsyendrāsana* (a seated twist) benefits the stomach, lungs, spine, gonads, adrenals, thymus, and thyroid glands and is prescribed for diabetes. There is a common belief that yoga was once a spiritual discipline without therapeutics, and that efforts to cure diseases through yoga is a new development. However, this ignores the fact that sickness was viewed as an obstacle to yoga as far back as Patañjali (*Yoga Sūtra* 1.30) and the therapeutic application of *āsana* is evident in the traditional *haṭha* texts, even the earliest, such as the *Vivekamārtaṇḍa*, which affirms: "Through *āsana*, diseases are removed" (2.11). This theme grew in prominence, and such later *haṭha* texts as the *Ṣaṭkarmasaṅgraha* and the fifth chapter of the *Haṭhapradīpikā* (in Kaivalyadhāma's edition) describe specific methods for overcoming a variety of different illnesses. Rather than "medicalizing" yoga, the Terāpanthīs and many Modern Indian yoga schools appear to be using medical and scientific knowledge to elaborate on a traditional aspect of *haṭha yoga*.

In a sense, the way the Terāpanthīs have adopted *haṭha yoga* reveals much about the history of *haṭha yoga* itself. Had it relied upon a particular tradition or lineage of gurus to perpetuate its teachings, it would have died out centuries ago. Instead, *haṭha yoga* is characterized by the constant adaptation of its techniques to suit the ambitions of yogins among various traditions. For example, in writing the *Haṭhapradīpikā*, Svātmarāma created a new system of practice by integrating a number of earlier systems of yoga (such as the *haṭha yoga* of the *Dattātreyayogaśāstra*, the *vāyu yoga* of the *Amṛtasiddhi*, the *vahni yoga* of the *Vivekamārtaṇḍa*, and so forth). Through its history, *haṭha yoga* has been combined with Advaita Vedānta (e.g., the *Yoga Upaniṣads*), Pātañjala Yoga (e.g., the sixteenth-century *Yogacintāmaṇi* of Śivānanda), and Ayurvedic concepts (e.g., Bhavadevamiśra's *Yuktabhavadeva*). It has also been practiced by a number of India's ascetic traditions (e.g., the Nāths, Rāmānandī Tyāgīs, etc.) as well as more orthodox brahmins (e.g., the *Vasiṣṭhasaṃhitā* and *Yogayājñavalkya*) and householders (e.g., *Śivasaṃhitā* and Godāvaramiśra's *Yogacintāmaṇi*). And in the twentieth century, the techniques of *haṭha yoga* survive in much the same way, as Indian yoga gurus combine them with the science of anatomy and physiology, various exercise regimes, relaxation therapies, physiotherapy, and so on. The survival of its techniques is a testimony to their efficacy and adaptability, and it is clear that the Terāpanthīs have adopted *haṭha yoga* in the same spirit. They regard *āsana*s as a necessary preparation for meditation, and the Samaṇīs report that yoga enables them to more successfully cope with the demands of their ascetic way of life. For example, *prāṇāyāma* can be used to alleviate thirst and hunger and this assists them to abide by their vow to fast daily from sunset until sunrise (which is a sixteen-hour interval during UK winters). The Samaṇīs claim that physical yoga also increases their pain threshold, which would certainly be an advantage when having their hair ritually plucked out (as an expression of their determination to successfully meet the rigorous demands of the ascetic life) and in wearing the same clothing all year round (indeed, they use the heating and cooling practices of *prāṇāyāma* to cope with this). Moreover, the capacity of physical yoga techniques to build strength of will and to quell passions such as anger, frustration, lust, greed, etc., enables the Terāpanthī monks to maintain their strict rules of conduct.

In their efforts to promote Jainism beyond the borders of India, the Terāpanthīs' knowledge of yoga has aided their missionary efforts. By promoting their yoga as a universal practice beneficial to all Jains and non-Jains alike, the public yoga class serves as a meeting place, so to speak, for people of all religions as well as the non-religious. Shankar Lal Mehta, director of the Tulsi Adhyatma Nidam, writes, "*Prekṣā*-dhyāna can be learnt and practiced by anybody without distinction of caste, colour, country and creed. There is no communal or theological bias, nor does it insist on any particular theological belief." By fostering harmony among diverse people and helping individuals through yoga, the Jain center has become prominent in the community, and this has generated interest from local people in the center's philosophy classes and religious activities.

Meditation in the Terāpanthī Tradition

The Terāpanthīs' system of meditation, *prekṣādhyāna*, is understood to mean the "meditation of seeing carefully and profoundly." It is not concerned with external perception, but rather looking inwards—as Acarya Mahaprajna says, "to perceive and realize the most subtle aspects of consciousness by your own conscious mind." It is a system of practice that consists of the following eight components (with Acarya Mahaprajna's translations):

1. Kāyotsarga (Total Relaxation)
2. Antaryātrā (The Internal Trip)
3. Śvāsaprekṣā (Perception of Breathing)
4. Śarīraprekṣā (Perception of Body)
5. Caitanyakendraprekṣā (Perception of Psychic Centers)
6. Leśyadhyāna (Perception of Psychic Colors)
7. Bhāvanā (Auto-Suggestion)
8. Anuprekṣā (Contemplation)

Unlike their physical yoga, *prekṣā* meditation is grounded more firmly in Jain tradition because it begins with the practice of *kāyotsarga* (literally, the "abandonment of the body"). *Kāyotsarga* was defined by Hemacandra (1089–1172 CE), the great exalter (*prabhāvaka*) of Śvetāmbara Jainism, as follows:

> The position in which one is indifferent towards the body [and in which] one is either seated or standing with both the arms hanging down, that is called kāyotsarga. (*Yogaśāstra* 4.133)

In both the Digambara and Śvetāmbara traditions of Jainism, *kāyotsarga* is one of the six obligatory duties of a mendicant (and a recommended practice for a layperson). This means that Jain ascetics were required to practice it daily, even though it was probably not performed separately but as an "adjunct" to the other rites. The Terāpanthīs tend to practice *kāyotsarga* either standing or in a seated position such as lotus (*padmāsana*), simple cross-legged (*sukhāsana*), or kneeling (*vajrāsana*). If seated, they place the hands on the knees, palms turned upward with the tip of the index fingers and thumbs touching, in a gesture called *jñānamudrā*. The spine is held upright, the eyes closed, and the posture free of strain. The practice begins with the recitation of the Sanskrit word *arhaṃ* nine times, thus venerating the "worthy" ones (*arhat*s) or Jinas. Then, the practitioner focuses on remaining motionless, alert, and free of muscular tension for the duration of the exercise. This involves scanning all parts of the body in a meticulous way, starting from the big toe and ending with the head. When breathing becomes minimal and the whole body completely relaxed, *kāyotsarga* is attained, and one may continue on to the other components of *prekṣā* meditation. *Kāyotsarga* is said to be "an essential precondition" and without it, the other components are inaccessible.

Acarya Mahaprajna explains *kāyotsarga* from both scientific and soteriological standpoints. In scientific language, he refers to it as the relaxation response and quotes from the work of the Swiss Nobel Laureate, Walter Hess, and the American cardiologist, Herbert Benson, who defined relaxation according to physiological conditions. Acarya Mahaprajna attributes the "healing power" of *kāyotsarga* to the "balancing" and "replenishing" effects it has on the nervous and endocrine systems. He believes that many illnesses, such as hypertension, are caused by the stress of modern living and he presents *kāyotsarga* as the "potent remedy" for them. He concludes that relaxation bestows physical, mental, and emotional well-being.

From a soteriological viewpoint, *kāyotsarga* is a means to "self realization." When the relaxation response has occurred and the body is free of movement and tension, then it is possible to "abandon the body" and see that the true, eternal Self is separate from the body. Acarya Mahaprajna writes, "total relaxation is that condition in which the separateness of the body and the soul is no longer a belief but a real experience. The awareness of the real Self apart from the body, apart from the tribulations, apart from the emotions and excitement is the real purpose of *kāyotsarga*."

Seen as a "simulation of death," *kāyotsarga* aims at affirming the Jain belief that the "real" Self is untouched by death and suffering. The relaxed state becomes a vantage point from which the practitioner can see that the root cause of suffering is, in fact, the subtle body (*karma śarīra*) because it keeps the gross body in a state of perpetual motion and agitation, thereby increasing the karmic matter that binds the Self. The stillness of relaxation loosens the grip of the subtle body over the gross, and opens the way for purification.

Acarya Mahaprajna's definition of *kāyotsarga* as the relaxation response is certainly another instance of his use of scientific terminology to explain a traditional teaching and to promote its health benefits. Singleton has argued convincingly that the "rotation of awareness" technique in Swami Satyananda's method of *yoganidrā* (which is similar to the method of scanning the body in *prekṣā* meditation) was adapted from Western relaxation methods such as Jacobson's *Progressive Muscle Relaxation*, Schultz's *Autogenic Training*, and Vittoz's *Brain Control Method*. Acarya Mahaprajna's scientific discussion on *prekṣā* appears to be no exception to this, and it has absorbed some of the ethos of Western "relaxationism," which Singleton identifies as discourse on the stress of modern living, the crippling effects of stress, and the panacean benefits of relaxation.

The willingness demonstrated by the creators of modern Indian yoga to incorporate Western innovations such as relaxation therapy can be explained to some extent by the similarities of these practices to traditional yoga techniques. The practice of rotating one's awareness or scanning the body is akin to the hathayogic technique of *pratyāhāra* described in the *Vasiṣṭhasaṃhitā*, the fourteenth- to fifteenth-century *Yogayājñavalkya* and the seventeenth-century *Yuktabhavadeva*, where the yogin mentally moves *prāṇa* from one vital point to another in a specific sequence that starts at the crown of the head and finishes at the big toes. The *Yogayājnavalkya* states that this practice is a means for destroying all diseases (7.21), purification from all vice, and ensuring a long life (7.31).

Acarya Mahaprajna has succeeded in combining the ethos of relaxationism with Jain soteriological aims in order to express the benefits of the practice in terms that would satisfy the monastic community of Terāpanthīs as well as its lay people. Indeed, the creators of modern Indian yoga may well believe that they have done the same, because beneath the rhetoric of relaxationism is the efficacy of its techniques for inducing the physiological conditions of profound meditative states. In teaching students to sit comfortably, release muscular tension, and remain still until the breath becomes subtle, Acarya Mahaprajna is following the fundamentals of many traditional Indian systems of meditation. The Jains incorporated such techniques through the work of Hemacandra, who borrowed verses from an earlier yoga text entitled *Amanaskayoga*, which describes the following practice:

> In an isolated, solitary, clean and beautiful place, the yogin sits comfortably on an even seat, having leaned slightly back [on something, for support]. The yogin, whose limbs are placed comfortably, who is very resolute, very still [and] whose gaze is held [on an empty space] the measure of an arm's length (in front), should practice [thus]. The yogin whose whole body is held relaxed from the tuft of hair on the crown of [his] head to the tip of [his] toenails, is free from all thoughts and movement, both internally and externally. (2.49–51)

The *Amanaskayoga* also reports the accompanying drop in the rate of respiration to the point where it disappears (AY 1.46), the abatement of thirst and hunger, a reduction in body temperature (AY 1.37), urine and feces, and greater softness of the body (i.e., reduced muscle tension) (AY 1.50), which are consistent with Benson's observations of a decreased rate of breathing and metabolism during the relaxation response. Just as Hemacandra adapted such yoga techniques to modernize Jainism at a time of great innovation in medieval yoga systems, so too Acarya Mahaprajna and other modern Indian yoga teachers have borrowed relaxation techniques for their broad appeal and efficacy in achieving traditional aims.

In the system of *prekṣā* meditation, *kāyotsarga* is followed by a series of meditative exercises that combine visualization techniques, manipulation of the breath, and auto-suggestion within the framework of an "insight" meditation practice. The visualization techniques are based on the Tantric physiology of psychic centers, which Acarya Mahaprajna refers to as "*kendra*s" rather than the term "*cakra*s" used by modern yoga schools. The use of psychic centers in the Jain tradition is not new, and can be traced back to the notion of *sandhi* (a point of connection in the body) in canonical texts such as the *Ācārāṅgasūtra*. In his *Yogaśāstra* (4.76–77), Hemacandra describes a meditation practice involving five "lotuses" (in the navel, heart, throat, mouth, and head). However, *prekṣā* meditation employs a system of thirteen centers, which includes the standard six (plus the crown of the head) that first appeared in later Kaula Tantra (as David Gordon White notes, in the tenth-century *Kubjikāmatatantra*) and was subsequently mentioned in some *haṭha* texts (such as the *Gorakṣaśataka* and *Śivasaṃhitā*). However, *prekṣā* has an additional six centers in the head, which relate to the senses and specific glands. For example, there is a psychic center at the tip of the tongue (the sense organ of taste) and one at the center of the forehead, which is said to affect the pineal gland.

The Terāpanthī system of thirteen psychic centers is a comprehensive attempt to connect the Tantric subtle body with the nervous and endocrine systems. Early Theosophists such as Leadbeater (1927) and, as Singleton notes, Cajzoran Ali (1928), made similar attempts, as did Sir John Woodroffe in his influential book, *The Serpent Power* (1931). However, there are differences in such opinions. For example, Acarya Mahaprajna aligns the middle of the eyebrows with the pituitary gland, whereas Leadbeater and Woodroffe align it with the pineal gland; and Acarya Mahaprajna aligns the pineal gland with the center of the forehead, whereas Ali and more recently, Mumford (1994) align it with *sahasrāra* (i.e., crown of the head). But such discrepancies have always characterized the subtle body. Tantras and yoga texts stipulate different numbers of *cakra*s, contradictory routes for the central channel (*suṣumnānāḍī*) and so on.

In contrast to elaborate Tantric visualizations of *cakra*s, the Terāpanthīs do not focus on an image, but the "subtle vibrations" produced by the flow of energy (*prāṇa*) in the area of a particular psychic center. Unlike the supernatural powers (*siddhi*s) promised by Tantra and *haṭha yoga*, the higher aims of *prekṣā*'s visualization practices are psychological. For example, the stage called the "internal trip" (*antaryātrā*), in which practitioners move their mind's focus from the base of the spine up to the crown of the head, is said to remove "psychological distortions" such as cruelty, greed, fear, hatred, and so forth, by turning vital energy upward (i.e., away from the sex organs and adrenals) to the higher psychic centers, which nurture virtues such as love, friendship, honesty, etc. The Terāpanthīs do not equate this practice with raising *kuṇḍalinī*, but instead value its role in creating their desired "attitudinal changes and integrated development of personality."

The third stage of *prekṣā*, called "perception of breathing," involves manipulating the breath in order to quell mental activity and to induce the calm needed for the visualization practices. A deliberate slowing of the breath and two types of alternate nostril breathing, the first performed manually by manipulating the nostrils with the fingers and the second performed mentally by alternating the breath through each nostril with the mind, are practiced for several rounds. This *prāṇāyāma* is performed without the three "locks" of *haṭha yoga* (i.e., *jālandharabandha*, etc.), and more closely resembles the descriptions of *prāṇāyāma* in traditions that are older than *haṭha yoga*, such as Patañjali's *Yoga Sūtra* (2.49–52), the *Mahābhārata* (6.26.29; 14.48.4, etc.), several of the Upaniṣads (*Śvetaśvātaropaniṣad*, 2.6–12; *Maitrāyaṇiyopaniṣad*, 6.18–19; etc.), the Dharmaśāstras (*Yājñavalkyasmṛti* 3.200; 3.275–77) and so on.

Another salient feature of *prekṣā* meditation is auto-suggestion (*bhāvanā*), which is listed as a separate stage and incorporated into three other stages, namely *kāyotsarga*, the *leśyādhyāna* (perception of psychic colors), and *bhāvanā* (contemplation). In Acarya Mahaprajna's words, "auto-suggestion or self-hypnosis may be seen as a special kind of hypnosis in which the patient himself controls the process. Auto-suggestion is the basic principle of the technique of relaxation. Each part of the body is relaxed, in turn, by coaxing auto-suggestion."

In Autogenic Training, "auto-suggestion" is used to induce relaxation and to gain a therapeutic aim such as quitting a bad habit, by a series of mental exercises and the repetition of an affirmative statement. This therapeutic use of auto-suggestion has been incorporated into *prekṣā* meditation and other systems of modern Indian yoga, such as Satyānanda Yoga, as Singleton notes. It is understandable that modern Indian yogins, whose traditions have long believed in the power of speech and mantra, would be willing to integrate the practice of repeating a few choice words while deeply relaxed, in light of the scientific authority behind such techniques.

While acknowledging the therapeutic aims of auto-suggestion, Acarya

Mahaprajna has used it extensively to further an aspirant's understanding of Jain doctrine. For example, the practice called "contemplating transitoriness," in which one reflects upon the impermanence of all things (physical, mental, good, bad, etc.) in light of the conscious Self's eternal nature, ends with the repetition of the phrases, the "body is transitory," "sickness is transitory," "mental problems are transitory," and "emotions and passions are transitory." It appears that auto-suggestion is being used here to affirm the anticipated result of the contemplative exercise. The question one might ask is what would be the outcome of this exercise if the aspirant's contemplation did not reveal that all things other than the Self are transitory. It seems that the auto-suggestive statements have been included to ensure the right outcome, regardless of the result of the contemplation. However, it is unlikely that the Terāpanthīs would ever see this as an act of indoctrination. Acarya Mahaprajna equates auto-suggestion with the Sanskrit word, *bhāvanā*, which may mean "to cultivate an attitude of mind or sentiment." Just as Patañjali (1.33) advises a yogin to cultivate feelings of friendliness, compassion, etc., in order to gain clarity of mind, so, Acarya Mahaprajna believes that the main benefit of auto-suggestion is to "produce a strong state of faith" in Jain beliefs that can cure illnesses and alleviate suffering.

In Jainism, the word *bhāvanā* (Digambaras use the term *anuprekṣā*) refers to the twelve themes of contemplation as well as twenty-five observances or supporting practices that strengthen the mendicant vows or *mahāvrata*s. It appears that Acarya Mahaprajna has translated auto-suggestion as *bhāvanā* because its practice is connected with the twelve themes of contemplation, which are attested in the Śvetāmbara Jain canon, systematized in the *Tattvārthasūtra*, and dealt with by Hemacandra as follows:

> Equanimity (*sāmya*) is attained through the state of non-attachment (*nirmamatva*). In order to attain that [state of non-attachment], one should cultivate the twelve themes of contemplation: on impermanence, helplessness, the cycle of transmigration, solitude, the distinction [of the Self and the body], the impurity [of the body], the influx of karmic matter, the stopping [of karmic influx], the elimination of karmic matter, the correctly expounded law, the universe, and the [difficulty of attaining] enlightenment (2.55–56).

The central practices of *prekṣā* meditation have been molded to fit its principal theme, which is encapsulated by the name *prekṣā* (i.e., perception). In particular, four components (perception of breathing, body, psychic centers, and psychic colors) are all concerned with seeing something that one would not normally see. For example, the practice called "perception of the body" aims at "seeing" what is inside the body. It resembles the body-scanning technique outlined in *kāyotsarga*, though its emphasis is on perception of the internal organs, so that the practitioner may "see" that the body is permeated by consciousness. Bodily sensations, which are designated as either pleasant or unpleasant, become the focus of attention. This practice is said to change one's sense of Self by creating a feeling of embodiment, in which the practitioner experiences and knows the Jain tenet that body and Self are separate.

Elements of the previous example as well as some of the slogans that go with it, such as "See the Self thyself" and "Perceive and know," would sound familiar to those who have practiced Buddhist systems of "insight meditation." Peter Flügel has observed that, "under the impression of the success of Goenka's *vipassanā* (meditation) classes in Rajasthan, [Acarya Mahaprajna] introduced a Jain version of insight meditation, *prekṣā dhyāna*, in 1975." There are certainly enough apparent similarities between *prekṣā* and modern *vipassanā* teachings to warrant a comparison. The following description of *vipassanā* by Goenka (at www.dhamma.org) will serve to illustrate this:

> Vipassanā is a way of self-transformation through self-observation. It focuses on the deep interconnection between mind and body, which can be experienced directly by disciplined attention to the physical sensations that form the life of the body, and that continuously interconnect and condition the life of the mind. It is this observation-based, self-exploratory journey to the common root of mind and body that dissolves mental impurity, resulting in a balanced mind full of love and compassion.

Prekṣā meditation appears to compete with *vipassanā* on a number of fronts. Firstly, they both trace back their system of meditation to a "founder." *Prekṣā* is said to be derived from the meditation practiced by the Jain saint, Mahāvīra, who lived around the same time as the historical Buddha. Both claim to be "non-sectarian" and it is worth noting that the main Jain center in Ladnun, Rajasthan, is called a "university." The Terāpanthīs teach *prekṣā* on eight-day retreats, which, like the ten-day Goenka retreats, require the participants to reside on campus and abide by a code of conduct. Both techniques claim to be "observation-based," and *prekṣā* has incorporated perception of the breath and body, the latter of which focuses on seeing bodily sensations and refining this perception until the subtlest sensations are seen. Both claim to bring an end to suffering. Goenka describes *vipassanā* as purifying the mind, and Acarya Mahaprajna says that *prekṣā* purifies the subtle body, which purifies both the subconscious and conscious mind. Though Buddhism is about seeing impermanence in everything, *prekṣā* aims at seeing all that is impermanent, so that the eternal Self is revealed. Both systems exhort practitioners to see these truths for themselves.

There is no doubt that the Terāpanthīs advertise their system with some of the same marketing as Goenka's *vipassanā* meditation. Yet, they also seem to say that *prekṣā* offers a great deal more, because it incorporates *kāyotsarga*, breathing exercises, relaxation techniques, contemplation, and auto-suggestion and is combined with an extensive range of physical yoga practices, whereas the Goenka technique relies solely on the experience of meditation. Indeed, Goenka asks his students to refrain from practicing anything other than *vipassanā* during a retreat, so that they may see its efficacy. Goenka meditation has a powerful simplicity to it and it is free from the metaphysics incorporated into *prekṣā*—such as the thirteen psychic centers, six psychic colors, and an eternal Self—which many Westerners may find difficult to accept. However, the eclectic mix of *prekṣā* has enabled Acarya Mahaprajna to claim a vast array of physical, physiological, psychological, and spiritual benefits and to endorse his claims with an extensive range of textual material (including Patañjali's *Yoga Sūtra*, the *Haṭhapradīpikā*, the *Bhagavad Gītā*, various Jain texts, as well as several scientific research articles).

Conclusion

The definition and semantic range of the term "yoga" in the textual traditions of Jainism, as well as in Jain practice, has changed and widened over time. This change was primarily the result of a historical development consisting in the increasing influence of classical and post-classical brahmanical yoga on both Śvetāmbara and Digambara Jainism. The influence was both of a rhetorical and structural nature and included the integration of practices previously unknown in Jainism, such as the Tantric yoga of various Śaiva provenances. One major reason why Jain authors incorporated these new elements and reformulated the Jain dogma was that they wished to participate in the pan-Indian debate on yoga as well as to contribute to the continuation and development of Jainism. The concept of yoga in the work of these classical Jain authors thus reflected the intertwined relationship with India's broad tradition of yoga as well as Jain innovations in the theory and practice of yoga.

The semantic range of the term "yoga" was further widened in modern times, notably in response to twentieth-century modernity in India, Europe, and the United States. Mendicant teachers such as Acarya Mahaprajna of the Terāpanthī sect constructed a universalistic and missionary Jainism, claiming compatibility with science and encompassing universal values. At its center is

"Jain Yoga," to borrow a term from Acarya Mahaprajna, based on ancient Jain doctrine and practice, but redesigned in accordance with modern forms of Indian yoga and meditative practices stemming from Buddhist *vipassanā* meditation. Alleged scientific and rational elements, along with a focus on meditation and promises of health benefits, are emphasized and conveyed in a medical and scientific language. Accordingly, in order to adapt to western modernistic discourses and to promote what are believed to be universal values, the practice of Jain yoga and meditation was moved out of its monastic context and transformed into a central lay practice. Consequently, it is becoming public property and is appearing in contexts, religious and profane, without any direct connection to Jainism as a religion. In such cases, the focus is on the worldly success and well-being of the individual, in line with the kind of therapy culture prevalent in the West, which highly values the well-being of the individual as well as his or her development toward self-realization and mental perfection. To borrow the analytical nomenclature of Torkel Brekke (in his analysis of the gradual development of the missionary Hinduism of Vivekananda), certain aspects of Jainism, in our case "yoga," have been objectified, individualized, and universalized by the Terāpanthī sect of Mahāprajñā. In other words, they can be separated from their earlier religious and social context, applied principally to the individual, and linked to human nature, opening the door for anyone, anywhere, at any time, to practice "Jain Yoga."

Suggestions for Further Reading

In order to appreciate the "Jain yoga" of the Śvetāmbara Terāpanthī tradition and to place its doctrines and practices accurately in the intellectual tradition from which they arise, as well as relate them to broader intellectual concerns of modern culture, the student is first of all advised to acquire some basic knowledge of Jainism and its development in and outside of India. Among the numerous introductory textbooks on Jainism, Paul Dundas's *The Jains* (London & New York: Routledge, 2002) is a very good introduction, because it emphasizes the importance of historical and geographical context in the attempt to understand the developing nature of the Jain tradition. The student will further advance his or her understanding of Jainism and much of the in-depth information given by Dundas by using Kristi Wiley's excellent and up-to-date *Historical Dictionary of Jainism* (Lanham, MD, Toronto, and Oxford: Scarecrow Press, 2004). The Tantric influence on Jainism prevalent in the Śvetāmbara Terāpanthī tradition, but with historical roots in medieval times, including postures and breathing exercises, physiology of psychic centers, etc., has been discussed by scholars such as Dundas, Cort, and Qvarnström, and is testified in texts like the *Yogaśāstra* of Hemacandra (Olle Qvarnström, *The Yogaśāstra of Hemacandra. A Twelfth Century Handbook on Jainism*, Harvard Oriental Series, Vol. 60 [Cambridge, MA: Harvard University Press, 2002]; Qvarnström, "Jain Tantra: Divinatory and Meditative Practice in the Twelfth-Century *Yogaśāstra* of Hemacandra," in *Tantra in Practice*, edited by David Gordon White [Princeton, NJ: Princeton University Press, 2000], pp. 595–604; and Qvarnström, "Losing One's Mind and Becoming Enlightened. Some Remarks on the Concept of Yoga in Śvetāmbara Jainism and its Relation to the Nāth Siddha Tradition," in *Yoga: The Indian Tradition*, edited by David Carpenter and Ian Whicher [London and New York: RoutledgeCurzon 2003], pp. 130–42).

In addition to acquiring a general knowledge of Jainism, the student is advised to become familiar with traditional *haṭha yoga* and its modern forms. The best overview of the Sanskrit literature on *haṭha yoga* is Christian Bouy's *Les Nātha-Yogin et les* Upaniṣads (Paris: Diffusion de Boccard, 1994). James Mallinson has added much to Bouy's work and has produced the most accurate translations of *haṭha* texts (*Khecarīvidyā* [London: Routledge, 2007]; *Gheraṇḍasaṃhitā* [Yogavidya.com, 2004], and *Śivasaṃhitā* [Yogavidya.com, 2007]). Elizabeth De Michelis (*A History of Modern Yoga: Patañjali and Western Esotericism* [London and New York: Continuum, 2004]) provides valuable guidelines on how to understand Modern Yoga; and Mark Singleton has shown the various ways modern Indian yoga has been influenced by Western culture, exercise regimes, and relaxation therapies (*Yoga Body: The Origins of Modern Posture Practice* [New York: Oxford University Press, 2010], and "Salvation Through Relaxation: Proprioceptive Therapy in Relation to Yoga," *Journal of Contemporary Religion* 20/3, 2005, 289–304).

The study of the "Jain yoga" of the Śvetāmbara Terāpanthī tradition may begin with Acarya Mahaprajna's own texts: *Prekṣā Dhyāna: Theory and Practice*, translated by Muni Mahendra Kumar and Jethalal Zaveri (Ladnun: Jain Vishva Bharati, 2004); the *Science of Living Series* I–X, translated by Muni Mahendra Kumar and Jethalal Zaveri (Ladnun: Jain Vishva Bharati, 1995–2003); and for those proficient in Hindi, *Jaina Yoga* (Curu [Rajasthan]: Adarśa Sahitya Sangha Praksashana, 1997). The Śvetāmbara Terāpanthī tradition has been studied by several Western scholars from a textual and anthropological perspective, notably Nalini Balbir ("Observations sur la Secte Jaina des Terāpanthī," *Bulletin D'Etudes Indiennes* 1 [1983]: 39–45); Anne Vallely (*Guardians of the Transcendent: An Ethnology of a Jain Ascetic Community* [Toronto: University of Toronto Press, 2002]); and the following works by Peter Flügel: "Terapanth Svetambara Jain Tradition," in *Religions of the World: A*

Comprehensive Encyclopedia of Beliefs and Practices, edited by J. Gordon Melton and G. Baumann (Santa Barbara: ABC-Clio, 2002), pp. 1266–67; "Jain Monastic Life: A Quantitative Study of the Terāpanth Śvetāmbara Mendicant Order," *Jaina Studies: Newsletter of the Centre of Jaina Studies* 4 (2009): 24–29; "The Codes of Conduct of the Terāpanth Samaṇ Order," *South Asia Research* 23:1 (2003): 7–53; "Protestantische und Post-Protestantische Jaina-Reformbewegungen: Zur Geschichte und Organisation der Sthānakavāsī I," *Berliner Indologische Studien* 13–14 (2000): 37–103; "The Ritual Circle of the Terāpanth Śvetāmbara Jains," *Bulletin d'Études Indiennes* 13 (1996): 117–76; and "Jain Monastic Life: A Quantitative Study of the Terāpanth Śvetāmbara Mendicant Order," *Jaina Studies* 4 (2009): 24–29.

GLOSSARY OF FOREIGN TERMS

[Unless otherwise indicated, all terms in this glossary are in Sanskrit.]

anusmṛti – "Recollection; remembrance"; in Buddhist meditation, the practice of recalling a deity to consciousness as a means to realizing one's intrinsic Buddha nature; the fifth limb of Buddhist forms of six-limbed yoga.

āsana – "Seated position"; yogic posture in which a practitioner holds himself immobile while practicing breath control and various forms of meditation. *Āsana* is the third limb of *aṣṭāṅga yoga.*

aṣṭāṅga yoga – "Eight-limbed yoga"; term denoting the yoga system of the *Yoga Sūtra*, comprising *yama*; *niyama*; *āsana*; *prāṇāyāma*; *pratyāhāra*; *dhāraṇā*; *dhyāna*, and *samādhi*. *See also* ṣaḍaṅga yoga.

ātmā/ātman – "Soul"; the individual self or soul, which leaves the body upon death; the inner, unchanging, immaterial essence of a living being. *See also* brahman; puruṣa.

avadhūtī – "She Who is Excluded"; a class of "outcaste" women who were the preferred consorts of Buddhist *mahāsiddha* practitioners. In tantric Buddhist mapping of the yogic body, the *avadhūtī* is the subtle central channel, into which *prāṇa* is forced through the emptying of the *lalanā* and *rasanā* side channels. *See also* suṣumnā.

āyurveda – "Science of Longevity"; the classical system of Indian medicine, which was later adapted into Tibetan Buddhism.

bandha – "Lock"; in *haṭha yoga*, a physical technique involving the contraction or constriction of various *nāḍī*s in combination with fixed postures. *See also* mudra.

bhāvanā – "Cultivation"; in Buddhist and Hindu meditation, a form of deep contemplation in which vivid visualization leads to a gnostic identity with a deity or principle. In classical Jainism, the twelve themes of contemplation and the twenty-five observances that strengthen the mendicant vows are called *bhāvanā*; in Jain Terāpanthī *prekṣa* meditation, *bhāvanā* is defined as a form of auto-suggestion or self-hypnosis.

bīja – "Seed"; according to the *Yoga Sūtra*, *bīja*s are the sources of thoughts, but also of the penultimate level of pure concentration (*sa-bīja samādhi*). In Tantra, a *bīja* is a monosyllabic "seed-syllable," the seminal essence of a sacred utterance or formula, which constitutes the energy or essence of the deity it acoustically embodies. *See also* bindu, mantra.

bindu – "Drop, dot, point"; in Indic scripts, the *anusvāra* mark written above a grapheme to denote a nasalization (as in the case of the mantra *oṃ* and the final *-ṃ* of *bīja* mantras); in the enunciation of mantras, the final silence that follows the recitation of a mantra, denoting the highest intensity of meditative focus. In Buddhist Tantra, the four *bindu*s are the subtle bases for the four states of the transmigratory mind, which are incinerated by the *cāṇḍālī*, the "fire of bliss" generated through sexo-yogic practice. See *also* nāda.

bodhisattva – "One Who Possesses the Essence of Enlightenment"; in Mahāyāna and later forms of Buddhism, a deified savior figure, a fully enlightened being who remains in the world in order to release all other creatures from suffering existence.

brahman – "Expansion"; in Hindu metaphysics, absolute Being; the self-existent, eternal, universal soul; the infinite power of beginningless being and becoming. *See also* ātmā/ atman.

buddhi – "Intellect, intelligence"; the capacity to apprehend facts and ideas and to reason about them. In Yoga philosophy, the *buddhi* is the highest of the cognitive faculties to devolve from *prakṛti*, and that faculty by means of which ordinary awareness (*citta*) is caused to cease, allowing for the arising of pure consciousness.

cakra – "Wheel, circle"; one of the energy centers, often reckoned as seven in number, aligned along the spinal column of the yogic body.

cāṇḍālī – "Outcaste Woman"; a class of women who were the preferred consorts of Buddhist *mahāsiddha* practitioners. In Buddhist Tantra, the "fire of bliss" generated through sexo-yogic practice, which incinerates the four "drops" (*binduṣ*), contained in the four *cakra*s. By means of the inner *cāṇḍālī*, the tantric practitioner purifies all of the mind-body constituents of their afflictive and cognitive obsuractions. *See also* kuṇḍalinī.

citta – "Thought"; ordinary experience or awareness; the process of thought; in Yoga philosophy, the functioning of a complex of mind, intellect, and ego, which is suppressed through practice, allowing for the arising of pure consciousness.

darśana – "Seeing, viewing"; a philosophical viewpoint; one of the six systems of orthodox Hindu thought: Sāṃkhya, Yoga, Nyāya, Vaiśeṣika, Mīmāṃsā, and Vedānta.

dhāraṇā – "Fixation; retention"; in the *Mahābhārata*, a "holding meditation" that ensures mental focus. In both *aṣṭāṅga* and *ṣaḍaṅga* yoga, the focusing of attention upon a specific location in space, either within or external to the body. In Buddhist Tantra, *dhāraṇā* is the entrance of the vital energies into the "drops" (*bindu*s) situated in the four *cakra*s, as well as their departure from them. *Dhāraṇā* is the fourth limb of six-limbed yoga and the fifth limb of eight-limbed yoga. *See also* saṃyama.

dharma (Pali: dhamma) – The teachings of a Buddha; the law, doctrine, or ethical precepts of Buddhism; a constituent element of reality; a phenomenon. In Hinduism, *dharma* is right action, duty, morality, or virtue; the complex of religious and social obligations a devout Hindu is required to fulfill.

dhyāna (Pali: *jhāna*; Ardhamagadhi: *jhāṇa*) – Unwavering attention to a single thread of thought, an unbroken flow of the same thought uninterrupted by any extraneous idea; yogic meditation, ritual visualization, inner vision; instructions for visualizing a Tantric deity. In Theravāda Buddhism, *jhāna* signifies a heightened but transient form of awareness akin to trance. In early Jain sources, the *jhāṇa*s were a series of contemplative exercises. *Dhyāna* is the second limb of six-limbed yoga and the sixth limb of eight-limbed yoga. *See also* saṃyama.

guṇa – "Strand"; in the Samkhyan metaphysics undergirding the system of the *Yoga Sūtra*, one of the three qualities, constituent processes, or dynamic strands pervading and constitutive of all levels of materiality (*prakṛti*). These are *sattva* (lucidity; the intelligibility or thinking process), *rajas* (passion; the energizing process), and *tamas* (dark inertia; the objectifying or objectification process).

guru – "Heavy; spiritual parent"; a religious preceptor or teacher; the person from whom a religious practitioner receives initiation and instruction.

haṭhayoga – "Forcible practice"; body of yogic practice that combines postures (*āsana*s), breath control (*prāṇāyāma*), seals (*mudrā*s), and locks (*bandhā*s) to reverse the normal downward flow of energy, fluids, and consciousness in the body, and thereby afford bodily immortality, supernatural powers, and liberation to the practitioner.

iḍā – "Refreshing draught"; in the Hindu mapping of the yogic body, the principal subtle channel, which, identified with the moon, runs the length of the spinal column, to the left of the medial *suṣūmnā* channel. Its homologue in Buddhist body mapping is the *lalanā*. *See also* nāḍī; suṣumnā; piṅgalā.

Iddhi. *See* siddhi.

indriya – "Sense faculty"; in Samkhyan metaphysics, one of the five *jñānendriyas* (sense faculties: smell, taste, touch, sight, hearing) to which are linked five *karmendriyas* (motor faculties: genitals, anus, feet, hands, mouth) as well as the mind (*manas*), the "sixth sense." Through the meditative techniques of *pātañjala yoga*, the *indriyas* become isolated from external stimuli, a primary stage in the disengagement of consciousness (*puruṣa*) from materiality (*prakṛti*).

īśvara – "Master; Lord of Yoga"; a master of yogic practice; in the *Yoga Sūtra*, Īśvara is identified as a distinct form of contentless consciousness (*puruṣa*) that has never been bound to matter, and as such is a model of eternal liberation worthy of devotion and as an object of meditiation. In the *Mahābhārata*, an *īśvara* is an empowered practitioner who has the godlike ability to control entities that are below him.

īśvara-praṇidhāna – "Deep longing for God; Dedication to the Lord of Yoga"; in the *Yoga Sūtra*, meditation on the yogic notion of God, who is visualized as dwelling in the heart.

jāgaraṇ (Hindi) – "Night vigil"; all-night ritualized sessions featuring Hindu devotional songs, often sung by professional musicians, on specific ritual occasions (funerals, weddings) or for purposes of pleasure and entertainment.

Jhāna. *See* dhyāna.

jina – "Conquerer"; title or epithet of a Jain *tīrthaṃkara*, one of the twenty-four saviors of the present world age. Mahāvīra, the sixth-century BCE Jain founder, is the last in this series.

jñāna – "Gnosis"; in Hindu epistemology, non-conceptual, spiritual knowledge of transcendent reality. *See also* prajñā.

kaivalyam – "Isolation"; in *pātañjala yoga*, the meditative isolation of *puruṣa*, consciousness, from *prakṛti*, materiality, which is tantamount to spiritual liberation. *See also* mokṣa.

kriyā – "Action; activity"; in the *Yoga Sūtras*, this term refers to the core practices of asceticism (*tapas*), study (*svādhyāya*), and devotion (*īśvarapraṇidhāna*); as well as to the first five of the eight limbs of *aṣṭāṅga yoga* (the last three limbs are collectively referred to as *saṃyama*). In *haṭha yoga*, a *kriyā* is one of the six preliminary practices undertaken to purify the body prior to *prāṇāyāma*.

kumbhaka – "Pertaining to the Water-pot"; in *haṭha yoga*, the retention of the vital breath below the diaphragm, by stopping the in-breath, closing off the nostrils, and forcing the breaths contained in the *iḍā* and *piṅgala* channels down into the lower abdomen.

kuṇḍalinī – "She Who is Coiled"; in Hindu *haṭha yoga* and Tantra, the female energy that descends through the yogic body to lie coiled in "sleep" in the lower abdomen. Through combined yogic techniques, she is "awakened" and made to rise through the cakras to the cranial vault. In Buddhist Tantra as well as certain Hindu traditions, the term *kuṇḍalī* ("ring") is used. *See also* avadhūtī; śakti.

mahāmudrā – "Great Seal"; in Tantric Buddhism, the direct experience of non-duality, the full and perfect awakening characterized by the gnosis of bliss. In the same tradition, the term is also applied to the sublime consort of the tantric practitioner, who is also identified with the bliss-induced heat arising in the region of the navel due to seminal non-emission in ritual intercourse with a human consort. In the Anuttara Tantras, *mahāmudrā* denotes meditation on empty space or a cloudless sky.

mahāsiddha – "Great Perfected Being"; a highly perfected and accomplished mystic; one of a class of legendary Buddhist tantric practitioners who propagated Tantra throughout South Asia, the Himalayan regions, and Tibet.

manas – "Mind"; the organ of cognition, which is considered to be a bodily sense faculty, a "sixth sense" that registers sense perceptions. These often lead the mind astray, until it is controlled and supplanted by the intellect.

mantra – "Mental device; instrument of thought"; an acoustic formula whose sound shape embodies the energy-level of a deity; a spell, incantation or charm employed in tantric ritual or sorcery.

māyā – "That which is measured out; cosmic illusion"; in nondualist metaphysics, the illusion that impedes human recognition of the unity underlying all apparent multiplicity. In Hindu tantric systems, the generative, procreative power of the divine feminine.

mokṣa – "Release, liberation"; the soteriological goal of Hinduism; definitive liberation from rebirth into the cycle of suffering existence. *See also* nirvāṇa.

mudrā – "Seal"; a ritually instrumental gesture of the hand or body. In *haṭha yoga*, an internal hermetic seal effected through breath control and other techniques. Among the Nāth Yogīs, *mudrās* are the great hoop earrings worn through the thick of the ear. In Buddhist Tantra, *mudrā* is one of the terms used for a male practitioner's female consort. See also *mahāmudrā*.

nāda – "Vibration, reverberation, sound"; in mantra practice, the *nāda* is the reverberation or humming sound that precedes the final fading into silence of an utterance. The fourth *cakra* of the yogic body, called the *anāhata* ("unstruck sound") is the point at which the practitioner begins to hear inner sounds that effect the absorption of his lower cognitive faculties into their divine, transcendent source.

nāḍī – In both Hindu and Buddhist mapping of the yogic body, one of an elaborate network of some 72,000 subtle ducts of the yogic body, through which breath and vital energy are channeled. Of these, the three that run through the center (*suṣumnā*; *avadhūtī*) and along the right (*piṅgalā*; *rasanā*) and left (*iḍā ; lalanā*) sides of the spinal column are most prominent. *See also* avadhūtī; iḍā; piṅgalā; suṣumnā.

nāth (Hindi; Sanskrit *nātha*) – "Master, lord"; member of a tantric order of yogis that traces its origins back to the twelfth-century founder Gorakhnāth, to whom several foundational haṭha yoga texts are attributed. Gorakhnāth and other fully realized members of the Nāth orders are referred to as Nāth Siddhas.

nibbāna. *See* nirvāṇa.

nirodha – "Cessation, stoppage"; in *pātañjala yoga*, the cessation of mental activities leads to the isolation (*kaivalyam*) of consciousness from materiality; in Buddhist meditation traditions, it leads to the extinction of suffering (*nirvāṇa*).

nirvāṇa (Pali: nibbāna) – "Extinction"; the soteriological goal of Buddhism; the definitive cessation of rebirth into suffering existence. *See also* mokṣa.

niyama – The "outer restraints" or personal purificatory ritual practices that comprise the second limb of eight-limbed yoga.

pātañjala – The philosophical system (*darśana*) based upon the fourth-century *Yoga Sūtra* of Patañjali. *Pātañjala yoga* denotes the application of the principles of Patañjali's Yoga philosophy through meditative practice.

piṅgalā – In Hindu yoga systems, principal subtle channel identified with the sun, which runs down the right side of the spinal column. Its homologue, in Buddhist body mapping, is the *rasanā*. *See also* avadhūtī; iḍā; nāḍī; suṣumnā.

prajnā – "Wisdom"; in Buddhist epistemology, non-conceptual, spiritual knowledge of the true nature of reality. *See also* jñana.

prakṛti – "Nature, materiality, feminine matter"; the material world as experienced in ordinary awareness. In Sāṃkhya and Yoga philosophy, the twenty-fourth principle (*tattva*), which encompasses the twenty-three lower principles as well as the three *guṇa*s. *See also* puruṣa; tattva.

prāṇa – "Breath"; the breath that animates and energizes the body, and which serves as the support for mantras and other speech acts. While *prāṇa* is an overarching term for breath, in Āyurveda and other systems it is counted as one of a set of five breaths: located in the heart, it is the up-breath. *See also* pūraka.

prāṇāyāma – "Breath control"; in both *pātañjala* and *haṭha yoga*, the body of techniques for regulating and stilling the breath, as a means to calming the mind. *Prāṇāyāma* is the third limb of six-limbed yoga and the fourth limb of eight-limbed yoga.

pratyāhāra – "Retraction"; the withdrawing and isolation of each of the senses from external stimuli, as a means to calming the mind. *Pratyāhāra* is the first limb of six-limbed yoga and the fifth limb of eight-limbed yoga.

pūraka – "Filling"; in tantric systems, the up-breath that fills the body with air. In *haṭha yoga*, the specific practice of closing the right nostril with the forefinger and drawing up air through the left, and then closing the left nostril and drawing up air through the right. *See also* recaka.

puruṣa – "Man"; the universal person or cosmic man; in Sāṃkhya and Yoga philosophy, the principle of consciousness, which realizes its transcendent subjectivity and intrinsic autonomy from *prakṛti* through meditation; the twenty-fifth and final principle of Samkhyan metaphysics. *See also* prakṛti; tattva.

rājayoga – "Royal yoga"; term used to designate the yoga system of the *Yoga Sūtra*, identified as "classical yoga" by Vivekananda and his successors in the twentieth century.

recaka – "Emptying, purging"; down-breath; in *haṭha yoga*, the practice of emptying of the lungs by expelling the breath out of one of the nostrils. *See also* pūraka.

śabda – "Word"; sound; words; language; primal vibration; the vibrational matrix of sound; the audible expression of thoughts.

sādhana – "Accomplishment; carrying out"; tantric ritual practice, including yoga, meditation, contemplation, visualization, worship, and ritual sex.

ṣaḍaṅga yoga – "Six-limbed yoga"; term denoting the yoga systems of certain Upaniṣads as well as of the Buddhist Tantras, comprising *pratyāhāra*, *dhyāna*, *prāṇāyāma*, *dhāraṇā*, *anusmṛti* (or *tarka*), and *samādhi*.

śakti – "Energy"; in Hindu Tantra, the power of the feminine that enlivens all of existence; the energy of a deity embodied in his female consort; a name of the great Goddess or any one of her subordinate goddesses/energies.

samādhi – "Composition; meditative concentration"; the final limb of practice in both six- and eight-limbed yoga. In the *Yoga Sutra*, *samādhi* is an integrated state of pure contemplation, in which consciousness is aware of its fundamental isolation from materiality, and its own absolute integrity. In Nāth Yogī traditions, a *samādhi* is the tumulus under which a Siddha is interred, seated in yogic posture.

samāpatti – "Coalescence"; term used in the *Yoga Sūtra* to denote the unique and single object encountered through the focused awareness of *samādhi*. There are eight types of *samāpatti*, which correspond to the eight levels of *samādhi*.

sāṃkhya – "Comprehensive Intuition; enumeration"; ancient Indian philosophical system involving a systematic, enumerative contemplation of the entire system of the world. Sāṃkhya metaphysics forms the basis for much of Yoga philosophy, the primary differences being that Sāṃkhya is atheistic (*nirīśvara*), while Yoga is theistic (*seśvara*), and that the meditative practices of Pātañjala Yoga are absent from Sāṃkhya.

saṃnyāsa – "Renunciation"; the fourth and final stage of life of a high-caste male Hindu, in which he renounces ties to family, society, and ritual practice by burning his sacrificial implements which he symbolically "lays up together" (*saṃnyāsa*) inside his body. Cultivating this inner fire of yoga and gnosis becomes the focus of his activity, as he lives a life of a hermit (if not of a forest animal) until his death.

saṃsāra – "Flowing together"; in all South Asian soteriologies, the cycle of transmigration; suffering existence; phenomenal reality.

saṃskāra – "Subliminal impression"; in the *Yoga Sūtra*, *saṃskāra* denotes an impression left in one's unconscious memory after any experience. In non-philosophical contexts, the *saṃskāra*s are ritual acts that transform and perfect the person or object toward which they are directed.

saṃyama – "Perfect discipline"; in the *Yoga Sūtra*, *saṃyama* is the term employed for the three final phases, taken together, of "inner practice": *dhāraṇā*, *dhyāna*, and *samādhi*.

sati. *See* smṛti.

siddha – "Perfected Being"; a tantric practitioner who has realized embodied liberation. In Hindu, Buddhist, and Jain soteriologies, the Siddhas form a class of liberated beings that inhabit the highest reaches of the cosmos, where they remain alive and intact during the cosmic dissolution. In Hindu and Buddhist Tantra, the Siddhas are a grouping of often antinomian culture heroes who founded lineages and traditions of teaching and practice. *See also* mahāsiddha; nāth.

siddhi (Pali: iddhi) – "Perfection"; one of the many supernatural powers possessed by Siddhas as a result of their practice, their *sādhana*. Included among the *siddhis* are the power of flight, invisibility, and the power to enter into other bodies. The *Yoga Sūtra* devotes much space to the *siddhi*s, but ultimately views them as an impediment to liberation.

smṛti (Pali: sati) – "That which has been recalled; tradition"; for Hindus, *smṛti* comprises the later, non-revealed scriptures of the sacred corpus: the epics, *Purāṇa*s, etc. *Smṛti* also denotes the power of recollection, to recall an object to memory. *See also* anusmṛti.

śūnyatā – "Emptiness, Voidness"; in Mahāyāna and Buddhist Tantra, the principle that all objects of the senses, mental concepts, metaphysical categories and language constructs are devoid of self-existence.

suṣumnā – In Hindu yoga systems, the principal subtle channel identified with fire, which runs down through the center of the spinal column. *See also* avadhūtī; iḍā; nāḍī; piṅgalā.

tapas – Asceticism, the heat generated through yogic practice; religious austerities.

tattva – "Reality; truth; essence"; In Sāmkyha and Yoga philosophy, one of the twenty-five irreducible basic principles of reality, ranging from the five gross elements to *puruṣa*.

vajra – "Diamond; thunderbolt"; in tantric Buddhism, adamantine symbol of the strength, immovability, and transcendent nature of the state of consciousness realized by perfected practitioners, *bodhisattva*s, and Buddhas.

vijñāna – Mundane or this-worldly knowledge, as opposed to gnosis, *jñāna*.

vipassanā (Pali: Sanskrit *vipaśyanā*) – "Penetrative insight"; a classical form of Buddhist meditation, issuing into insight into the true nature of reality.

yama – "Restraint"; the various ethical rules and behavioral restraints comprising the first limb of eight-limbed yoga.

INDEX